Histiocytic Disorders of Children and Adults

As the first comprehensive reference on all aspects of the histiocytic disorders, *Histiocytic Disorders of Children and Adults* stands out as the definitive text on the genetics, pathophysiology, and clinical management of this wide range of disease. The chapters, written by acknowledged experts in the field, cover all aspects of histiocytic disorders, from Langerhans cell histiocytosis and hemophagocytic lymphohistiocytosis, to the uncommon cutaneous and extracutaneous histiocytic disorders. Current views on the function of normal histiocytes in the immune system, the pathogenesis, underlying genetic defects, clinical presentation, treatment, controversies in therapy, salvage therapies and the late consequences are discussed in detail. This book will be a valuable resource to clinicians and researchers who wish to learn more about histiocytic disorders.

Sheila Weitzman is Professor of Paediatrics at the Hospital for Sick Children, University of Toronto, Toronto, Canada.

R. Maarten Egeler is Professor of Paediatrics at the University of Leiden, Leiden, The Netherlands.

T0213327

Histiocytic Disorders of Children and Adults

Edited by

Sheila Weitzman

and

R. Maarten Egeler

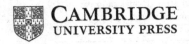
CAMBRIDGE
UNIVERSITY PRESS

CAMBRIDGE UNIVERSITY PRESS
Cambridge, New York, Melbourne, Madrid, Cape Town, Singapore,
São Paulo, Delhi, Dubai, Tokyo, Mexico City

Cambridge University Press
The Edinburgh Building, Cambridge CB2 8RU, UK

Published in the United States of America by Cambridge University Press, New York

www.cambridge.org
Information on this title: www.cambridge.org/9780521184168

© Cambridge University Press 2005

First published 2005
First paperback edition 2010

A catalogue record for this publication is available from the British Library

ISBN 978-0-521-83929-7 Hardback
ISBN 978-0-521-18416-8 Paperback

Contents

List of contributors

Nicola E. Annels
Immunology Laboratory
Dept of Paediatrics
Leiden University Medical Center
The Netherlands

Maurizio Aricò
Director, Paediatric Haematology/Oncology
Ospedale dei Bambini
Palermo, Italy

Robert Arceci
Director, Paediatric Oncology
Johns Hopkins Oncology Centre
Baltimore, MD, USA

Cristiana E.T. da Costa
Immunology Laboratory
Dept of Pediatrics
Leiden University Medical Center
Leiden, The Netherlands

Cesare Danesino
Genetica Medica
Università di Pavia
Pavia, Italy

Emanuela De Juli
Chairman, Rare Pulmonary Diseases Unit
Co-Chairman, Lung Transplant Program
Ospedale Niguarda – Ca' Granda
Milano, Italy

Giulio John D'Angio
Emeritus Professor of Radiation Oncology,
Radiology and Pediatrics
University of Pennsylvania School of
Medicine
Philadelphia, PA, USA

Jean Donadieu
Haematology/Oncology
Hopital Trousseau
Paris, France

R. Maarten Egeler
Past President Histiocyte Society
Director, Immunology, Haematology,
Oncology
Bone Marrow Transplantation and Auto
immune diseases
Leiden University Medical Center
Leiden, The Netherlands

Kim Ericson
Division of Clinical Genetics
Department of Molecular Medicine and
Child Cancer Research Unit
Karolinska Institute
Stockholm, Sweden

Bengt Fadeel
Member, Scientific Committee, Histiocyte
Society
Division of Molecular Toxicology
Institute of Environmental Medicine
Karolinska Institute
Stockholm, Sweden

Helmut Gadner
Past President Histiocyte Society
Director Paediatric Oncology
St Anna Children's Hospital
Vienna, Austria

Thierry Généreau
Dept Internal Medicine
Hôpital Saint-Antoine
Paris, France

Nicole Grois
Consultant Paediatric Oncologist
St Anna Children's Hospital
Vienna, Austria

Riccardo Haupt
Consultant Paediatric
Haematologist/Oncologist
Gaslini Children's Hospital
Genova, Italy

Jan-Inge Henter
President Histiocyte Society
Professor of Pediatrics
Pediatric Hematology/Oncology
Karolinska University Hospital and
Child Cancer Research Unit
Karolinska Institute
Stockholm, Sweden

T. Jeroen N. Hiltermann
Department of Pulmonology
Deventer Ziekenhuis
Deventer, The Netherlands

Shinsaku Imashuku
Director, Kyoto City Institute of Health
Kyoto, Japan

Ronald Jaffe
Director, Dept of Pathology
Children's Hospital
Pittsburgh, PA, USA

Gritta Janka
Consultant Pediatric Hematology/Oncology
Children's University Hospital
Hamburg, Germany

Bernice Krafchik
Emeritus Professor of Paediatrics
Consultant Dermatologist
Toronto, Canada

Elizabeth Kuh
Consultant Psychiatrist
Bala Cynwyd, PA, USA

Stephan Ladisch
Past President Histiocyte Society,
Scientific Director
Children's National Medical Center
Washington DC, USA

Hans Lassmann
Institute for Brain Research
University of Vienna
Vienna, Austria

Ronald Laxer
Vice-President Medical Affairs
Consultant Rheumatologist
The Hospital for Sick Children
Toronto, Canada

Pieter J.M. Leenen
Lecturer in Immunology and Histology
Erasmus MC
Rotterdam, The Netherlands

Kenneth L. McClain
Past President Histiocyte Society
Director: Histiocytosis Center
Texas Children's Cancer Center/
Hematology Service
Houston, Texas, USA

Vasanta Nanduri
Consultant Paediatric Oncologist
Watford General Hospital
Honorary Consultant Paediatric Oncologist
Great Ormond Street Hospital
London, UK

Tatjana Nikolić
Dept of Pulmonary and Critical Care
Medicine
Erasmus MC
University Medical Centre, Rotterdam
The Netherlands

Elena Pope
Director, Division of Dermatology
The Hospital for Sick Children
Toronto, Canada

Daniela Prayer
University Clinic for Radiology
Vienna, Austria

Jon Pritchard
Consultant Paediatric Oncologist
Royal Hospital for Sick Children and
University of Edinburgh
Edinburgh, UK

Helmut Prosch
Paediatric Haematology/Oncology
St Anna Children's Hospital
Vienna, Austria

Athimalaipet Ramanan
Consultant Paediatric Rheumatologist
North Bristol NHS Trust and
Royal National Hospital for
Rheumatic Diseases
Bath, UK

Alan Saven
Head, Division of Haematology/Oncology
Scripps Clinic
Director, Scripps Cancer Centre
La Jolla, CA, USA

Susi Scappaticci
Genetica Medica
Università di Pavia
Pavia, Italy

Rayfel Schneider
Director, Division of Rheumatology
The Hospital for Sick Children
Toronto, Canada

Steve Simms
Consultant Psychologist
Gladwyne
Pennsylvania, USA

Abdellatif Tazi
Professor of Medicine
Université de Médecine Paris
Head of Pulmonary department
Hôpital Saint-Louis
Paris, France

Roberto Vassallo
Division of Pulmonary and Critical
Care Medicine
Mayo Clinic
Rochester, MN, USA

Scott R.A. Walsh
Consultant Dermatologist
Sunnybrook and Womens Health
Sciences Centre
Toronto, Canada

David K.H. Webb
Consultant Paediatric
Haematologist/Oncologist
Great Ormond St Hospital for Sick Children
London, UK

Sheila Weitzman
Associate Director Clinical Affairs
Division of Haematology/Oncology
The Hospital for Sick Children
Toronto, Canada

James Whitlock
Director, Paediatric Haematology/Oncology
Vanderbilt University Medical Centre
Nashville, TN, USA

Preface

This book, the only current comprehensive text on the histiocytic disorders, is intended to be a useful source of information for all those who care for patients with one of the histiocytoses, for clinicians with primary responsibility for patient management, physicians concerned with laboratory medicine, and all who are involved with research in the field. Furthermore, patients with histiocytosis and/or their families may well find it useful to have the book as a standard reference for themselves and for every caregiver who tells them that histiocytosis is rare and that they know nothing about the condition and do not feel comfortable managing it.

Patients with histiocytoses, especially with Langerhans cell histiocytosis (LCH) and hemophagocytic lymphohistiocytosis (HLH), are sufficiently common that they constitute an important problem but, on the other hand, are sufficiently uncommon that it has been difficult for many/most physicians to gain experience in their care.

In particular, research into the special problems of adults with histiocytic disorders has not kept pace with that in paediatrics except in certain areas such as adult lung histiocytosis. One of the goals of this book is to encourage the same comprehensive care of adult patients as has become the standard for children.

In this book, you will find discussion of all aspects of the histiocytic disorders, written by some 50 international experts in the field. The discussion includes a chapter on histiocyte function in the normal immune system as well as the most recent research into genetic predisposition, pathogenesis, clinical features, modern and salvage therapy and the late permanent consequences. The section on LCH includes separate chapters on the commonest disease manifestations in bone, skin and adult lung, while the HLH section includes discussion of Epstein–Barr virus (EBV)-HLH, lymphoma-associated hemophagocytosis and HLH associated with rheumatic diseases. In addition, chapters on the malignant histiocytic diseases and the psychologic aspects of histiocytosis have been included, as well as a detailed discussion of the less common histiocytic disorders, the non-LCH, including an up-to-date review of current therapy.

There has been great progress in the understanding of the basic biology and clinical features of the histiocytoses over the last few decades. We hope that sharing the experience of the experts through the medium of this book will be of value to all caregivers confronted with these difficult but fascinating problems, as well as to the patients and their families.

Sheila Weitzman
R. Maarten Egeler

Histiocytic disorders of children and adults: introduction to the problem, overview, historical perspective and epidemiology

Sheila Weitzman and R. Maarten Egeler

The histiocytic disorders are defined as disorders due to an abnormal accumulation of cells of the mononuclear phagocytic system (MPS), consisting of dendritic cells (DCs) and macrophages. They comprise a wide variety of diverse conditions that affect both children and adults, and have been difficult to classify and to treat.

Figure 1.1 is a simplified schematic representation of the development of various components of the MPS from the primitive CD34+ hematopoietic stem cell.

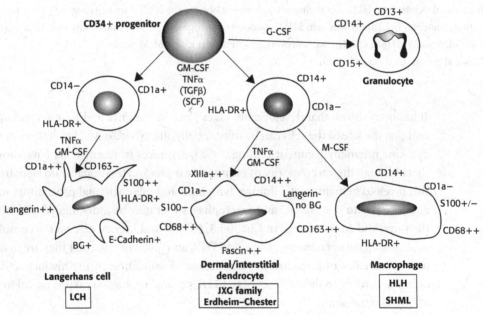

Figure 1.1   Schematic representation of histiocyte developmental pathway. Development along alternate pathways such as from monocytes or even lymphocytes has been shown to be possible; BG: Birbeck granule; GM-CSF: granulocyte–macrophage colony stimulating factor; HLA: human leukocyte antigen; JXG: juvenile xanthogranuloma; SCF: stem cell factor; TNFα: tumour necrosis factor α; TGFβ: transforming growth factor β. Reprinted with permission from John Wiley & Sons

Table 1.1 Characteristics of histiocytes in health and disease*

Clinical	LCH	Interdigitating cell sarcoma	JXG family	HLH	SHML
	LC	IDC	DD	M/M	SHML
HLA-DR	++	+	−	+	+
CD1a	++	−	−	−	−
CD14	−	−	++	++	++
CD68 (KP-1, PGM-1)	+/−	+/−	++	++	++
CD163	−	−	−	++	++
Factor XIIIa	−	−	++	−	−
Langerin	++	−	−	−	−
Fascin	−	++	++	+/−	+
S100	+	++	−	+/−	+
Lysozyme	−	−	−	++	++
Birbeck granules	+	−	−	−	−
Hemophagocytosis				+/−	
Emperipolesis					+

DD: dermal dendrocyte; HLH: hemophagocytic lymphohistiocytosis; IDC: interdigitating cell; JXG: juvenile xanthogranuloma; LC: Langerhans cell; M/M: monocyte/macrophage; SHML: sinus histoctosis with massive lymphadenopathy (SHML cellular markers overlap with dendritic and M/M markers).
*Personal communication of R. Jaffe.

It has been shown that development takes place in response to different cytokines, and that the fate of the cells can be substantially altered or skewed by changes in the cytokine microenvironment (Young, 1999). Advances in recent years have shown that although the vast majority of mononuclear phagocytes probably do stem from this myeloid hematopoietic lineage, lymphoid and mesenchymal progenitors may also give rise to mature DC and macrophages that may be indistinguishable from their myeloid counterparts. In Chapter 3, Nikolić and Leenen discuss the complex relationship between macrophages and DCs, and give evidence that they are in fact on the extremes of a spectrum. Nonetheless, classification of the histiocytic disorders according to their relationship to DCs or macrophages remains useful from a clinical standpoint.

The histiocytic disorders are generally defined by their constitutive cell, on the basis of well-established pathologic and immunohistochemical criteria (Table 1.1). It has become obvious that establishment of the correct individual diagnosis requires the fulfillment of these classic criteria, but also requires the correct clinical context. The diagnostic criteria are, therefore, correctly termed 'clinicopathologic' (Jaffe, Chapter 2).

Table 1.2 Classification of histiocytic disorder

---

1 **Disorders of varying biologic behavior**
  a. *Dendritic cell related*
    Langerhans cell histiocytosis
    Juvenile xanthogranuloma and related disorders including:
    – Erdheim–Chester disease
    – Solitary histiocytomas with juvenile xanthogranuloma phenotype
    Secondary dendritic cell disorders
  b. *Monocyte/macrophage related*
    Hemophagocytic lymphohistiocytosis
      Familial and sporadic
    Secondary hemophagocytic syndromes:
    – Infection associated
    – Malignancy associated
    – Autoimmune associated
    – Other
    Sinus histiocytosis with massive lymphadenopathy (Rosai–Dorfman disease)
    Solitary histiocytoma of macrophage phenotype

2 **Malignant disorders**
  Dendritic cell related
  Histiocytic sarcoma (localized or disseminated)
  Monocyte/macrophage related
  Leukemias:
  – Monocytic leukemias M5A and B
  – Acute myelomonocytic leukemia M4
  – Chronic myelomonocytic leukemias
  Extramedullary monocytic tumors or sarcoma (monocytic counterpart of granulocytic sarcoma)
  Macrophage-related histiocytic sarcoma (localized or disseminated)
  (specify phenotype: follicular dendritic cell, interdigitating dendritic cell, etc.)

Adapted from Favara *et al.* (1997).

In 1987, the Writing Group of the Histiocyte Society attempted to bring some order into the chaos surrounding these diseases, by classifying them according to their relationship to normal histiocyte subsets (Chu *et al.*, 1987). The classification was revised in 1997 (Favara *et al.*, 1997) to take into account the biologic behavior of the various disorders (Table 1.2). In this system, the major histiocytic disorders are divided into two broad groups, those of varying biologic behavior and those that are truly malignant. Within each category the disorders are subclassified according to their affiliation with DCs or with the macrophage/monocyte pathway. At present the uncommon histiocytic disorders – the non-Langerhans cell histiocytoses (non-LCH) – are divided between the two classes, with disorders thought possibly to arise from the dermal dendrocyte, such as the juvenile xanthogranuloma family, being classified with the DC disorders, while those disorders such as sinus histiocytosis with massive lymphadenopathy (SHML) (Rosai–Dorfman disease) being assigned to the macrophage line. When dealing with such varying clinical behavior, no classification system is likely to be perfect, but the system does provide a method of standardizing the nomenclature, and giving a 'universal histiocytic language' (Egeler and D'Angio, 1998). This together with the guidelines for diagnosis and for uniform follow-up provided by the Histiocyte Society (Chapter 6) have made possible the large international cooperative studies which have shed light on the epidemiology, natural history and therapeutic outcomes of the major histiocytic disorders, LCH and hemophagocytic lymphohistiocytosis (HLH). Over the past decade, a vast amount of research has improved understanding of the basic science of normal and abnormal histiocytes, and the clinical aspects of LCH and HLH as well as the uncommon histiocytic disorders (the non-LCH).

In the following chapters, the biology, genetics, histopathology, clinical presentation, diagnosis, natural history, therapy and prognosis of the 'classic' histiocytic disorders, LCH, HLH and the non-LCH will be reviewed in depth.

Langerhans cell histiocytosis

LCH is by far the commonest of the histiocytoses, characterized by excess accumulation of CD1a+ Langerhans cells (LCs) at various tissue sites.

The disease manifests in a variety of ways, ranging from spontaneously regressing single lesions, to repeated reactivations with the risk of permanent long-term disabilities, to a life-threatening multisystem (MS) disorder with rapid progression and death.

LCH has been variously classified as a neoplasm, a reactive disorder or an aberrant immune response (Bhatia et al., 1997). As will be described in later chapters, LCH cells are pathologic cells, but the granulomatous lesion includes the accumulation of normal inflammatory cells such as eosinophils, lymphocytes and macrophages. The cellular infiltration and the clinical features are all explicable as a result of aberrant secretion of cytokines by lesional cells and activated T-cells, leading to a unique clinicopathologic picture (Egeler et al., 1999). Recent advances suggest that clonal changes in LCH cells underlie the aberrant immune interaction with T-cells (Laman et al., 2003), nonetheless the exact etiology and pathogenesis remains uncertain. The following chapters will describe the function of normal LCs in the immune system, the large body of literature regarding pathologic LCH cells, its cytokine microenvironment, and the evidence for and against LCH being a neoplastic, genetic or infectious disorder.

Investigators in the field have long been aware that LCH in adults is at least as significant as in the pediatric population. While pediatric histiocytoses have found a base in the world of pediatric oncology, adult LCH patients have for the most part no such niche, being variously looked after by dermatologists, pulmonologists, surgeons and neurologists. Therefore this book includes chapters on adult LCH written by experts in the field, while other chapters on LCH of skin, bone, uncommon histiocytic disorders and HLH will include sections dedicated to issues specific to adult patients.

Historical aspects of LCH

In 1868, Paul Langerhans, then a 21-year-old student, published the landmark manuscript describing the non-pigmentary DCs in the epidermis which now bear his name. The sketches he made and his quantification (500–900/cm^2) are still valid today (Lampert, 1998). The first clear description of a patient with impetigo and holes in the cranium is by Smith in 1865 (Coppes-Zantinga and Egeler, 2002), although there is a description of a non-fatal disease associated with painful skull lesions by Hippocrates (about 400–450 BC) (Donadieu and Pritchard, 1999).

In 1893, Hand described a child with polyuria and exophthalmos which he attributed to tuberculosis (Hand, 1893). Schüller (1915), and Christian (1920), described similar patients with skull defects, exophthalmos and diabetes insipidus (DI), and eventually the eponym Hand–Schüller–Christian disease was given to a disease with a characteristic triad of exophthalmos, skull lesions and DI (Coppes-Zantinga and Egeler, 2002). In 1933, Siwe grouped previously reported cases (including one by Letterer in 1924) of organomegaly, lymphadenopathy, localized tumors in bone, secondary anemia, a hemorrhagic tendency and hyperplasia of non-lipid storing macrophages, into the disease that later became known as Letterer–Siwe disease (Siwe, 1933). In 1941, Farber noted that these two conditions, plus the newly diagnosed eosinophilic granuloma of bone, described the previous year in two separate articles (Lichtenstein and Jaffe, 1940; Otani and Ehrlich, 1940), represented variations of the same disease process (Farber, 1941). Later Lichtenstein introduced the concept that the three entities were part of a spectrum of the same disorder which he called histiocytosis X (Lichtenstein, 1953). In 1961, Birbeck *et al.* described the characteristic granules seen on electron microscopy (EM), thus introducing a distinctive recognition marker (Lampert, 1998) (Figure 1.2). During the next few years several investigators described the finding of Birbeck granules in different forms of LCH, and in 1973 Nezelof published a report that showed that histiocytosis X was the result of proliferation of pathologic LCs (Nezelof, 1992), a manuscript (and concept) that took many years to be accepted (Coppes-Zantinga and Egeler, 2002). In 1983, it was suggested that the name histiocytosis X be changed to Langerhans cell histiocytosis (Risdall *et al.*, 1983), in recognition of the key role of LCs in all forms of the disease (Risdall *et al.*, 1983). Finally in 1985,

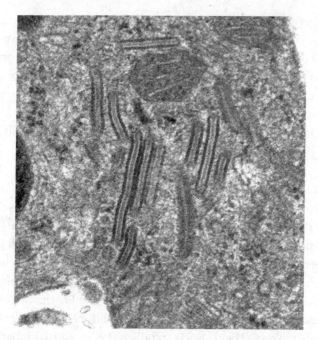

Figure 1.2   Electron microscopic view of characteristic granules as described by Birbeck *et al.* (1961)

Dr. Giulio D'Angio convened the first workshop on histiocytosis leading to the formation of the Histiocyte Society, an international society dedicated to the understanding of all aspects of the histiocytic disorders (Coppes-Zantinga and Egeler, 2002). An important step which soon followed was the formation by the Toughill family of the parent support group, now the very successful Histiocytosis Association of America, which together with similar groups from other countries, is a major supporter of research, as well as parent and patient support. Together with the 'Nikolas Symposium' an annual 'think-tank' supported by the Kontoyannis family, at which basic researchers and clinicians interested in these diseases are brought together to formulate new ideas, they have been responsible for many of the advances that have been made over the last two decades.

Epidemiology of LCH

Age and gender

LCH can present at any age from the neonatal period until old age. The estimated prevalence in children is 1:50,000 (Carstensen and Ornvold, 1993) with an annual incidence of $2–5/10^6$/year in children under 15 years of age. A more recent study from Sweden, however, found a higher incidence of $8.9/10^6$/year in children with the increase seen in MS as well as single system (SS) disease (Karis *et al.*, 2003).

Moreover, since 30–50% of cases occur in patients over the age of 15 years (Berry and Becton, 1984), the actual incidence figures for all age groups is probably closer to $11–12/10^6$/year. These figures almost certainly underestimate the scope of the problem, as many patients, particularly those with localized bone or skin LCH, are likely to go un-referred and undiagnosed.

In one study of 346 LCH patients less than 15 years of age, the median age at diagnosis was 30.2 months (The French LCH Study Group, 1996). A slight male preponderance was reported similar to that in other studies, although some series have reported a male predominance as high as 2:1 (Carstensen and Ornvold, 1993). In the overall pediatric age range, almost 70% have SS disease of which the commonest system involved is bone (Stuurman et al., 2003). However MS LCH usually occurs in children less than 2 years of age, multifocal SS in children between 2 and 5 years, while 50% of unifocal bone disease occurs in children over the age of 5 years (Huang and Arceci, 1999).

Analysis of patients over the age of 18 years, reported to the Histiocyte Society Adult Registry, showed a mean age at diagnosis of 35 with 10% being older than 55 years. Five percent of adults had a delay of more than 10 years between onset of symptoms and diagnosis. Over two-thirds (68.6%) had MS disease with skin and lung involvement in 51% and 62%, respectively (Aricò et al., 2003). Of the 86 adults (31%) with SS LCH, SS bone was seen in 38%, SS skin in 14.3% and SS lung in 51%, most of whom were smokers. A more detailed discussion of adult LCH can be found in Chapters 7–10.

Genetic and ethnic factors

The only histiocytic disorder unequivocally due to an underlying genetic abnormality is familial HLH. Evidence of familial clustering of LCH and higher concordance in monozygotic twins than would be expected by chance suggest that a genetic predisposition may also exist for LCH (Aricò et al., 2001).

Evaluation of 84 Nordic patients found no association between human leukocyte antigen (HLA) subtypes and the occurrence of LCH; however, stratification into SS and MS disease showed that SS patients more often had the phenotype DRB1*03 and the deduced haplotype HLA-A*01, B*08, DRB1*03 was found only in SS patients. The possibility was raised that HLA-DRB1*03 plays a protective role against developing MS disease. Further studies of this interesting concept are required (Bernstrand et al., 2003). McClain et al. (2003) found a high incidence of DR4 or Cw7 in Caucasian LCH patients, particularly those with single bone disease and suggested possible associations with immune dysfunction leading to LCH.

The genetics of LCH and of HLH will be discussed in detail in Chapters 5 and 17.

The increased incidence reported in white children is likely to be due to reporting bias, as there is no known racial bias for the development of LCH.

Risk factors for LCH

Defective immune function has long been suggested as being central to the pathogenesis of LCH. Recent studies described in detail in Chapter 3, discuss the possibility of genetic abnormality in LC function which may underlie the immune disorder.

An alternative hypothesis is that this is a reactive disease, resulting from environmental or other triggers which lead to the aberrant reaction between LCs and T-cells (Glotzbecker *et al.*, 2002). The association between LCH and malignancy described in Chapter 14 may give some credence to this hypothesis.

Alternatively, environmental and other factors may act as initiating events on the background of immune dysregulation.

An epidemiologic study compared 459 children with LCH to matched case–controls from the normal population and to children with cancer. Risk factors associated with MS-LCH in the study (Bhatia *et al.*, 1997) were an increase in infections and use of antibiotics in the first 6 months of life and a family history of thyroid disease, while SS-LCH was significantly associated with diarrhea and vomiting in the postnatal period. Both MS and SS disease were associated with a history of thyroid disease in the proband. A history of smoking pre-conception and *in utero*, maternal infections or medication use during pregnancy, did not appear to be associated with a higher risk of LCH even in early onset MS disease. Patients with LCH were consistently under-immunized compared to controls. It is interesting to speculate that lack of immunization rendered the children more susceptible to infection leading to LCH, but the association could simply be due to deferral of immunizations in ill children (Bhatia *et al.*, 1997).

Studies for an infectious origin in LCH have produced varying results. An analysis for nine different viruses by *in situ* hybridization (ISH) and polymerase chain reaction (PCR) failed to demonstrate an association (McClain *et al.*, 1994); however, more recently human herpes virus (HHV)-6 has been found in a high percentage of LCH lesional tissue by immunohistochemistry and ISH by investigators from Philadelphia, who suggest that all the manifestations of LCH could be secondary to a viral infection of lymphocytes (Glotzbecker *et al.*, 2002). Further studies to clarify the role of HHV-6 and other viruses are necessary.

In adults, cigarette smoking has been shown to be a clear risk factor for the development of pulmonary LCH. The exact relationship of this sometimes polyclonal lung disease to the monoclonal forms of the disease remains to be elucidated, particularly in view of a Swedish study which raised the possibility of an increased risk for the development of lung LCH in adult survivors of pediatric LCH who smoke (Bernstrand *et al.*, 2000).

No other environmental risk factors for the development of LCH have been found to date.

Hemophagocytic lymphohistiocytosis

The hemophagocytic syndromes are subdivided into primary and secondary forms.

Primary HLH appears to arise *de novo* without any known preceding conditions. A major subdivision of primary HLH is the autosomal recessive form of the disease, now mainly called familial hemophagocytic lymphohistiocytosis (FHL). Recent studies suggest that 20–40% of FHL is due to perforin gene mutations (Goransdotter Ericson *et al.*, 2001) but, as discussed in Chapter 17, several gene mutations may underlie the deficiency in the triggering of apoptosis which results in the HLH phenotype. As more genetic defects are discovered, the diagnosis of non-familial primary HLH will be made correspondingly less often, and it may well be that all primary HLH will eventually be shown to have a genetic basis.

In secondary forms of HLH, hemophagocytosis occurs as a result of macrophage activation by a known stimulus which can be infectious, malignant, autoimmune or physical. A number of infections have been shown to be associated with secondary HLH, of which Epstein–Barr virus (EBV) is the commonest (discussed in detail in Chapter 18); but other viruses, bacteria and fungal infections may also be found (Fisman, 2000).

Whatever the etiology, the pathogenesis involves production of high levels of proinflammatory cytokines by T-helper cells, excessive activation of monocytes and macrophages leading to the phagocytosis of blood cells which is the hallmark of the disease (see Chapters 18 and 19).

Historical perspectives on HLH

The first publication describing FHL is usually said to be that of Farquhar and Claireaux (1952). They reported two siblings with unexplained fevers, progressive panhematopenia, hepatosplenomegaly and terminal bruising. At autopsy a proliferation of histiocytes were found, many of which showed erythrophagocytosis (Filipovich, 1997). As pointed out, however (Fisman, 2000), the syndrome also called histiocytic medullary reticulosis was first described in 1939 (Scott and Robb-Smith, 1939). In 1979, Risdall *et al.* described 19 patients with similar findings, most of whom proved to have virus-associated HLH (Risdall *et al.*, 1979). In 1980, successful treatment of two children with etoposide was described (Ambruso *et al.*, 1980); however in 1983, a review of FHL still showed a median survival of less than 2 months, and a 1-year survival close to 0% (Janke, 1983). In 1986, an important breakthrough occurred when Fischer *et al.* demonstrated that allogeneic bone marrow transplant could affect a cure in some patients (Fischer *et al.*, 1986). In 1994, the HLH-94 protocol of the Histiocyte Society was developed, combining immunotherapy with chemotherapy and recommending bone marrow transplantation for all primary HLH patients for whom a donor could be found.

Recently published results of this protocol provide unequivocal evidence of the value of international collaboration in uncommon disorders (Henter et al., 2002).

This improvement in clinical management was paralleled by the rapidly increasing understanding of the underlying biology. Many studies show that the clinical syndrome was due to an excess of proinflammatory cytokines (Henter et al., 1991b; Imashuku et al., 1991; Osugi et al., 1997), and suggested that the familial form of HLH was due to faulty triggering of apoptosis (Henter et al., 1996). This led to the discovery that many of the cases were due to defects in the perforin gene (Dufourcq-Lagelouse et al., 1999; Ohadi et al., 1999; Stepp et al., 1999), and the subsequent finding of several other gene defects which result in the same phenotype.

Epidemiology of HLH

The estimated incidence of FHL is 1/50,000 live births (Henter et al., 1991a), but this figure will almost certainly increase as more genetic defects are discovered.

The male to female ratio is 1:1. There is an increased incidence of the disease in ethnic groups with higher rates of consanguinity (Henter et al., 1998), and this holds true even within the same ethnic group. In Japan, FHL is significantly commoner in Western Japan where the rate of consanguinity is higher (Ishii et al., 1998). The majority of patients present before the age of 1 year; however, with the finding of the perforin and other gene mutations, family members presenting with the disease in their 20s have been described.

The association of secondary HLH with EBV infection has been well described, more than 50% of the patients coming from the Far East Japan, China or Taiwan (Janke et al., 1998). At least in the childhood population, EBV-associated HLH appears to occur in young children, with more than 50% being less than 3 years of age (Janke et al., 1998), and with a mortality that has been estimated to be as high as 41% (Imashuku, 2000). Although a few cases of FHL present in young adults, the majority of adult cases are due to secondary HLH. A recent review from Japan, of 52 adults with HLH, showed underlying lymphomas in 26 (lymphoma-associated hemophagocytic syndrome, LAHS), virus-associated hemophagocytic syndrome (VAHS) in 17, bacterial disease in 6 and autoimmune disease (all systemic lupus erythematosus (SLE)) in 3. LAHS had the highest median age at diagnosis and the highest mortality in this study (Takahashi et al., 2001), which confirmed previous reports that lymphoma is the commonest cause of adult-onset HLH.

Conclusion

After a prolonged period of inertia following the original description of LCH, the last few decades has seen major gains in knowledge regarding the underlying defects, clinical presentation, therapy and outcome of the histiocytic disorders.

This book, written by experts in the field, will provide readers with an understanding of the state of the art in LCH, HLH and the less common histiocytoses. It is our hope that this will also serve to raise interest and spark further research into these fascinating disorders.

REFERENCES

Ambruso, D.R., Hays, T., Zwartjes, W.J., et al. (1980). Successful treatment of lymphohistiocytic reticulosis with phagocytosis with epipodophyllotoxin VP-16-213. Cancer, 45, 2516–2520.

Aricò, M., Haupt, R. and Russotto, V.S., et al. (2001). Langerhans cell histiocytosis in two generations: a new family and review of the literature. Med Pediatr Oncol, 36, 314–316.

Aricò, M., Girschikofsky, M., Généreau, T., et al. (2003). Langerhans cell histiocytosis in adults report from the International Registry of the Histiocyte Society. Eur J Cancer, 39, 2341–2348.

Bernstrand, C., Cederlund, K., Åhstrom, L., et al. (2000). Smoking preceded pulmonary involvement in adults with Langerhans cell histiocytosis diagnosed in childhood. Acta Paediatr, 89, 1389–1392.

Bernstrand, C., Carstensen, H., Jakobsen, B., et al. (2003). Immunogenetic heterogeneity in single-system and multisystem Langerhans cell histiocytosis. Pediatr Res, 54, 30–36.

Berry, D.H. and Becton, D.L. (1984). Natural history of histiocytosis X. Hematol Oncol Clin North Am, 1, 23–24.

Bhatia, S., Nesbit, M.E., Egeler, R.M., et al. (1997). Epidemiologic study of Langerhans cell histiocytosis in children. J Pediatr, 130, 774–784.

Birbeck, M.S., Breathnach, A.S. and Everall, J.D. (1961). An electron microscopy study of basal melanocytes and high-level clear cells (Langerhans cells) in vitiligo. J Invest Dermatol, 37, 51–63.

Carstensen, H. and Ornvold, K. (1993). The epidemiology of Langerhans cell histiocytosis in children in Denmark, 1975–89. Med Pediatr Oncol, 21, 387–388.

Christian, H. (1920). Defects in membraneous bones, exophthalmos and diabetes insipidus: an unusual syndrome of dyspituitarism. Med Clin North Am, 3, 849–871.

Chu, T., D'Angio, G.J., Favara, B., et al. (1987). Histocytosis syndromes in children. Lancet, 1, 208–209.

Coppes-Zantinga, A. and Egeler, R.M. (2002). The Langerhans cell histiocytosis X files revealed. Historical review. Br J Haematol, 116, 3–9.

Donadieu, J. and Pritchard, J. (1999). Langerhans cell histiocytosis – 400BC? Med Pediatr Oncol, 33, 520.

Dufourcq-Lagelouse, R., Jabado, N., Le Deist, F., et al. (1999). Linkage of familial hemophagocytic lymphohistiocytosis to 10q21-22 and evidence for heterogeneity. Am J Hum Genet, 64, 172–179.

Egeler, R.M. and D'Angio, G.J. (1998). Langerhans cell histiocytosis, Preface. Hematol Oncol Clin North Am, 12, XV–XVii.

Egeler, R.M., Favara, B.E., van Meurs, M., et al. (1999). Differential in situ cytokine profiles of Langerhans-like cells and T cells in Langerhans cell histiocytosis: abundant expression of cytokines relevant to disease and treatment. Blood, 94, 4195–4201.

Farber, S. (1941). The nature of 'solitary or eosinophilic granuloma' of bone. Am J Pathol, 17, 625–629.

Farquhar, J. and Claireaux, A. (1952). Familial haemophagocytic reticulosis. Arch Dis Child, 27, 519–525.

Favara, B.E., Feller, A.C., Pauli, M., *et al.* (1997). Contemporary classification of histiocytic disorders. Reclassification Working Group of the Histiocyte Society. *Med Pediatr Oncol*, 29, 157–166.

Filipovich, A.H. (1997). Hemophagocytic lymphohistiocytosis: a lethal disorder of immune regulation. *J Pediatr*, 130, 337–338.

Fischer, A., Cerf-Bensussan, N., Blanche, S., *et al.* (1986). Allogeneic bone marrow transplantation for erythrophagocytic lymphohistiocytosis. *J Pediatr*, 108, 267–270.

Fisman, D.N. (2000). Hemophagocytic syndromes and infection. *Emerg Infect Dis*, 6, 601–608.

Glotzbecker, M.P., Carpentieri, D.F. and Dormans, J.P. (2002). Langerhans cell histiocytosis: clinical presentation, pathogenesis, and treatment from the LCH etiology research group at the Children's Hospital of Philadelphia. *UPOJ*, 15, 67–73.

Goransdotter Ericson, K.G., Fadeel, B., Nilsson-Ardnor, S., *et al.* (2001). Spectrum of perforin gene mutations in familial hemophagocytic lymphohistiocytosis. *Am J Hum Genet*, 68, 590–597.

Hand, A. (1893). Polyuria and tuberculosis. *Arch Pediatr*, 10, 673–675.

Henter, J.-I., Elinder, G., Söder, O., *et al.* (1991a). Incidence in Sweden and clinical features of familial hemophagocytic lymphohistiocytosis. *Acta Paediatr Scand*, 80, 428–435.

Henter, J.-I., Elinder, G., Söder, O., *et al.* (1991b). Hypercytokinemia in familial hemophagocytic lymphohistiocytosis, *Blood*, 78, 2918–2922.

Henter, J.-I., Andersson, B., Elinder, G., *et al.* (1996). Elevated circulating levels of interleukin-1 receptor antagonists but not IL-1 agonists in hemophagocytic lymphohistiocytosis. *Med Pediatr Oncol*, 27, 21–25.

Henter, J.-I., Aricò, M., Elinder, G., *et al.* (1998). Familial hemophagocytic lymphohistiocytosis. *Hematol Oncol Clin North Am*, 12, 417–433.

Henter, J.-I., Samuelsson-Horne, A., Arico, M., *et al.* (2002). Treatment of hemophagocytic lymphohistiocytosis with HLH-94 immunochemotherapy and bone marrow transplantatation. *Blood*, 100, 2367–2373.

Huang, F. and Arceci, R. (1999). The histiocytoses of infancy. *Semin Perinatol*, 23, 319–331.

Imashuku, S. (2000). Advances in the management of hemophagocytic lymphohistiocytosis. *Int J Hematol*, 72, 1–11.

Imashuku, S., Ikushima, S., Esumi, N., *et al.* (1991). Serum levels of interferon-gamma, cytotoxic factor and soluble interleukin-2 receptor in childhood hemophagocytic syndromes. *Leukemia lymphoma*, 3, 287–292.

Ishii, E., Ohga, S., Tanimura, M., *et al.* (1998). Clinical and epidemiologic studies of familial hemophagocytic lymphohistiocytosis in Japan. Japan LCH Study Group. *Med Pediatr Oncol*, 30, 276–283.

Janke, G.E. (1983). Familial hemophagocytic lymphohistiocytosis. *Eur J Pediatr*, 140, 230.

Janke, G., Imashuku, S., Elinder, G., *et al.* (1998). Infection- and malignancy-associated hemophagocytic syndromes: secondary hemophagocytic lymphohistiocytosis. *Hematol Oncol Clin North Am*, 12, 435–444.

Karis, J., Bernstrand, C., Fadeel, B., *et al.* (2003). The incidence of Langerhans cell histiocytosis in children in Stockholm County, Sweden 1992–2001. *Proceedings of the XIX Meeting of Histiocyte Society*, Philadelphia, p. 21.

Laman, J.D., Leenen, P.J., Annels, N.E., *et al.* (2003). Langerhans-cell histiocytosis 'insight into DC biology'. *Trend Immunol*, 24, 190–196.

Lampert, F. (1998). Langerhans cell histiocytosis. Historical perspectives. *Hematol Oncol Clin North Am*, **12**, 213–219.

Letterer, E. (1924). Aleukamische retikulose (ein Beitrag zu den proliferativen Erkrankungen des reticuloendothelialapparates). *Frankfurter Zeitschritte Pathol*, **30**, 377–394.

Lichtenstein, L. (1953). Histiocytosis X: integration of eosinophilic granuloma of bone, Letterer–Siwe disease and Schüller–Christian disease as related manifestations of a single nosologic entity. *AMA Arch Pathol*, **56**, 84–102.

Lichtenstein, L. and Jaffe, H. (1940). Eosinophilic granuloma of bone. *Am J Pathol*, **16**, 595–604.

McClain, K., Jin, H., Gresik, V., *et al.* (1994). Langerhans cell histiocytosis: lack of a viral etiology. *Am J Hematol*, **47**, 16–20.

McClain, K.L., Laud, P., Wu, W-S., *et al.* (2003). Langerhans cell histiocytosis patients have HLA CW7 and DR4 types associated with specific clinical presentations and no increased frequency in polymorphisms of the tumor necrosis factor alpha promoter. *Med Pediatr Oncol*, **41**, 502–507.

Nezelof, C. (1992). The histiocytoses of childhood. *Histopathology*, **21**, 395–396.

Ohadi, M., Lalloz, M.R.A. and Sham, P. (1999). Localization of a gene for familial hemophago-cytic lymphohistiocytosis at chromosome 9q21.3-22 by homozygosity mapping. *Am J Hum Genet*, **64**, 165–171.

Osugi, Y., Hara, J., Tagawa, S., *et al.* (1997). Cytokine production regulating Th-1 and Th-2 cytokines in hemophagocytic lymphohistiocytosis. *Blood*, **89**, 4100–4103.

Otani, S. and Ehrlich, J. (1940). Soliary granuloma of bone, simulating primary neoplasm. *Am J Pathol*, **16**, 479–490.

Risdall, R.J., McKenna, R.W., Nesbit, M.E., *et al.* (1979). Virus-associated hemophagocytic syndrome: a benign histiocytic proliferation distinct from malignant histiocytosis. *Cancer*, **44**, 993–1002.

Risdall, R.J., Dehner, L.P., Duray, P., *et al.* (1983). Histiocytosis X (Langerhans cell histiocytosis). Prognostic role of histopathology. *Arch Pathol Lab Med*, **107**, 59–63.

Schüller, A. (1915). Uber eigenartige schadeldefekte im jugendalter. *Fortschritte Auf der Gebiete Rontgenstrahlen*, **23**, 12–18.

Scott, R. and Robb-Smith, A. (1939). Histiocytic medullary reticulosis. *Lancet*, **2**, 194–198.

Siwe, S. (1933). Die Reticuloendotheliose-ein neues krankheitsbild unter den hepatospleno-megalien. *Zeitschrift fur Kinderheilkunde*, **55**, 212–247.

Stepp, S.E., Dufourq-Lagelouse, R., Le Deist, F., *et al.* (1999). Perforin gene defects in familial hemophagocytic lymphohistiocytosis. *Science*, **286**, 1957–1959.

Stuurman, K.E., Lau, L., Doda, W., *et al.* (2003). Evaluation of the natural history and long term complications of patients with Langerhans cell histiocytosis of bone. *Proc XIX meeting Histiocyte Society*, Philadelphia.

Takahashi, N., Chubachi, A., Kume, M., *et al.* (2001). A clinical analysis of 52 adult patients with hemophagocytic syndrome: the prognostic significance of the underlying disease. *Int J Hematol*, **74**, 209–213.

The French LCH Study Group (1996). A multicentre retrospective survey of LCH: 348 cases observed between 1983 and 1993. *Arch Dis Child*, **75**, 17–24.

Young, J.W. (1999). Cell fate development in the myeloid system. In: Lotze, M.T. and Thomson, A.W. eds., *Dendritic Cells*, Academic Press, San Diego, Calfornia, pp. 29–49.

2

The diagnostic histopathology of Langerhans cell histiocytosis

Ronald Jaffe

Introduction

Langerhans cell (LC) disease covers a wide range of clinical presentations with peaks of incidence in early and later life. What ties these disparate conditions together is their histopathology, which has as its bedrock the identification, in the tissues or fluids, of a population of abnormal Langerhans cell histiocytosis cells (LCH cells). Like all other laboratory tests, biopsy pathology must be subjected to the rules of sensitivity and specificity. Sensitivity relates to the incidence of false negative samples. Sampling is always an issue in biopsy pathology, but considerations of sensitivity relate to those features that are essential to the diagnosis so that ideally, all patients with LCH will be identified. Specificity in a diagnostic biopsy is concerned with false positive results, and deals with the differential diagnosis of those conditions most likely to be mistaken for LCH. Since LCH involves a multitude of different anatomical sites, each of which has unique issues of access, intrinsic anatomy and cell populations, as well as the other lesions characteristic to that site, the sensitivity and specificity of LCH diagnosis must be considered for each site.

The diagnostic criteria for LCH have been a moving target. Birbeck and colleagues first described intracytoplasmic inclusions in dermal LCs (Birbeck et al., 1961). Soon after Birbeck granules were found in histiocytosis X (Basset and Nezelof, 1966), tying histiocytosis X and dermal LCs together (Nezelof et al., 1973). Later CD1a was identified as a useful diagnostic marker for LCs and later for histiocytosis X (Murphy et al., 1983). S100 was also identified as a useful tissue marker but with lower specificity for the LC since melanocytes and nevus cells also stain positive (Nakajima et al., 1982).

In 1987, the Histiocyte Society (Writing Group, 1987) defined levels of confidence in the diagnosis of LCH. A 'definitive' diagnosis required classical histopathology, confirmed by the ultrastructural presence of Birbeck granules or by demonstration of CD1a on the lesional cells, which could be done only on frozen tissue at that time. Anything less was regarded as 'presumptive'. Since then, antibodies have become available that are applicable to fixed LCH tissues for the demonstration of CD1a (Emile *et al.*, 1995) and for Langerin (CD207)[1] (Geissmann *et al.*, 2001). The current gold standard for the diagnosis is a lesion that is morphologically appropriate for LCH, in which lesional cells demonstrate CD1a and Langerin positivity or Birbeck granules. There are important limits to the sensitivity and specificity of these diagnostic markers that warrant caution, and these exceptions are noted where relevant in the discussion of the various sites of disease.

Langerhans cell histiocytosis – the prototype

A current, but incomplete, model of dendritic cell (DC) biology supposes a bone marrow precursor that gives rise to cells of the myeloid lineage that become sentinel immature DCs (see Chapter 3). The epidermal and mucosal population of LCs are the best characterized subset of DCs but there are others. Once activated the immature DCs undergo maturation. LCH appears to represent a proliferative, clonal population of immature myeloid DC arrested in the pre-maturation state (Laman *et al.*, 2003). LCH cells may, however, retain a limited capacity to mature (Geissmann *et al.*, 2001).

Despite their affiliation to the 'DC' system, LCH cells do not have 'dendritic' morphology *in situ*, or in body fluid cytology, but are round to oval in shape. In tissues, they are most commonly found in aggregates and are about 20–25 μm in size, 2–3 times as large as intervening lymphocytes. Although the coffee-bean groove of the nucleus has been emphasized, the most characteristic nuclei have complex angular and elaborate folds (Figure 2.1). Cytoplasm is generous, rarely spindled. In a prototypical lesion (soft tissue or bone), LCH cells are interspersed with eosinophils, albeit unevenly. The eosinophil presence can be extreme, with eosinophilic microabscess formation containing abundant Charcot–Leyden crystals, but eosinophils can be absent and are not a required diagnostic feature. Small lymphocytes may be sprinkled through or more commonly, around the periphery of lesions, sometimes even in dense sheets, but lymphoid activation and plasma cells are not usual. Macrophages, both phagocytic and giant cell forms, can be found in many sites. Osteoclast-like giant cells, are conspicuous in any lesion involving bone. They are generally CD1a/S100 negative and have characteristics of macrophages (Figure 2.2). In contrast, binucleate forms often carry nuclei with characteristic LCH folds and a partial surface rim of CD1a/Langerin.

[1] Langerin is a type II lectin that has mannose specificity and is represented on the cell surface and in the cytoplasm of LCs. It is responsible for Birbeck granule formation by superimposing and zippering of membranes (Valladeau *et al.*, 2000).

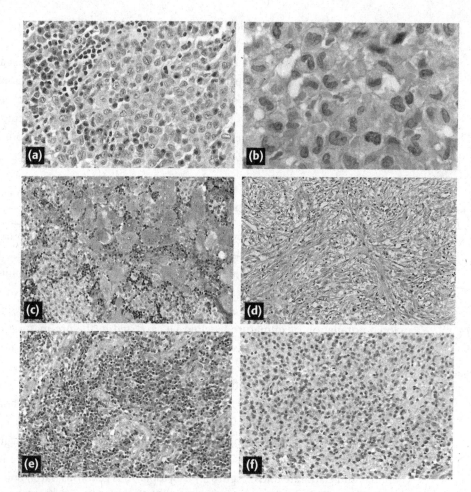

Figure 2.1   LCH histology. (a) LCH in its most classical form has sheets of cytoplasm-rich pale
histiocytes interspersed with inflammatory cells, eosinophils and lymphocytes.
(b) Nuclear morphology is typical and consists of monocytoid, grooved and complexly
folded forms in a pale-staining cytoplasm. (c) Giant cells can be of different types.
Osteoclast-like giant cells are most common in and around bone lesions. This picture
shows osteoclast-type giant cells with multiple round nuclei in a lymph node. (d) LCH can
adopt a spindle-cell form. The LCH phenotype of these spindled forms is preserved.
(e) Eosinophils can be overwhelming, forming eosinophilic micro-abscesses that contain
Charcot–Leyden crystals. (f) Eosinophils are not a required component. Some lesions are
devoid of eosinophils (same patient as Figure 2.1(e)). See also color plates

By definition, LCH cells have a surface rim of CD1a and a granular cyto-
plasmic/surface staining for Langerin (Figure 2.3). S100 immunostain will give
a nuclear and cytoplasmic blush to the cells, and fascin is demonstrable in
low to moderate amount in only few of the cells (Figure 2.2). HLA-II (LN3

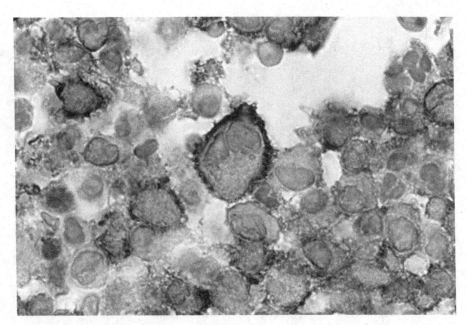

Figure 2.2   LCH giant cells. Giant and multinucleated forms can occur by cell fusion of LCH cells. A binucleated cell has classical complex LCH nuclei and strong surface CD1a staining. Most giant cells are CD1a−. See also color plates

antibody) and CD68 (KP-1) display punctate paranuclear Golgi-like intracytoplasmic staining.

In aspirated or cytospin preparations, the cells are also oval (not dendritic), and have a folded nucleus that is less obvious because the cells are flattened. The generous cytoplasm, often with azurophilic granules, is conspicuous. S100 is not applicable to unfixed cells, but CD1a and Langerin are well demonstrated by immunocytochemistry (Figure 2.3).

Sensitivity and specificity of diagnostic features at various sites

Bone and adjacent soft tissue

The histopathology and corresponding imaging studies can be markedly influenced by the stage of the disease. Early and expanding proliferating lesions will have a more confluent and generous representation of LCH cells and corresponding imaging will reflect a lytic, rapidly growing process with poorly defined margins – mimicking a malignant process (Meyer and DeCamargo, 1998). Hence the differential diagnosis of early and evolving bone lesions is Ewings' sarcoma, osteosarcoma, neuroblastoma in children and metastatic disease in adults. In this phase of the disorder, the diagnosis can be made by needle aspiration cytology, needle or trephine biopsy or

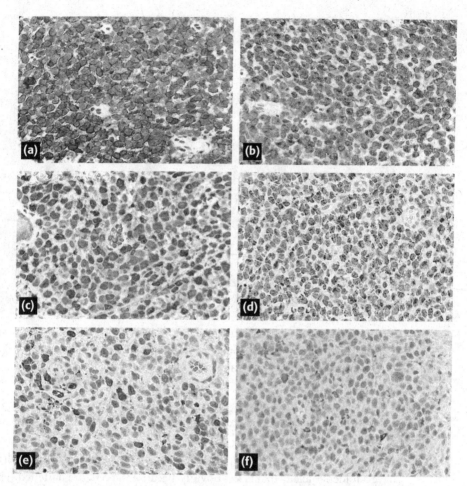

Figure 2.3   LCH prototypical phenotype. (a) The LCH cells have surface and some paranuclear staining for CD1a. (b) Granular cytoplasmic staining for Langerin. (c) Diffuse cytoplasmic/nuclear staining for S100. (d) HLA Class II (LN3 antibody) reveals intracytoplasmic, often paranuclear staining. (e) Fascin is variable and ranges from none to light staining on a minority of cells. (f) CD68, KP-1 antibody, has light granular cytoplasmic staining only. See also color plates

open biopsy. Active bone LCH has a dominant population of oval cells, CD1a+, Langerin+, S100+ with an interspersed population of osteoclast-type giant cells. Lymphocyte and phagocytic macrophages are commonly found, plasma cells and neutrophils are not in uncomplicated lesions. The diagnosis can be made with assurance on cytologic or histopathologic features, and confirmed by immunocytology or immunohistochemistry since none of the competing possibilities mentioned share the morphology or phenotype of LCH. Decalcification has only a minor effect, in most instances, on the ability to demonstrate clear surface-pattern staining for

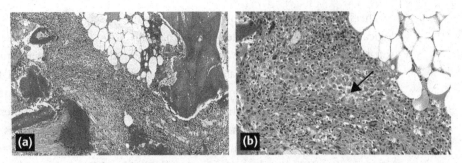

Figure 2.4   LCH bone, regressing. LCH lesions of bone can appear like those in Figure 2.1 in the active phase. (a) In the regressing phase there is progressive fibrosis, scarring and involution of the LCH cells. (b) The cluster of cells (arrow) was the only residual found after two unsuccessful needle biopsies. See also color plates

CD1a and for Langerin reactivity. Since cartilage and fat are also S100-reactive, care must be taken to ensure that it is the lesional cells that stain, S100 alone is insufficient for the definitive diagnosis of LCH in bone. Sensitivity and specificity of the diagnosis are very high.

The natural history of bony LCH is to involute. Involuting lesions may give rise to diagnostic problems not shared by earlier expanding ones, and diagnosis can be more difficult. The differential diagnosis in children is osteomyelitis, most specifically multifocal recurrent chronic osteomyelitis which is culture-negative, and mycobacterial infections (Edgar et al., 2001). Sampling is the single most important issue, because as lesions regress, the clusters of LCH cells decrease and become more dispersed until they disappear completely. Aspiration and needle biopsy may fail to confirm the diagnosis, and larger, repeated biopsies should be considered when clinical suspicion is compelling. Pathologic fracture can compound diagnostic difficulties: the presence of necrosis, hemorrhage and a macrophage component can mimic chronic recurrent multifocal osteomyelitis or fibrohistiocytic lesions of bone. Multiple sections are sometimes required, until CD1a immunostains eventually reveal small clusters or aggregates of LCH cells (Figure 2.4). Sensitivity of the diagnosis is much lower because of sampling problems.

Osteomyelitis, conventional and mycobacterial is best confirmed by culture. Rosai–Dorfman disease of bone may mimic the lesions of healing or involuting LCH. The histopathology showing large, pale, cytoplasm-rich cells with emperipolesis is distinctive (see Figure 15.8, Chapter 15). Since Rosai–Dorfman cells are S100+, CD1a−, CD1a staining is used to resolve the differential diagnosis. Erdheim–Chester disease (ECD) in adults is a radiologic diagnosis (see Figure 15.7). Bone histopathology is poorly characterized (Ivan et al., 2003) but has typical features of juvenile xanthogranuloma (JXG) (see below).

There is a small group of soft-tissue lesions that closely resemble LCH morphologically but are CD1a−, Langerin− and have no Birbeck granules. These skin and soft-tissue non-LC lesions are not well characterized. In the contemporary classification of histiocytoses (Favara *et al.*, 1997) these lesions are listed under DC-related disorders as 'solitary histiocytomas of various DC phenotypes'. This serves to indicate that there is considerable variation in the nuances of the phenotypes of these lesions. There are a number of published case reports of lesions that could fit this category, but phenotyping is usually insufficient to distinguish them from better-defined lesions such as JXG (see discussion under 'Skin'). Non-LC lesions may have features of DCs that have matured beyond the LC stage (Jaffe, 1999; Jaffe and Favara, 2002).

The index case presented at age 6 with a classical LCH lesion in the clavicle. A soft-tissue lesion which developed at the same site 6 years later, looked similar but lacked CD1a, Langerin or Birbeck granules, hence, was now a non-LC lesion. The phenotype was that of a maturing DC lesion with high surface expression of HLA-DR (LN3 antibody), S100+ and higher fascin expression. The features are different from interdigitating cell (IDC) lesions that have spindle cell morphology and very high S100/fascin expression. These non-LCH DC lesions appear to have some predeliction for the meninges in the cranium or spinal canal and the clinical behavior is unlike LCH. The lesions are mostly unifocal without systemic involvement (except very rarely) and local recurrence is a feature, unlike classical LCH (Jaffe and Favara, 2002).

Skin

Skin involvement is present in over 50% of LCH patients (Munn and Chu, 1998). Papular skin lesions in the newborn have been referred to as self-healing reticulohistiocytosis or Hashimoto–Pritzker disease (Hashimoto *et al.*, 1986). Neither term is satisfactory. Some of Hashimoto and Pritzker's original cases (Hashimoto and Pritzker, 1973, 1986) according to the illustrations, were congenital reticulohistiocytomas, a different disorder, and 'self-healing' is a diagnosis best made in retrospect because some infants with skin-only lesions have gone on to disseminate and even die of disease (Longaker *et al.*, 1994; Stein *et al.*, 2001).

Congenital LCH lesions show large, disaggregated LCH cells, rich in CD1a and Langerin (Figure 2.5), the lesions may urticate, ulcerate or appear as vesiculopustules. It is claimed (Geissmann *et al.*, 2001) that cells of 'self-healing' or isolated cutaneous LCH have a more mature phenotype than those in disseminated disease, being CD86+ and CD14−. This limited ability to mature *in situ* is also encountered in lymph nodes and liver. A prior suggestion (Geissmann *et al.*, 1997) that loss of E-cadherin from LCH cells was a marker of dissemination, was not confirmed prospectively. At present there is no validated way to prognosticate on the basis of LCH histopathology. In the newborn, important differential diagnoses include solitary reticulohistiocytoma, JXG, urticaria pigmentosa and cutaneous monoblastic leukemia (Figure 2.6). Sensitivity and specificity of the diagnosis are

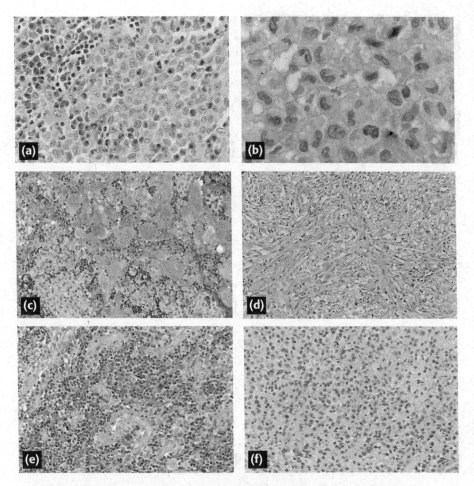

Fig. 2.1 LCH histology. (a) LCH in its most classical form has sheets of cytoplasm-rich pale histiocytes interspersed with inflammatory cells, eosinophils and lymphocytes. (b) Nuclear morphology is typical and consists of monocytoid, grooved and complexly folded forms in a pale-staining cytoplasm. (c) Giant cells can be of different types. Osteoclast-like giant cells are most common in and around bone lesions. This picture shows osteoclast-type giant cells with multiple round nuclei in a lymph node. (d) LCH can adopt a spindle-cell form. The LCH phenotype of these spindled forms is preserved. (e) Eosinophils can be overwhelming, forming eosinophilic micro-abscesses that contain Charcot–Leyden crystals. (f) Eosinophils are not a required component. Some lesions are devoid of eosinophils (same patient as Figure 2.1(e))

Figures 2.1-7.15 in this section are available for download in colour from www.cambridge.org/9780521184168

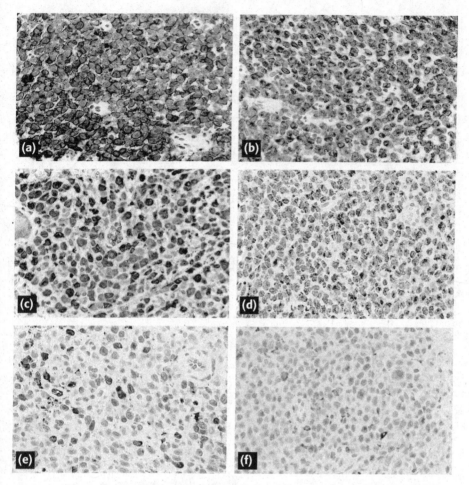

Fig. 2.3 LCH prototypical phenotype. (a) The LCH cells have surface and some paranuclear staining for CD1a. (b) Granular cytoplasmic staining for Langerin. (c) Diffuse cytoplasmic/nuclear staining for S100. (d) HLA Class II (LN3 antibody) reveals intracytoplasmic, often paranuclear staining. (e) Fascin is variable and ranges from none to light staining on a minority of cells. (f) CD68, KP-1 antibody, has light granular cytoplasmic staining only

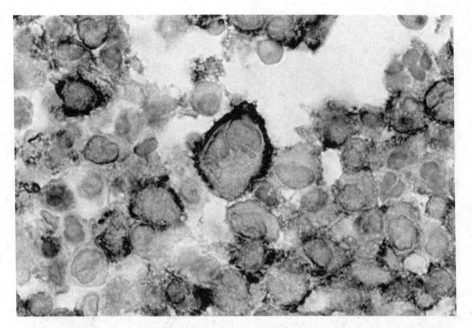

Fig. 2.2 LCH giant cells. Giant and multinucleated forms can occur by cell fusion of LCH cells. A binucleated cell has classical complex LCH nuclei and strong surface CD1a staining. Most giant cells are CD1a−

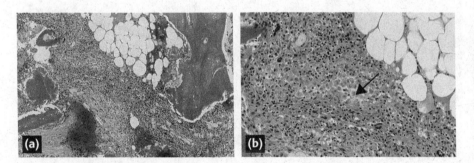

Fig. 2.4 LCH bone, regressing. LCH lesions of bone can appear like those in Figure 2.1 in the active phase. (a) In the regressing phase there is progressive fibrosis, scarring and involution of the LCH cells. (b) The cluster of cells (arrow) was the only residual found after two unsuccessful needle biopsies

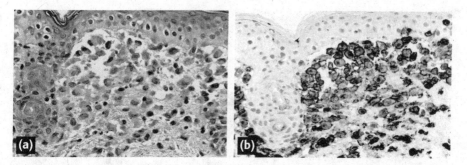

Fig. 2.5 LCH of skin. LCH is described as 'epidermotropic' and fills the papillary dermis in classical LCH. Note (a) that the LCH cells are oval to round not dendritic and (b) that the CD1a+ infiltrate is not perivascular (see also Figure 2.6(f))

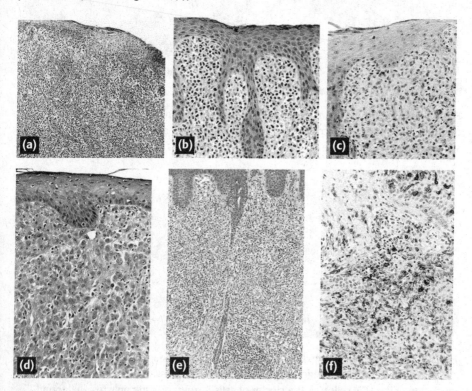

Fig. 2.6 Skin, LCH and look-alikes. (a) Congenital LCH, papular and ulcerated lesion, fills the dermis to the sub-dermal fat. (b) Urticaria pigmentosa. The epidermal saw-tooth hyperplasia and rounded papillae are a feature of mast cell lesions that lack the nuclear complexity. (c) JXG can look very similar when Touton cells are not prominent and can even have a high content of CD1a cells in the sub-epidermal area. Phenotyping (S100−/FXIIIa/fascin/CD163) may be required. (d) Solitary reticulohistiocytomas can be congenital and have large cells with abundant cytoplasm that contain round nuclei with prominent nucleoli. (e) and (f) Some chronic dermatitides contain a substantial dendritic-cell component (S100+/CD1a+). The DCs in these conditions are perivascular in distribution (e) and are generally spindled or dendritic in shape (f) (CD1a stain), unlike LCH cells (see Figure 2.5(a))

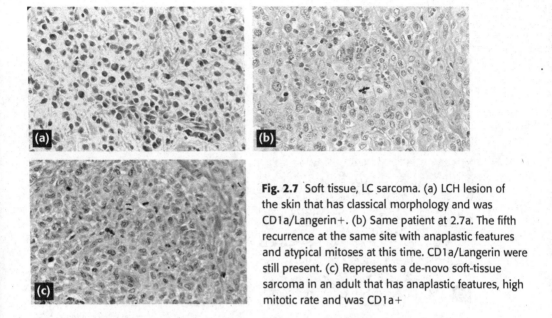

Fig. 2.7 Soft tissue, LC sarcoma. (a) LCH lesion of the skin that has classical morphology and was CD1a/Langerin+. (b) Same patient at 2.7a. The fifth recurrence at the same site with anaplastic features and atypical mitoses at this time. CD1a/Langerin were still present. (c) Represents a de-novo soft-tissue sarcoma in an adult that has anaplastic features, high mitotic rate and was CD1a+

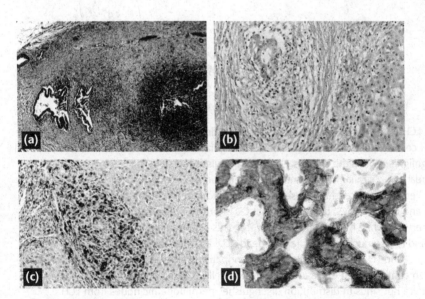

Fig. 2.9 LCH in the liver. (a) The extra-hepatic biliary tree and major bile ducts may be a site of predeliction for LCH involvement of the liver (S100). (b) Intra-hepatic bile ducts can have epithelial damage, periductal LCH infiltration and concentric fibrous scarring. (c) Langerin staining reveals the portal nature of the infiltrate centered around a bile duct. (d) Double-staining with CD1a (black) and cytokeratin (blue) shows the LCH cells in black as they infiltrate proliferating bile ductules and remain confined within the biliary basement membrane. LCH cells can be overlooked unless immunostains are used

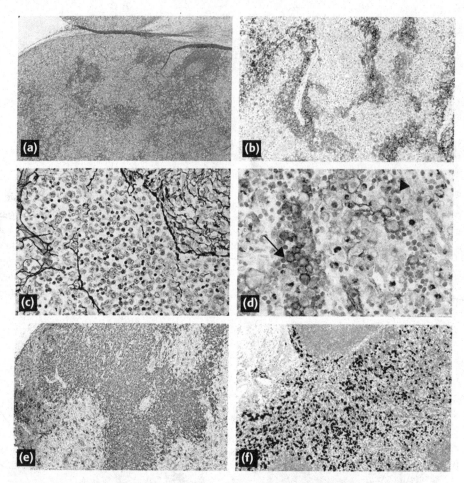

Fig. 2.8 LCH in the lymph node. (a) The lymph node that harbors LCH appears to be filled with LCH cells and only residual follicles are recognized. (b) CD1a immunostain in lymph node highlights cells in the sinuses. Paracortical cells fail to stain for CD1a even though they appear to be similar in appearance. (c) Reticulin stain confirms that much of the LCH infiltrate lies within distended sinuses. (d) Paracortical areas double-stained for CD1a (brown) and HLA-11 (LN3, blue) show that CD1a brown-stained LCH cells in clusters fill sinuses (arrow) while many of the paracortical cells express high levels of HLA-11 on their surface and in paranuclear zones (arrow head) CD1a is presumably lost as these cells 'mature'. (e) and (f) Dermatopathic lymphadenopathy can be confused with LCH because of the high content of (e) CD1a and (f) Langerin cells. A high content of fascin-staining cells that are not sinus in distribution distinguishes dermatopathic nodes from LCH

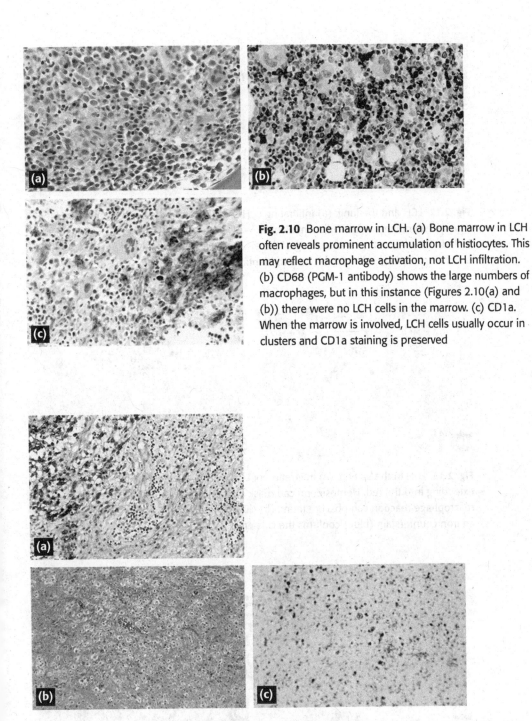

Fig. 2.10 Bone marrow in LCH. (a) Bone marrow in LCH often reveals prominent accumulation of histiocytes. This may reflect macrophage activation, not LCH infiltration. (b) CD68 (PGM-1 antibody) shows the large numbers of macrophages, but in this instance (Figures 2.10(a) and (b)) there were no LCH cells in the marrow. (c) CD1a. When the marrow is involved, LCH cells usually occur in clusters and CD1a staining is preserved

Fig. 2.11 LCH in the brain. (a) Posterior-pituitary and hypothalamic lesions represent LCH infiltration and the cells can be identified (CD1a). (b) and (c) By contrast, the late 'demyelinating' type lesions like this one in the cerebellum do not have identifiable infiltrate (b) and the high content of microglial macrophages is highlighted by CD68 (c)

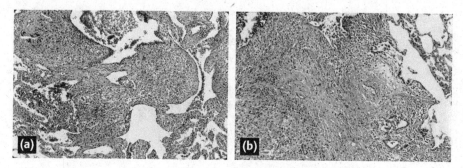

Fig. 2.12 LCH and the lung. (a) Infiltrating LCH cells form nodular aggregates around the airways extending out into adjacent alveolar walls in the active disease. (b) Later effects include the obliteration and scarring of the airways with surrounding inflammatory cells but the sparse LCH cells may be hard to identify

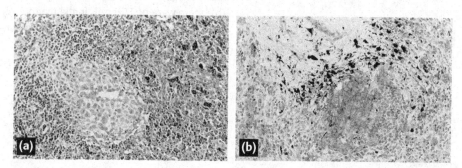

Fig. 2.13 LCH in the spleen. (a) Infiltration of LCH cells is at the margins of the white pulp extending into the red. Hemosiderin can mask the infiltrate and the common presence of macrophage reaction can obscure them. (b) CD1a immunostain (red) in the presence of an iron counterstain (blue) confirms the clusters of LCH cells

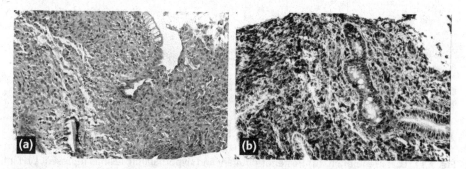

Fig. 2.14 LCH and the intestine. (a) LCH infiltration involves and can fill the lamina propria with superficial epithelial damage. (b) S100 immunostain confirms the nature of the infiltrate

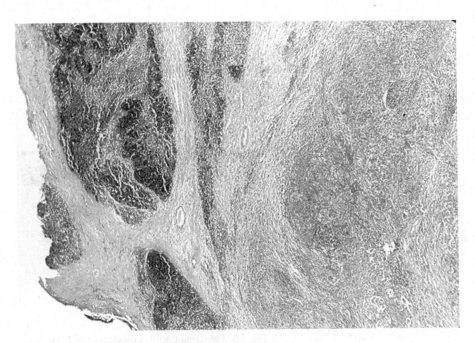

Fig. 2.15 Thymic LCH. LCH in the thymus forms eosinophilic granulomas similar to those at soft-tissue sites and there is often reactive cystic change of the thymus

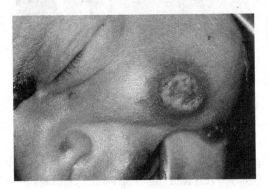

Fig. 7.1 Necrotic papule in a 3-month-old baby with congenital self-healing reticulohistiocytosis

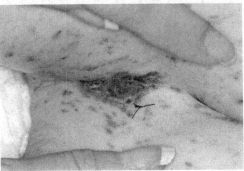

Fig. 7.2 Ulceration, petechiae and papules in 6-month-old baby with disseminated LCH

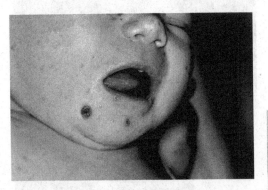

Fig. 7.3(a) Neonate born with deep ulceration on cheek

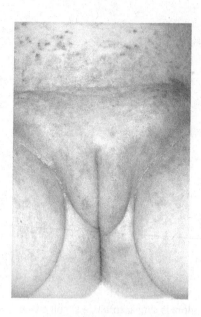

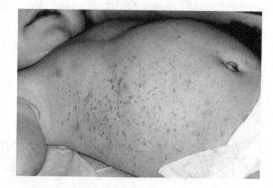

Fig. 7.4 Seborrheic pattern of histiocytosis with petechiae at peripheral edge

Fig. 7.5 Petechial papules diagnostic of LCH

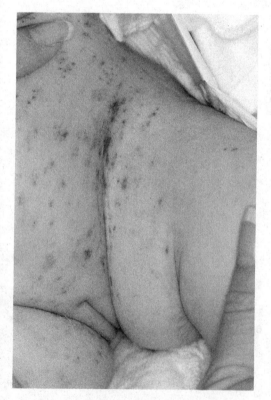

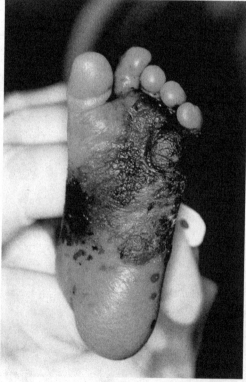

Fig. 7.6 Scattered petechiae in LCH in diaper area

Fig. 7.7 Deep hemorrhagic bulla in a child with skin-only LCH who later progressed to fatal MS disease

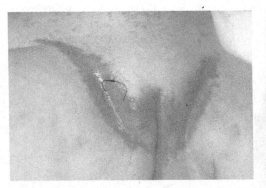

Fig. 7.8 Typical deep seborrheic pattern of LCH in diaper area

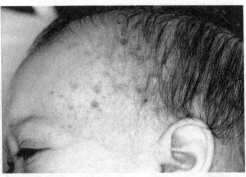

Fig. 7.9 LCH crusting and petechiae on scalp

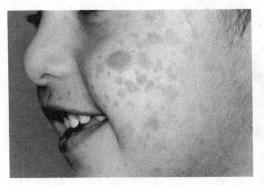

Fig. 7.10 Micronodular lesions of JXG

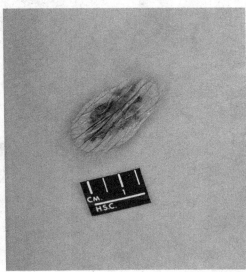

Fig. 7.13 Wrinkling after disappearance of large JXG

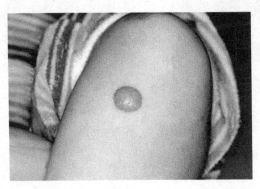

Fig. 7.14 Xanthogranuloma: a typical red-yellow nodule

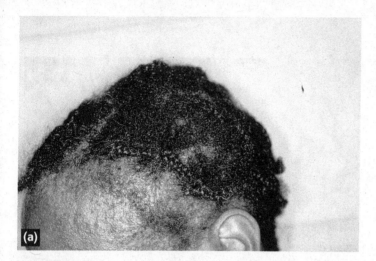

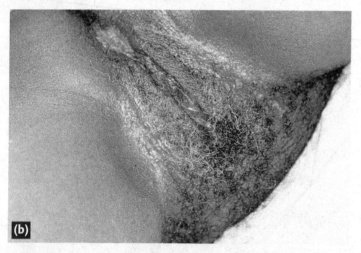

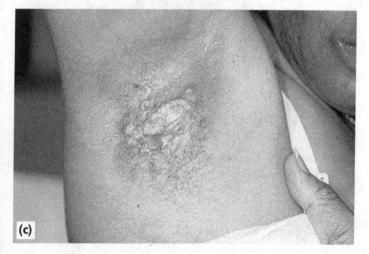

Fig. 7.15 Adult with skin LCH.
(a) Involving scalp,
(b) vulva and (c) axillary lesion
(Figures courtesy of Algin B.
Garrett, MD., Richmond, VA.)

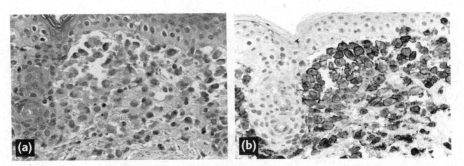

Figure 2.5   LCH of skin. LCH is described as 'epidermotropic' and fills the papillary dermis in classical LCH. Note (a) that the LCH cells are oval to round not dendritic and (b) that the CD1a+ infiltrate is not perivascular (see also Figure 2.6(f)). See also color plates

high since these conditions do not share the LCH phenotype. It should be remembered that congenital nevoid lesions are S100+ and that myelomonocytic leukemias may occasionally exhibit some CD1a positivity.

In children outside the neonatal period, the differential diagnosis includes seborrheic dermatitis, diaper rash, dermatophyte disease and scabies, both acute and chronic. Sampling is generally not an important issue as skin lesions can be visualized, but it is important to recall that LCs and so-called CD1a+ dermal inflammatory DCs (Wollenberg et al., 2002) are normally present in the epidermis and dermis. These cells can increase substantially along with other inflammatory cells in the superficial perivascular plexus and upper dermis in other chronic dermatitides, most notably chronic scabies. Reactive DCs are spindled or dendritic in shape unlike LCH cells, and perivascular in distribution (Figure 2.6).

The LCH infiltrate is epidermotropic with clusters of large oval cells filling the papillary dermis, some extending into the overlying epidermis. Intrinsic LCs are often decreased. A sparse T cell infiltrate, occasional eosinophils and very rare giant cells are identifiable, and may on occasion mask the LCH in small lesions. Parakeratosis, neutrophils in the horny layer, ulceration and secondary infection can complicate diagnosis. Definitive diagnosis is made by demonstrating a population of large, oval cells that have strong membrane expression of CD1a, Langerin and S100. As lesions resolve, the CD1a+ positive cells disappear, xanthomatous macrophages increase in number and definitive diagnosis may not be possible, or lesions may be mistaken for JXG.

JXG is the most common diagnostic confounder in children. The phenotype is consistent, Factor XIIIa+/CD68+/CD163+/CD14+/Fascin+/CD1a−/S100− even in the absence of characteristic Touton cells at non-dermal sites (Dehner, 2003).

Lesions that are CD1a+ but without Birbeck granules on electron microscopy (EM), have been termed 'indeterminate-cell lesions' (Rosenberg and Morgan, 2001). Better phenotyping will more correctly identify this group of lesions under the heading of 'solitary histiocytomas of various DC phenotypes'.

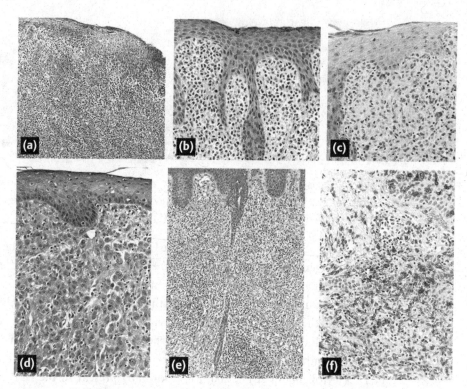

Figure 2.6   Skin, LCH and look-alikes. (a) Congenital LCH, papular and ulcerated lesion, fills the
dermis to the sub-dermal fat. (b) Urticaria pigmentosa. The epidermal saw-tooth
hyperplasia and rounded papillae are a feature of mast cell lesions that lack the nuclear
complexity. (c) JXG can look very similar when Touton cells are not prominent and can
even have a high content of CD1a cells in the sub-epidermal area. Phenotyping
(S100−/FXIIIa/fascin/CD163) may be required. (d) Solitary reticulohistiocytomas can
be congenital and have large cells with abundant cytoplasm that contain round nuclei
with prominent nucleoli. (e) and (f) Some chronic dermatitides contain a substantial
dendritic-cell component (S100+/CD1a+). The DCs in these conditions are perivascular
in distribution (e) and are generally spindled or dendritic in shape (f) (CD1a stain), unlike
LCH cells (see Figure 2.5(a)). See also color plates

In adults, the differential diagnosis and the character of the lesion are of special
concern. Specifically, other skin infiltrates can be S100+ and/or CD1a+ mimicking
LCH, and there are instances of malignant disease best characterized as 'DC-related
histiocytic sarcoma of LC-phenotype' in the 'contemporary classification' (Favara
et al., 1997) or as LC sarcoma by the International Lymphoma Study Group (Pileri
et al., 2002). Lesions that may mimic LCH are myelo-monocytic leukemias or myeloproliferative syndromes that have dermal or subcutaneous masses consisting of large
oval or round cells with strong CD1a expression (Segal *et al.*, 1992; Lauritzen *et al.*,

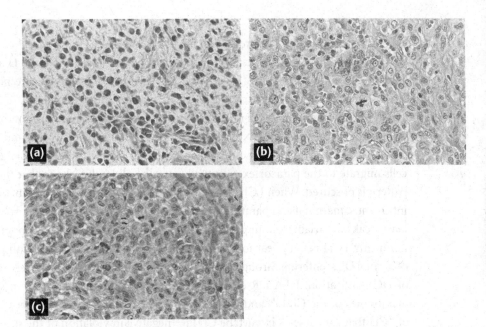

Figure 2.7   Soft tissue, LC sarcoma. (a) LCH lesion of the skin that has classical morphology and was CD1a/Langerin+. (b) Same patient as 2.7a. The fifth recurrence at the same site with anaplastic features and atypical mitoses at this time. CD1a/Langerin were still present. (c) Represents a de-novo soft-tissue sarcoma in an adult that has anaplastic features, high mitotic rate and was CD1a+. See also color plates

1994; Hermanns-Le *et al.*, 1998; Baikian *et al.*, 1999). In the few cases examined, S100 staining has been variable or absent and Langerin is negative.

Primary LC sarcoma can present in skin and is associated with widespread tumoral disease, distant metastases and poor outcome. The lesions are character-ized by cells that are often more spindled and not typical of LCH (Pileri *et al.*, 2002) but are phenotypically CD1a+, have Birbeck granules and are Langerin+. There is prominent nuclear pleomorphism, a feature not seen in childhood or even adult LCH, with atypical mitoses (Figure 2.7) (Wood *et al.*, 1984; Ben-Ezra *et al.*, 1991; Tani *et al.*, 1992; Itoh *et al.*, 2001; Yagita *et al.*, 2001).

There are very rare examples of LCH that have progressed over time to sarcoma. The recurrences get increasingly more bizarre and pleomorphic with anaplastic progression but retain CD1a positivity that may be lost only in advanced disease (Figure 2.7) (Elleder *et al.*, 1986).

The diagnostic specificity of these disorders will depend on the familiarity of pathologists with the cytologic features of LCH versus its malignant counterparts, since phenotyping alone does not distinguish them.

Lymph node

A lymph node may be the presenting and only site of LCH, but nodal disease is more commonly seen in association with skin or bone (osteolymphatic) LCH or as part of disseminated disease (Favara and Steele, 1997). Since nodes are not routinely sampled, the incidence of nodal disease may be underestimated.

LCH involvement in lymph nodes is primarily sinusoidal, an important differential diagnostic observation (Nezelof, 1979; Motoi et al., 1980; Favara and Steele, 1997). As the disease progresses, the paratrabecular sinuses fill with LCH and the cells migrate to the paracortex, eventually effacing all landmarks so that the sinus pattern is obscured. When LCH nodes are stained for CD1a and Langerin, only the intra-sinus, marginal and paratrabecular LCH cells stain strongly. Paracortical cells have weak or variable staining. S100, however, stains the entire LCH population uniformly. LCH cells appear to recapitulate the migration and maturation pattern of dermal DCs, entering through the sinuses and losing their CD1a/Langerin as part of DC maturation. HLA-DR expression is correspondingly increased on surface membranes of the CD1a^{lo} and CD1a$-$ paracortical cells. This is another example of LCH that can, at least in part, be CD1a$-$ negative in violation of the strict definition of the disease. In lymph nodes, Langerin staining should be substituted for CD1a with caution, since there is a normal population of Langerin$+$ cells in the medullary sinuses that are however, CD1a$-$ (Figure 2.8) (Chikwava and Jaffe, 2004).

Macrophage activation syndrome can accompany disseminated LCH and involved nodes may have large numbers of macrophages (with variable hemophagocytosis) (Favara et al., 2002). The absence of CD1a on paracortical LCH cells and S100 positivity on activated macrophages, can confound the diagnosis. Appropriate histopathology and CD1a$+$ staining of sinus LCH cells is the most reliable feature.

If eosinophil-rich micro-abscesses are present, the nodes can mimic visceral larva migrans but the sinus CD1a$+$ population is diagnostic. Occasional nodes have very heavy hemosiderin deposition that can obscure LCH. An iron counterstain on a node immunostained for CD1a can still be diagnostic.

The sensitivity of the diagnosis, therefore, depends on the ability to identify LCH cells in situations in which the diagnostic markers are vulnerable, or where they may be masked by other similar, confounding cells. There are two situations in which the diagnosis of LCH, though suggestive, is probably not warranted.

There are reports of LCH occurring in the same lymph node as lymphoma or leukemia. Since none of these patients has had LCH at any other site, before or after, the finding might best be regarded as localized reactive LC hyperplasia (Neumann and Frizzer, 1986; Li and Borowitz, 2001).

The other pattern was described as epithelioid granulomas within abdominal nodes that have high CD1a surface expression on the epithelioid cells (Favara and Steele, 1997). It is likely that this represents the enteric counterpart of 'dermatopathic' lymphadenopathy. The cells do not have the sinus pattern typical

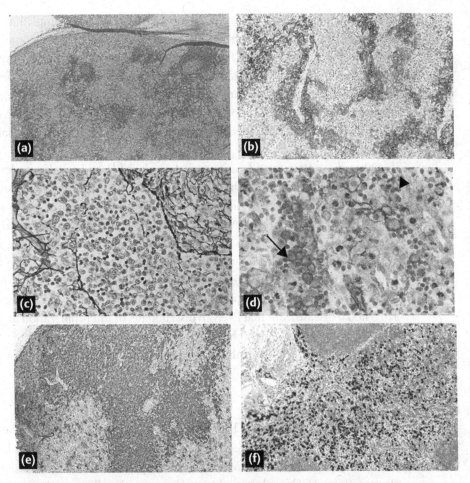

Figure 2.8   LCH in the lymph node. (a) The lymph node that harbors LCH appears to be filled with
LCH cells and only residual follicles are recognized. (b) CD1a immunostain in lymph
node highlights cells in the sinuses. Paracortical cells fail to stain for CD1a even though
they appear to be similar in appearance. (c) Reticulin stain confirms that much of the
LCH infiltrate lies within distended sinuses. (d) Paracortical areas double-stained for CD1a
and HLA-11 (LN3) show that CD1a$^+$ LCH cells in clusters fill sinuses (arrow) while many of
the paracortical cells express high levels of HLA-11 on their surface and in paranuclear zones
(arrow head). CD1a is presumably lost as these cells 'mature'. (e) and (f) Dermatopathic
lymphadenopathy can be confused with LCH because of the high content of (e) CD1a and
(f) Langerin cells. A high content of fascin-staining cells that are not sinus in distribution
distinguishes dermatopathic nodes from LCH. See also color plates

of LCH, nor has disease been seen outside of those nodes in the patients described
to date.

The specificity of the findings in lymph nodes relates to conditions that can
mimic LCH. Dermatopathic lymphadenopathy is the most important of these

because lymph nodes draining LCH-involved skin may be sampled as part of a 'staging' procedure. While dermatopathic nodes may have conspicuous numbers of CD1a+/Langerin+ DC in the expanded paracortex, they lack the sinus involvement typical of LCH. Fascin, a marker present in LCH cells in small amounts only, is highly expressed in paracortical maturing DC and interdigitating DC, and high paracortical expression of fascin in the paracortical cells favors the diagnosis of dermatopathic reaction even in patients with LCH (Figure 2.8) (Jaffe et al., 1998).

Other diagnostic considerations are less plausible and involve nodes that are partially or totally replaced by histiocytic infiltrates or granulomatous disease. Kikuchi disease and histiocytic-rich malignant disorders such as some anaplastic large cell lymphomas may simulate LCH, but can be excluded by their own characteristic phenotypes and the lack of CD1a/Langerin on the histiocytes, as well as their lack of a sinus pattern. Eosinophil-rich lymph nodes, such as some instances of Hodgkins' disease or Churg–Strauss disease, lack the diagnostic LCH infiltrate.

As in the skin, there are no features that predict outcome and distinguish isolated nodal disease from that likely to disseminate. In situ proliferation as seen with Ki-67 immunostain can be high within the CD1a+ population, up to 48% (Schmitz and Favara, 1998). Pleomorphism, anaplasia and atypical mitoses, however, are features of sarcoma.

Liver

Liver 'involvement' in LCH is best defined as LCH infiltration into the liver. Some children with LCH at other sites have hepatomegaly and hypoalbuminemia and this reversible phenomenon may represent macrophage activation without infiltration (Favara, 1996). LCH involving only liver is an exceptionally rare phenomenon (Finn and Jaffe, 1997; Kaplan et al., 1999) and most patients who have liver disease have multisystem LCH (French LCH Study Group, 1996; Braier et al., 2002). LCH has a unique tropism for the bile ducts of the liver, affecting mostly the larger bile channels, and for this reason, hyperbilirubinemia and a raised gammaglutamyl peptidase (GGT) serum level are sensitive indicators of hepatic infiltration.

Sensitivity of the diagnosis is influenced by the confusion as to what, exactly, constitutes liver 'involvement'. The problems of percutaneous sampling of a process that involves the central biliary tree and the subtlety of the features of LCH on biopsy have led to the belief that pre-treatment liver biopsies are only rarely diagnostic (Heyn et al., 1990; Braier et al., 2002). LCH usually infiltrates major bile ducts (this can be seen on imaging studies). There is involvement of major bile ducts with mucosal damage leading to scarring and sclerosing cholangitis. The LCH infiltrate can extend into small peripheral bile radicals, creeping between the biliary epithelial cells and their basement membrane. Recognition of this subtle feature, seen in

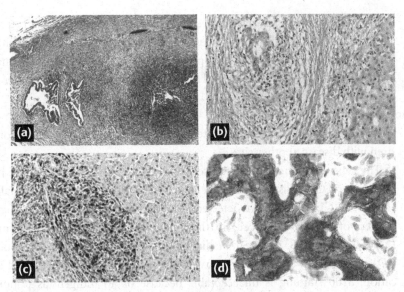

Figure 2.9   LCH in the liver. (a) The extra-hepatic biliary tree and major bile ducts may be a site of predeliction for LCH involvement of the liver (S100). (b) Intra-hepatic bile ducts can have epithelial damage, periductal LCH infiltration and concentric fibrous scarring. (c) Langerin staining reveals the portal nature of the infiltrate centered around a bile duct. (d) Double-staining with CD1a and cytokeratin shows the darkly stained LCH cells as they infiltrate proliferating bile ductules and remain confined within the biliary basement membrane. LCH cells can be overlooked unless immunostains are used. See also color plates

some instances in the absence of extrabiliary LCH cells, will increase the sensitivity of liver biopsy (Figure 2.9).

LCH cells within the walls of small bile ducts can be demonstrated with CD1a, Langerin or S100 stains, but may be almost invisible without these. Affected portal areas are usually expanded with some degree of edema and bile ductular proliferation. In some instances, there is extravasation of LCH cells outside the bile ducts into adjacent portal areas, and, when large enough, into the lobules. This is another example of *in situ* maturation: the extrabiliary cells may be S100+ but relatively poor in CD1a. Active LCH can regress after having caused sclerosing cholangitis and cirrhosis, so that sensitivity of the diagnosis is affected by the stage of disease. In most instances of livers explanted for transplantation of LCH-related cirrhosis, no active disease is found (Braier *et al.*, 2002).

The major pathology in the liver, even in the absence of demonstrable LCH, is that of biliary obstruction, with a pattern common to other causes of sclerosing cholangitis (LeBlanc, 1981; Favara, 1996; Kaplan *et al.*, 1999; Braier *et al.*, 2002). The specificity of the diagnosis can be affected by the presence of non-Langerhans macrophages since macrophage activation syndrome may lead to an increase in

S100+ activated sinus macrophages (Jaffe, 2004). Owing to the very predictable pattern of hepatic involvement, a pattern of biliary obstruction/sclerosing cholangitis should be regarded as presumptive evidence of LCH-mediated damage even in the absence of demonstrable LCH cells in a patient with LCH at other sites.

Bone marrow

Marrow involvement by LCH is often a critical element in the evaluation of children with disease at other sites.

The sensitivity and risk of a falsely negative diagnosis are influenced by sampling since LCH cells may be present in small numbers. Under normal circumstances, no CD1a+ cells are detected in bone marrow. The presence of groups or clusters of CD1a+ large cells in the marrow is diagnostic of LCH infiltration (McClain et al., 1983) and can be diagnosed using the 010 or MTB1 antibodies to CD1a in formalin or B5-fixed biopsy samples, even after most forms of decalcification. S100 staining is unacceptable because of an indigenous population of S100+ spindle and DC in the marrow, as well as fat, and because activated macrophages can stain for S100 (Schmitz and Favara, 1998). On occasion heavy hemosiderin deposition can obscure the presence of small numbers of LCH cells, but CD1a immunostain with an iron counterstain can resolve this difficulty. Specificity is affected by the presence of non-LCH macrophage histiocytosis. Macrophage activation and frank hemophagocytic syndrome are not uncommon in children with disseminated LCH, and the marrow can be filled with activated macrophages even in the absence of LCH cells. Immunostains for CD163 (or CD68, PGM-1 antibody) will highlight the macrophages with minimal cross-reactivity against LCH cells (Figure 2.10). Anemia and pancytopenia in LCH is hardly ever attributable to marrow infiltration or to myelofibrosis/depletion, but is most likely to be a manifestation of macrophage activation syndrome (Favara et al., 2002). After treatment with chemotherapeutic agents, the marrow of patients with LCH can have sheets of foamy macrophages and stromal disruption with fibrosis. This macrophage histiocytosis can be misinterpreted as LCH, as can granulomas.

Central nervous system

Three types of central nervous system (CNS) involvement have been described in LCH, direct infiltration, space occupying lesions of the ventricles, choroid or meninges, and neurodegenerative lesions (Grois et al., 1998; Schmitz and Favara, 1998).

Hypothalamic-posterior pituitary and pineal involvement is by direct infiltration leading to local destruction, the usual outcome is irreversible diabetes insipidus (DI) (Dunger et al., 1989; Broadbent and Pritchard, 1997) (Figure 2.11). DI can precede the other manifestations of LCH and in such circumstances, a tissue diagnosis may be warranted. Sensitivity and specificity are high because biopsy can be imaging

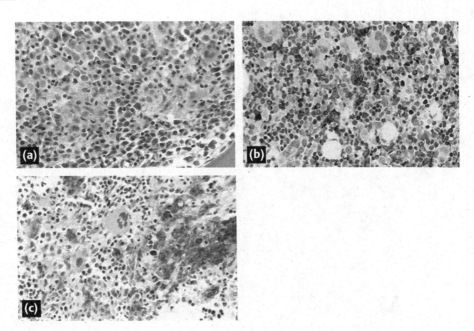

Figure 2.10 Bone marrow in LCH. (a) Bone marrow in LCH often reveals prominent accumulation of histiocytes. This may reflect macrophage activation, not LCH infiltration. (b) CD68 (PGM-1 antibody) shows the large numbers of macrophages, but in this instance (Figures 2.10(a) and (b)) there were no LCH cells in the marrow. (c) CD1a. When the marrow is involved, LCH cells usually occur in clusters and CD1a staining is preserved. See also color plates

(CT scan)-directed, and because the damage is caused by direct LCH infiltration. CD1a is the marker of choice because of endogenous S100 positivity. The differential diagnosis rests between craniopharyngioma/Rathke pouch cyst, granulomatous inflammation and germ cell lesions, each of which has distinguishing morphologic and phenotypic characteristics. The space occupying lesions can be intracerebral, within the meninges, or intraventricular in the choroid plexus. Intracerebral lesions are rare, and may be difficult to confirm because of sampling problems, paucity of LCH cells, and the relatively prominent inflammatory, macrophage and astroglial components (Kepes and Kepes, 1969). Timing affects the sensitivity, earlier lesions are more likely to contain aggregates of CD1a+ LCH cells and the major differential is that of other macrophage containing cerebral lesions. Space occupying lesions may involve the choroid plexus or leptomeninges, and in these sites, the specificity of the histologic features of LCH is reduced because there is often a striking xanthomatous response with foamy macrophages that may dominate the picture, obscuring the few LCH cells that are present (Schmitz and Favara, 1998). Choroid plexus involvement and meningeal involvement can mimic JXG although the foamy cells are generally Factor XIIIa negative.

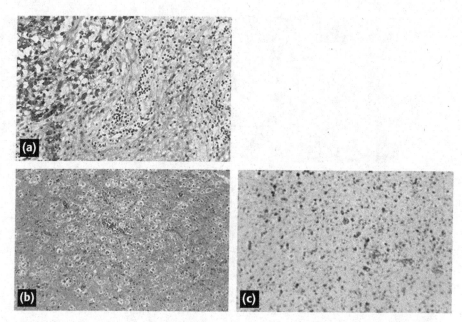

Figure 2.11   LCH in the brain. (a) Posterior-pituitary and hypothalamic lesions represent LCH infiltration
and the cells can be identified (CD1a). (b) and (c) By contrast, the late 'demyelinating'
type lesions like this one in the cerebellum do not have identifiable infiltrate (b) and the
high content of microglial macrophages is highlighted by CD68 (c). See also color plates

Teenagers and young adults can develop another late form of LCH-related CNS
disorder. These neurodegenerative lesions can involve cerebellum bilaterally and
the imaging reveals magnetic resonance imaging (MRI) signals that simulate multisystem atrophy in dentate nuclei and basal ganglia. These lesions have never been
shown to harbor LCH directly, and biopsy is of no value in diagnosis. The lesions
contain inflammatory cells, edema and axonal degeneration like those seen in
other immune-mediated and paraneoplastic lesions (Figure 2.11).

Lung

Lung involvement in LCH differs in children and adults and may represent a different pathophysiological process. Isolated lung involvement is virtually never seen
in children in whom lung disease accompanies multivisceral or disseminated disease. Lung LCH is commoner in adults, over 90% are smokers and lung is the only
disease-site (Vassallo *et al.*, 2000). Lung nodules taken from adults were shown to
be non-clonal in 70%, and even in the 30% that are clonal, a given patient may
have different clones in separate nodules or non-clonal nodules (Yousem *et al.*,
2001). Thus in contrast to pediatric disease, in which LCH appears to be clonal,
adult pulmonary LCH associated with smoking behaves more like the outgrowth

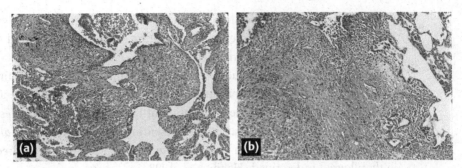

Figure 2.12 LCH and the lung. (a) Infiltrating LCH cells form nodular aggregates around the airways extending out into adjacent alveolar walls in the active disease. (b) Later effects include the obliteration and scarring of the airways with surrounding inflammatory cells but the sparse LCH cells may be hard to identify. See also color plates

of clonal nodules on a background of non-clonal LC hyperplasia. Allelic loss of heterozygosity using polymorphic satellite markers on this same population revealed tumor-suppressor-gene loss especially for those on chromosomes 9p and 22q in 8/14 patients (Dacic *et al.*, 2003). Smoking can increase the number of LC in lung and even induce LCH in the lungs of adults who previously had LCH (of any form) in childhood (Casolaro *et al.*, 1988; Bernstrand *et al.*, 2000).

High resolution computed tomography reveals the interstitial pattern of nodular and cystic changes mostly in middle and upper lobes, bilateral and symmetric (Sundar *et al.*, 2003). Pulmonary lesions are bronchocentric and intervening lung is usually normal. Bronchial obstruction can lead to the accumulation of intra-alveolar macrophages that are not very different from LCH cells in appearance, and lymphocytes, eosinophils and plasma cells can contribute to the peribronchial nodules. CD1a and S100 are effective in revealing the LCH cells in lung biopsies (Figure 2.12). As the disease advances, there is regression of the LCH cells, with peribronchial fibrosis and progressive cystic change peripheral to the retracting nodules. At some point, the LCH cells may no longer be detectable and the diagnostic distinction between advanced LCH and other causes of honeycombing can be lost (Travis *et al.*, 1993).

The major differential diagnostic considerations of active LCH, given the characteristic imaging features, are sarcoidosis and hypersensitivity pneumonitis, both of which lack the large and oval-shaped CD1a+ S100+ LCH cells.

Broncho-alveolar lavage (BAL) cytology has been used, in conjunction with clinical and imaging features, to diagnose LCH. Although LCs are a prominent component of many interstitial and even some neoplastic pulmonary processes, a BAL with greater than 5% CD1a+ large cells is highly suggestive of childhood lung-LCH in the active stage (Réfabert *et al.*, 1996). This is not true for adults, in whom the sensitivity is much lower due to the many conditions (including smoking) in which reactive LC hyperplasia is a feature (Tazi *et al.*, 2000), and would be true for neither in the late 'fibrosis' stage.

Pulmonary LCH can produce pleural bullae that rupture with resulting pneumothoraces. Rupture of pleural bullae in non-LCH patients can evoke a striking eosinophil response, so that demonstration of LCH cells is required to establish a diagnosis when pneumothorax is the presenting feature (Gervais *et al.*, 1993). Lung transplantation has been used for advanced late-stage disease and recurrence in the allograft is described (Habib *et al.*, 1998).

Spleen

The true incidence of LCH in the spleen is unknown. Splenomegaly *per se* is not sufficient for diagnosis of splenic involvement because it can be a manifestation of macrophage activation that accompanies some instances of multifocal or disseminated disease (Favara *et al.*, 2002). Splenic puncture to confirm the presence of LCH is not widely practiced.

LCH in the spleen can take two forms. The more common is a subtle involvement of the red pulp with clusters of LCH cells; diagnosis can be difficult because this form is usually accompanied by hyperplasia of other splenic macrophages and diagnosis requires the demonstration of CD1a/Langerin on the surface of candidate cells. There is no endogenous Langerin in the spleen. S100 reactivity is insufficient for diagnosis since there are endogenous cells and activated macrophages that stain for S100. Excessive hemosiderin can confound the immunostains but can be circumvented by application of Perl's iron stain following the immunostain (Figure 2.13). Less commonly, nodular, tumoral splenic aggregates can occur in disseminated LCH. These may be spindled and morphologically not typical of LCH elsewhere, but CD1a/S100 positivity is maintained (Figure 2.13) (Yagita *et al.*, 2001).

In splenic LCH, sensitivity of the diagnosis is impacted by the difficulty of getting tissue, while specificity is compromised by the presence of reactive splenic macrophages that confound the diagnosis.

Gastrointestinal tract

Gastrointestinal involvement is seen in children and adults. Only rarely is the intestine the presenting site and it is even more unusual for it to be the only site (Geissmann *et al.*, 1996).

In children, the infiltrate is part of multivisceral involvement and can lead to diarrhea, protein-losing enteropathy and anemia due to widespread mucosal disease (Egeler *et al.*, 1990; Boccon-Gibod *et al.*, 1992). The diagnosis is made by confirming that the large pale cells that fill the superficial mucosa, beneath the surface epithelium (Figure 2.14), display CD1a and S100 (Egeler *et al.*, 1990; Schmitz

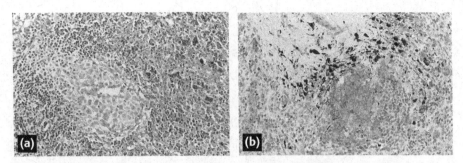

Figure 2.13 LCH in the spleen. (a) Infiltration of LCH cells is at the margins of the white pulp
extending into the dark area. Hemosiderin can mask the infiltrate and the common
presence of macrophage reaction can obscure them. (b) CD1a immunostain in the
presence of an iron counterstain confirms the clusters of LCH cells. See also color plates

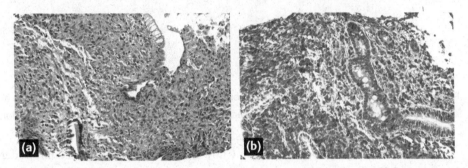

Figure 2.14 LCH and the intestine. (a) LCH infiltration involves and can fill the lamina propria with
superficial epithelial damage. (b) S100 immunostain confirms the nature of the
infiltrate. See also color plates

and Favara, 1998). Adult disease is more likely to involve stomach and large bowel
and can present with obstruction (Iwafuchi *et al.*, 1990; Hofman *et al.*, 2002).
Pancreatic involvement is exceptionally rare (Yu *et al.*, 1993).

Thymus

The thymus can harbor clusters of CD1a+ large DC in myasthenia gravis and other
conditions, and this is best regarded as focal LC hyperplasia since no disease is
encountered elsewhere (Gilcrease *et al.*, 1997). The thymus is commonly enlarged
in systemic LCH (Junewick and Fitzgerald, 1999) but the true incidence of involvement is unknown. The thymus can be partially or wholly involved with LCH as a
solitary site in childhood or adults and this is usually accompanied by cystic
change (Siegal *et al.*, 1985; Wakely and Suster, 2000). The cystic change with necrosis and xanthomatous reaction rich in macrophages may mask the sheets of LCH
cells. Confirmation using CD1a and S100 is required, and the fact that the small

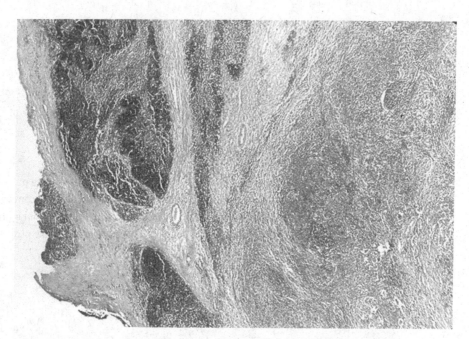

Figure 2.15 Thymic LCH. LCH in the thymus forms eosinophilic granulomas similar to those at soft-tissue sites and there is often reactive cystic change of the thymus. See also color plates

cortical lymphocytes are also CD1a positive should not be a confounder (Figure 2.15). Langerin is expressed on very rare intralobular spindled and oval cells and in some Hassal's corpuscles, and can be used for the diagnosis of LCH in the thymus.

Thyroid

LCs may participate in the immune reactions in thyroid conditions and increased number of S100+ DCs are reported in papillary carcinomas of the thyroid. The thyroid is uncommonly involved in childhood LCH, but can be involved as a solitary site in adults (Behrens *et al.*, 2001). Because it presents as a thyroid swelling, thyroid LCH is especially amenable to needle aspiration, and confirmation as a relatively pure population by CD1a/Langerin immunocytology (Sahoo *et al.*, 1998). Rare instances of symptomatic parathyroid involvement are encountered (Yap *et al.*, 2001).

Sites at which LCH is not found

There are sites in the body in which LCH is hardly ever found (except, perhaps at autopsy of patients with disseminated disease). The gonads, testis in particular, less so the ovary, seem to be resistant to LCH (Axiotis *et al.*, 1991). The kidney is another site in which LCH is not described. Understanding the local phenomena that govern resistance to LCH would be of great interest.

Other histiocytic lesions in the differential diagnosis of LCH

Rosai–Dorfman disease (sinus histiocytosis with massive lymphadenopathy)

Sinus histiocytosis with massive lymphadenopathy (SHML) is distinguished from LCH primarily by very large pale histiocytes with abundant cytoplasm, a central large, round and not folded nucleus and intracytoplasmic emperipolesis of lymphocytes, neutrophils and plasma cells. The cells have a characteristic phenotype, S100+ Fascin+, as well as CD68+ and CD163+. Thus caution is needed when using S100 to differentiate this condition from LCH (Jaffe *et al.*, 1998; Middel *et al.*, 1999). Coexistance of LCH and SHML is described (Wang *et al.*, 2002).

Juvenile xanthogranuloma

JXG can mimic LCH quite closely in a number of tissue sites as well as being multifocal with visceral involvement on occasion (Dehner, 2003). The characteristic Touton cells are not invariably seen, but the phenotype of the infiltrate appears to be consistent in most lesions, Factor XIIIa+/Fascin+/CD68+/CD163+/CD14+/CD1a−/S100−. There is a connection between LCH and JXG with dermal JXG lesions being seen in children after LCH. This can cause confusion when recurrence is suspected since dermal JXG is usually self-limiting (Hoeger *et al.*, 2001).

REFERENCES

Axiotis, C.A., Merino, M.J. and Duray, P.H. (1991). Langerhans' cell histiocytosis of the female genital tract. *Cancer*, **67**, 1650–1660.

Baikian, B., Descamps, V., Grossin, M., *et al.* (1999). Langerhans' cell histiocytosis and myelomonocytic leukemia: a non-fortuitous association. *Ann Dermatol Venereol*, **126**, 409–411.

Basset, F. and Nezelof, C. (1966). Presence en microscopic electronique de structures filamenteuses originals dans le lesions pulmonaries et osseuses de l'histiocytose-X. *Bull Mem Soc Med Hop* (Paris), **117**, 413–426.

Behrens, R.J., Levi, A.W., Westra, W.H., *et al.* (2001). Langerhans' cell histiocytosis of the thyroid: a report of two cases and review of the literature. *Thyroid*, **11**, 697–705.

Ben-Ezra, J., Bailey, A., Azumi, N., *et al.* (1991). Malignant histiocytosis X. A distinct clinicopathologic entity. *Cancer*, **68**, 1050–1060.

Bernstrand, C., Cederlund, K., Ashtrom, L., *et al.* (2000). Smoking preceded pulmonary involvement in adults with Langerhans' cell histiocytosis diagnosed in childhood. *Acta Paediatr*, **89**, 1389–1392.

Birbeck, F., Breathnach, A.S. and Everall, J.D. (1961). An electron microscopic study of basal melanocytes and high-level clear cells (Langerhans' cells) in vitiligo. *J Invest Dermatol*, **37**, 51–64.

Boccon-Gibod, L.A., Krichen, H.A., Carlier-Mercier, L.M., *et al.* (1992). Digestive tract involvement with exudative enteropathy in Langerhans' cell histiocytosis. *Pediatr Pathol*, **12**, 515–524.

Braier, J., Ciocca, M., Latella, A., *et al.* (2002). Cholestasis, sclerosing cholangitis, and liver transplantation in Langerhans' cell histiocytosis. *Med Pediatr Oncol*, **38**, 178–182.

Broadbent, V. and Pritchard, J. (1997). Diabetes insipidus associated with Langerhans' cell histiocytosis. Is it reversible? *Med Pediatr Oncol*, **28**, 289–293.

Casalaro, M.A., Bernaudin, J.F., Saltini, C., *et al.* (1988). Accumulation of Langerhans' cells on the epithelial surface of the lower respiratory tract in normal subjects in association with cigarette smoking. *Am Rev Respir Dis*, **137**, 406–411.

Chikwava, K. and Jaffe, R. (2004). Langerin (CD207) staining in normal pediatric tissues, reactive lymph nodes and childhood histiocytic disorders. *Pediatr Dev Pathol*, **7**, 607–614.

Dacic, S., Trusky, C., Bakker, A., *et al.* (2003). Genotypic analysis of pulmonary Langerhans cell histiocytosis. *Hum Pathol*, **34**, 1345–1349.

Dehner, L.P. (2003). Juvenile xanthogranulomas in the first two decades of life: a clinicopathologic study of 174 cases with cutaneous and extracutaneous manifestations. *Am J Surg Pathol*, **27**, 579–593.

Dunger, D.B., Broadbent, V., Yeoman, E., *et al.* (1989). The frequency and natural history of diabetes insipidus in children with Langerhans-cell histiocytosis. *New Engl J Med*, **321**, 1157–1162.

Edgar, J.D., Smyth, A.E., Pritchard, J., *et al.* (2001). Interferon-gamma receptor deficiency mimicking Langerhans' cell histiocytosis. *J Pediatr*, **139**, 600–603.

Egeler, R.M., Schipper, M.E. and Heymans, H.S. (1990). Gastrointestinal involvement in Langerhans' cell histiocytosis (histiocytosis X): a clinical report of three cases. *Eur J Pediatr*, **149**, 325–329.

Elleder, M., Fakan, F. and Hula, M. (1986). Pleiomorphous histiocytic sarcoma arising in a patient with histiocytosis X. *Neoplasm*, **33**, 117–128.

Emile, J.F., Wechsler, J., Brousse N., *et al.* (1995). Langerhans' cell histiocytosis. Definitive diagnosis with the use of the monoclonal antibody O10 on routinely paraffin-embedded samples. *Am J Surg Pathol*, **19**, 636–641.

Favara, B.E. (1996). Histopathology of the liver in histiocytosis syndromes. *Pediatr Pathol Lab Med*, **16**, 413–433.

Favara, B.E. and Steele, A. (1997). Langerhans' cell histiocytosis of lymph nodes. A morphological assessment of 43 biopsies. *Pediatr Pathol Lab Med*, **17**, 769–787.

Favara, B.E., Feller, A., Pauli, M., *et al.* (1997). For the Reclassification Work Group of the Histiocyte Society. Contemporary classification of histiocyte disorders. *Med Pediatr Oncol*, 157–166.

Favara, B.E., Jaffe, R. and Egeler, R.M. (2002). Macrophage activation and hemophagocytic syndrome in Langerhans' cell histiocytosis. A report of 30 cases. *Pediatr Dev Pathol*, **5**, 130–140.

Finn, L.S. and Jaffe, R. (1997). Langerhans' cell granuloma confined to the bile duct. *Pediatr Pathol Lab Med*, **17**, 461–468.

Geissmann, F., Thomas, C., Emile, J.F., *et al.* (1996). Digestive tract involvement in Langerhans' cell histiocytosis. The French Langerhans' Cell Histiocytosis Study Group. *J Pediatr*, **129**, 836–845.

Geissmann, F., Emile, J.F., Andry, P., *et al.* (1997). Lack of expression of E-cadherin is associated with dissemination of Langerhans' cell histiocytosis and poor outcome. *J Pathol*, **181**, 301–304.

Geissmann, F., Leppelletier, Y., Fraitag, S., *et al.* (2001). Differentiation of Langerhans' cells in Langerhans cells histiocytosis. *Blood*, **97**, 1241–1248.

Gervais, D.A., Whitman, G.J. and Chew, F.S. (1993). Pulmonary eosinophilic granuloma. *Am J Roentgenol*, **161**, 1158.

Gilcrease, M.Z., Rajan, B., Ostrowski, M.L., *et al.* (1997). Localized thymic Langerhans' cell histiocytosis and its relationship with myasthenia gravis. Immunohistochemical, ultrastructural and cytometric studies. *Arch Pathol Lab Med,* **121,** 134–138.

Grois, N.G., Favara, B.E., Mostbeck, G.H., *et al.* (1998). Central nervous system disease in Langerhans' cell histiocytosis. *Hematol Oncol Clin North Am,* **12,** 287–305.

Habib, S.B., Congleton, J., Carr, D., *et al.* (1998). Recurrence of recipient Langerhans' cell histiocytosis following bilateral lung transplantation. *Thorax,* **53,** 323–325.

Hashimoto, K. and Pritzker, M.S. (1973). Electron microscopic study of reticulohistiocytoma. An unusual case of self-healing reticulohistiocytosis. *Arch Dermatol,* **107,** 263–270.

Hashimoto, K., Bale, G.F., Hawkins, H.K., *et al.* (1986). Congenital self-healing reticulohistiocytosis (Hashimoto–Pritzker type). *Int J Dermatol,* **25,** 516–523.

Hermanns-Le, T., Arrese, J.E. and Pierard, G.E. (1998). Langerhans cell histiocytosis and acute monoblastic leukemia type LMA4. *Ann Dermatol Venereol,* **125,** 124–126.

Heyn, R.M., Hamoudi, A. and Newton Jr, W.A. (1990). Pretreatment liver biopsy in 20 children with histiocytosis X: a clinicopathologic correlation. *Med Pediatr Oncol,* **18,** 110–118.

Hoeger, P.H., Diaz, C., Malone, M., *et al.* (2001). Juvenile xanthogranuloma as a sequel to Langerhans cell histiocytosis: a report of three cases. *Clin Exp Dermatol,* **26,** 391–394.

Hofman, V., Hourseau, M., Musso, S., *et al.* (2002). Langerhans' cell histiocytosis of the large bowel. *Ann Pathol,* **22,** 461–464.

Itoh, H., Miyaguni, H., Kataoka, H., *et al.* (2001) Primary cutaneous Langerhans' cell histiocytosis showing malignant phenotype in an elderly woman: report of a fatal case. *J Cutan Pathol,* **28,** 371–378.

Ivan, D., Neto, A., Lemos, L., *et al.* (2003). Erdheim–Chester disease. A unique presentation with liver and vertebral osteolytic lesions. *Arch Pathol Lab Med,* **127,** e337–e339.

Iwafuchi, M., Watanabe, H., Shiratsuka, M., *et al.* (1990). Primary benign histiocytosis X of the stomach. A report of a case showing spontaneous remission after 5½ years. *Am J Surg Pathol,* **14,** 489–496.

Jaffe, R. (1999). The histiocytoses. *Clin Lab Med,* **19,** 135–155.

Jaffe, R. (2004). Liver involvement in the histiocytic disorders of childhood. *Pediatr Devel Pathol,* **7,** 214–225.

Jaffe, R. and Favara, B.E. (2002). Non-Langerhans' dendritic cell histiocytosis (abstract). *Pediatr Dev Pathol,* **5,** 99.

Jaffe, R., DeVaughn, D. and Langhoff, E. (1998). Fascin and the differential diagnosis of childhood histiocytic lesions. *Pediatr Dev Pathol,* **1,** 216–221.

Junewick, J.J. and Fitzgerald, N.E. (1999). The thymus in Langerhans' cell histiocytosis. *Pediatr Radiol,* **29,** 904–907.

Kaplan, K.J., Goodman, Z.D. and Ishak, K.G. (1999). Liver involvement in Langerhans' cells histiocytosis: a study of nine cases. *Mod Pathol,* **12,** 370–378.

Kepes, J.J. and Kepes, M. (1969). Predominantly cerebral forms of histiocytosis X. A reappraisal of 'Gagel's hypothalamic granuloma' 'granuloma infiltrans of the hypothalamus' and 'Ayala's disease' with report of four cases. *Acta Neuropathol* (Berlin), **14,** 77–98.

Laman, J.D., Leenen, P.J., Annels, N.E., *et al.* (2003). Langerhans-cell histiocytosis, 'insights into DC biology'. *Trend Immunol,* **24,** 190–196.

Lauritzen, A.F., Delsol, G., Hansen, N.E., *et al.* (1994). Histiocytic sarcomas and monoblastic leukemias. A clinical, histologic and immunophenotypical study. *Am J Clin Pathol*, **102**, 45–54.

LeBlanc, A., Hadchouel, M., Jehan, P., *et al.* (1981). Obstructive jaundice in children with histiocytosis X. *Gastroenterology*, **80**, 134–139.

Li, S. and Borowitz, M.J. (2001). CD79a(+) and T cell lymphoblastic lymphoma with co-existing Langerhans' cell histiocytosis. *Arch Pathol Lab Med*, **125**, 958–960.

Longaker, M.A., Frieden, I.J., LeBoit, P., *et al.* (1994). Congenital 'self-healing' Langerhans' cell histiocytosis: the need for long-term follow-up. *J Am Acad Dermatol*, **31**, 910–916.

McClain, K., Ramsay, N.K., Robinson, L., *et al.* (1983). Bone marrow involvement in histiocytosis X. *Med Pediatr Oncol*, **11**, 167–171.

Meyer, J.S. and DeCamargo, B. (1998). The role of radiology in the diagnosis and follow-up of Langerhans-cell histiocytosis. *Hematol Oncol Clin North Am*, **12**, 307–326.

Middel, P., Hemmerlein, B., Fayyazi, A., *et al.* (1999). Sinus histiocytosis with massive lymphadenopathy: evidence for its relationship to macrophages and for cytokine-related disorder. *Histopathology*, **35**, 525–533.

Motoi, M., Helbron, D., Kaiserling, E., *et al.* (1980). Eosinophilic granuloma of lymph nodes – a variant of histiocytosis X. *Histopathology*, **4**, 585–606.

Munn, S. and Chu, A.C. (1998). Langerhans' cell histiocytosis of the skin. *Hematol Oncol Clin North Am*, **12**, 269–286.

Murphy, G.F., Harrist, T.J., Bhan, A.K., *et al.* (1983). Distribution of cell surface antigens in histiocytosis X cells. Quantitative immunoelectron microscopy using monoclonal antibodies. *Lab Invest*, **48**, 90–97.

Nakajima, T., Watanabe, S., Sato, Y., *et al.* (1982). S-100 protein in Langerhans' cells, interdigitating reticulum cells and histiocytosis X cells. *Gann*, **73**, 429–432.

Neumann, M.P. and Frizzera, G. (1986). The coexistence of Langerhans' cell granulomatosis and malignant lymphoma may take different forms: report of seven cases with review of literature. *Hum Pathol*, **17**, 1060–1065.

Nezelof, C. (1979). Histiocytosis X: a histological and histogenetic study. *Perspect Pediatr Pathol*, **5**, 153–178.

Nezelof, C., Basset, F. and Rousseau, M.F. (1973). Histiocytosis X: histogenetic arguments for a Langerhans' cell origin. *Biomedicine*, **18**, 365–371.

Pileri, S.A., Grogan, T.M., Harris, N.L., *et al.* (2002). Tumours of histiocytes and accessory dendritic cells: an immunohistochemical approach to classification from the International Lymphoma Study Group based on 61 cases. *Histopathology*, **41**, 1–29.

Réfabert, L., Rambaud, E., Mamou-Mani, T., *et al.* (1996). CD1a-positive cells in bronchoalveolar lavage samples from children with Langerhans' cell histiocytosis. *J Pediatr*, **129**, 913–915.

Rosenberg, A.S. and Morgan, M.B. (2001). Cutaneous indeterminate cell histiocytosis: a new spindle cell variant resembling dendritic cell sarcoma. *J Cutan Pathol*, **28**, 531–537.

Sahoo, M., Karak, A.K. and Bhatnagar, D. (1998). Fine-needle aspiration cytology in a case of isolated involvement of thyroid with Langerhans' cells histiocytosis. *Diagn Cytopathol*, **19**, 33–37.

Schmitz, L. and Favara, B.E. (1998). Nosology and pathology of Langerhans' cell histiocytosis. *Hematol Oncol Clin North Am*, **12**, 221–246.

Segal, G.H., Mesa, M.V., Fishleder, A.J., *et al.* (1992). Precursor Langerhans' cell histiocytosis. An unusual histiocytic proliferation in a patient with persistent non-Hodgkin lymphoma and terminal acute monocytic leukemia. *Cancer*, **70**, 547–553.

Siegal, G.P., Dehner, L.P. and Rosai, J. (1985). Histiocytosis X (Langerhans' cell granulomatosis) of the thymus. A clinicopathologic study of four childhood cases. *Am J Surg Pathol*, **9**, 117–124.

Stein, S.L., Paller, A.S., Haut, P.R., *et al.* (2001). Langerhans cell histiocytosis presenting in the neonatal period: a retrospective series. *Arch Pediatr Adolesc Med*, **155**, 778–783.

Sundar, K.M., Gosselin, M.V., Chung, H.L., *et al.* (2003). Pulmonary Langerhans' cell histiocytosis: emerging concepts in pathobiology, radiology, and clinical evolution of disease. *Chest*, **123**, 1673–1683.

Tani, M., Ishii, N., Kumagai, M., *et al.* (1992). Malignant Langerhans' cell tumour. *Br J Dermatol*, **126**, 398–403.

Tazi, A., Soler, P. and Hance, A.J. (2000). Adult pulmonary Langerhans' cell histiocytosis. *Thorax*, **55**, 405–416.

The French Langerhans' Cell Histiocytosis Study Group (1996). A multicentre retrospective survey of Langerhans' cell histiocytosis: 348 cases observed between 1983 and 1993. *Arch Dis Child*, **75**, 17–24.

Travis, W.D., Borok, Z., Roum, J.H., *et al.* (1993). Pulmonary Langerhans' cell granulomatosis (histiocytosis X). A clinicopathologic study of 48 cases. *Am J Surg Pathol*, **17**, 971–986.

Valladeau, J., Ravel, O., Dezutter-Dambuyant, C., *et al.* (2000). Langerin, a novel C-type lectin specific to Langerhans cells, is an endocytic receptor that induces the formation of Birbeck granules. *Immunity*, **12**, 71–81.

Vassallo, R., Ryu, J.H., Colby, T.V., *et al.* (2000). Pulmonary Langerhans-cell histiocytosis. *New Engl J Med*, **342**, 1969–1978.

Wakely, P. and Suster, S. (2000). Langerhans' cell histiocytosis of the thymus associated with multilocular thymic cyst. *Hum Pathol*, **31**, 1532–1535.

Wang, K.H., Cheng, C.J., Hu, C.H., *et al.* (2002). Coexistence of localized Langerhans cell histiocytosis and cutaneous Rosai–Dorfman disease. *Br J Dermatol*, **147**, 770–774.

Wollenberg, A., Mommaas, M., Oppel, T., *et al.* (2002). Expression and function of the mannose receptor CD206 on epidermal dendritic cells in inflammatory skin diseases. *J Invest Dermatol*, **118**, 327–334.

Wood, C., Wood, G., Deneau, D.G., *et al.* (1984). Malignant histiocytosis X. Report of a rapidly fatal case in an elderly man. *Cancer*, **54**, 347–352.

Writing Group of the Histiocyte Society. (1987). Histiocytosis syndromes in children. *Lancet*, **1**(8526), 208–209.

Yagita, K., Iwai, M., Yagita-Toguri, M., *et al.* (2001). Langerhans' cell histiocytosis of an adult with tumors in liver and spleen. *Hepatogastroenterology*, **48**, 581–584.

Yap, W.M., Chuah, K.L. and Tan, P.H. (2001). Langerhans cell histiocytosis involving the thyroid and parathyroid glands. *Mod Pathol*, **14**, 111–115.

Yousem, S.A., Colby, T.V., Chen, Y.Y., *et al.* (2001). Pulmonary Langerhans' cell histiocytosis: molecular analysis of clonality. *Am J Surg Pathol*, **25**, 630–636.

Yu, R.C., Attra, A., Quinn, C.M., *et al.* (1993). Multisystem Langerhans' cell histiocytosis with pancreatic involvement. *Gut*, **34**, 570–572.

3

Histiocyte function and development in the normal immune system

Tatjana Nikolić and Pieter J.M. Leenen

Introduction

Histiocytes, represent the cells of the mononuclear phagocyte system (MPS) that can give rise to histiocytoses when they accumulate pathogenically in tissues due to dysregulation of proliferation or survival. This nomenclature may be somewhat misleading as histiocytes, in the strict sense, are macrophages located in connective tissue. However, macrophages and dendritic cells (DC) of different origins, which now are joined in the MPS, can give rise to different forms of histiocytosis, and this deviation is not restricted to connective tissue macrophages. As no alternative term exists that better describes the aberrant accumulation of mononuclear phagocytes, the term 'histiocytes' in the current context thus indicates mononuclear phagocytes in general.

Heterogeneity of the MPS

The MPS consists of hematopoietic cells with very diverse characteristics, originally recognized as related cells on the basis of a common lineage derivation and primary function of endocytosis (van Furth *et al.*, 1972; van Furth, 1980). In general, cells of the MPS originate in bone marrow and migrate as monocytes through the blood to peripheral tissues, where they develop into mature cells with different features depending on tissue-specific environmental conditions. Macrophages occur virtually in all organs. Moreover, each organ contains multiple, phenotypically different macrophage subpopulations. For example, lung hosts at least two different macrophage types: alveolar macrophages in alveolar spaces and interstitial macrophages integrated in the tissue. Microglia are phagocytes of the nervous tissue, osteoclasts of bone and Kupffer cells of liver. As many of these cells were identified before their relationship to the MPS was established, their names often do not identify them as macrophages. Apart from these resident macrophages, exudate macrophages develop at acute inflammation sites (van Furth, 1985). In chronic inflammation, granuloma macrophages and epitheloid cells are present and can fuse to form multinucleated giant cells (Turk and Narayanan, 1982; Williams and Williams, 1983).

Soon after the identification of the DC, by Steinman and co-workers (Steinman and Cohn, 1973; Tew *et al.*, 1982), members of this family were considered as candidates for the MPS (van Furth, 1980; Diebold, 1986). Initially this notion was not broadly accepted. The more recent observation that DC as well as macrophages can be generated *in vitro* from peripheral blood monocytes, has increased the awareness that both cell types are closely related and are justly unified in a single system (Kabel *et al.*, 1989; Peters *et al.*, 1991; Sallusto and Lanzavecchia, 1994; Goerdt *et al.*, 1996; Hume *et al.*, 2002).

A conceptual difficulty, discussed further later, is raised by the relatively recent findings that DC and macrophages may originate from myeloid- or lymphoid-related progenitors (Borrello *et al.*, 2001; Shortman and Liu, 2002). In addition, some populations of mononuclear phagocytes may be maintained in the steady state independently from bone marrow precursors (Merad *et al.*, 2002), while others are strictly marrow dependent. Thus, despite similarities in morphologic and molecular phenotype observed in the various MPS populations, a common developmental origin might not be true for all MPS cells.

Similar to their developmental diversity, the various MPS members have widely diverse functions and cannot be unified by a single functional characteristic. The commonest feature of mononuclear phagocytes is their significant ability to endocytose different substances, hence their name. However, DC are only strongly endocytic in an immature state and downregulate this activity upon final maturation. Furthermore, DC and macrophages fulfill different functions through endocytosis. Macrophages use endocytosis for clearance of pathogens or other unwanted material, with least consequences for the host. Dendritic cell, however, employ endocytosis to collect antigens for presentation to the adaptive immune system. Thus, although these cell types share the capacity to engulf substances of foreign or self-origin, they employ this feature in different manners to perform distinct functions.

The best-known functions ascribed to macrophages – clearance by phagocytosis and digestion, and to DC – primary activation of the adaptive immune system – have long been the leading principle in distinguishing between these cell types. We will retain this convention here, despite the fact that this distinction is strongly biased by the initial, historical characterization of these cell types, while the biologic reality is much more complex. In this review we hope to make clear that mononuclear phagocytes comprise a large family of functionally and/or developmentally related cells that form a continuum in which the cells recognized as prototypical 'macrophages' and 'DC' are the extremes of a spectrum.

Given the lack of conclusive selective criteria that unequivocally characterize all cells of the MPS, we propose that mononuclear phagocytes are leukocytes that lack specific criteria found in other leukocytes such as polymorphonuclear morphology, specific granularity or unique antigen-specific receptor expression realized by gene rearrangement. Mononuclear phagocytes have specialized in certain functions that are shared by large groups in the family, such as endocytosis, antigen presentation and sentinel function for exogenous stimuli. Their functional diversity, however, goes far beyond these tasks and justifies the notion that mononuclear phagocytes are crucial cells in the maintenance of homeostasis.

Taken together, the heterogeneity of mononuclear phagocytes can be defined at several levels. They are extremely versatile and heterogeneous in function, depending on factors such as cell type, tissue localization, maturation or activation status. In conjunction with their functional heterogeneity, the phenotype of the different mononuclear phagocytes, reflected in morphology, ultrastructural features, and surface and intracellular molecule expression, varies significantly. This has enabled the demarcation of a plethora of cell types that belong to the MPS. Finally, cells can be segregated based on their developmental relationship and hematopoietic origin. In the subsequent sections, we will elaborate these aspects of mononuclear phagocyte heterogeneity.

Functional heterogeneity of macrophages and DC

Macrophages and DC have long been considered separate cell types, specialized in particle uptake and degradation on the one hand, and antigen presentation and immune activation on the other. However, the dichotomy between macrophages and DC regarding these primary functions has proven to be unrealistic, as DC phagocytose considerably, while macrophages may also activate the immune system. Moreover, macrophages and DC perform many more homeostatic functions than the ones mentioned (Table 3.1). In general, these can be separated into functions related to endocytosis and digestion, and those related to tissue regulation. The production of cytokines and other mediators plays an important role in these regulatory functions.

Endocytosis

The common characteristic of macrophages and DC is their extensive ability to endocytose particulate and soluble substances. Based on the nature of the endocytosed substance and the mechanism of uptake, endocytosis has been subdivided into pinocytosis and phagocytosis (reviewed by Conner and Schmid (2003)). Phagocytosis starts with recognition of the material via surface receptors that facilitate the full enclosure of the particle by the phagocyte membrane in a zipper-like fashion. Albeit mononuclear phagocytes lack antigen-specific receptors as expressed by T- and B-lymphocytes, they display an impressive array of less selective receptors that enable them to sample their environment continuously. These receptors are involved in

Table 3.1 Overview of mononuclear phagocyte functions

Function	Cell type (example)
Endocytosis and digestion	
Effete cells	Splenic red pulp macrophages
Bone and cartilage degradation	Osteoclasts
Killing and degradation of micro-organisms*	Monocytes/inflammatory macrophages
Tissue regulation	
Regulation of inflammation	Resident tissue macrophages
Regulation of immune responses	Mature DC in the lymph node
Regulation of hematopoiesis	Hematopoietic island macrophages in bone marrow
Regulation of endocrine function	Folliculo-stellate cells in pituitary
Tissue remodeling	Embryonic macrophages
Wound healing and tissue regeneration	Histiocytes (connective tissue macrophages)
Killing or support of tumor cells	Macrophages and DC in the tumor

* Depending on the activation stage of mononuclear phagocytes, they support microbial growth as well.

endocytosis, but also lend the cells their sentinel function, depending on the signaling cascade triggered by occupation of the receptor. Phagocyte receptors can be segregated into several groups depending on their ligands, their overall molecular structure, the structure of the recognition site or a common function that phagocytes performs by employing them (reviewed by Aderem and Underhill (1999)).

Different *lectin*-like receptors recognize carbohydrate structures and play an important role in host defense (Linehan *et al.*, 2000; Marshall and Gordon, 2004). They include distinct families of receptors which enable complex interactions with pathogens as well as (modified) self-molecules. The most extensive family comprises the C-type lectins that require calcium ions for carbohydrate recognition. A number of these C-type lectins, such as CD205/DEC-205, CD207/Langerin and CD209/DC-SIGN are expressed more specifically on DC and are used as markers for these cells (Figdor *et al.*, 2002). The versatility of these lectins is well illustrated by the variety of functions identified for CD209/DC-SIGN. This lectin is involved in the recognition of a variety of micro-organisms, including HIV and mycobacteria, but also in transendothelial migration of DC precursors as well as interaction with T cells (Geijtenbeek *et al.*, 2002).

The *Toll-like receptors* (TLRs) represent another family of structurally homologous receptors that mediate the recognition of primarily microbial structures (reviewed by Akira and Hemmi (2003)). The most thoroughly studied is TLR4, essential in binding lipopolysaccharide (LPS) and initiating the subsequent signaling cascade. TLRs are also present on DC and provide a means for diversification of different DC types as they express specific sets of TLRs differentially (Muzio and Mantovani, 2000; Akira and Hemmi, 2003). Interestingly, this differential expression of TLRs by different mononuclear phagocytes implies that distinct cell types will respond initially depending on the nature of the infective agent.

Additional mononuclear phagocyte receptors involved in recognition of potentially hazardous substances are *Fc receptors* which bind immunoglobulin-opsonized particles (Fanger *et al.*, 1996; Ravetch and Bolland, 2001), *complement receptors* (Barrington *et al.*, 2001) or *scavenger receptors*, which recognize a wide variety of mostly poly-anionic molecules (Peiser *et al.*, 2002). In addition to a phosphatidylserine receptor, the scavenger receptors also mediate phagocytosis of apoptotic cells (Geske *et al.*, 2002). This homeostatic clearance function is probably the primary role of these receptors. Uptake of apoptotic cells does not activate mononuclear phagocytes, unless they are simultaneously triggered by a danger signal, such as those delivered by TLRs.

The fate of endocytosed substances depends highly on their nature, as well as the mononuclear phagocyte type that engulfs them. Prototypical scavenger macrophages have an extensive lysosomal machinery that mostly facilitates elimination. DC have different subcellular features allowing them to contain many microbes, such as Mycobacteria, in a live but inactive stage and extends their ability to process microbial molecules for presentation to the adaptive immune system (Tailleux *et al.*, 2003).

Antigen presentation

DC and macrophages share, together with B cells, the function of antigen presentation that leads to the activation of T cells. In general, DC are claimed to be unique in their capacity to activate naïve T cells, while macrophages and B cells primarily stimulate memory responses (Banchereau and Steinman, 1998). *In vivo* models in which DC were depleted experimentally, leading to a significant decrease in immune activation, support this view (Salomon *et al.*, 1997; Jung *et al.*, 2002). However, this generalization should be viewed cautiously, since multiple studies show that cells with unequivocal features of macrophages may also activate naïve T cells (Askew *et al.*, 1995; Cappello *et al.*, 2004).

Activation of T cells requires that at least two signals are transferred by antigen-presenting cells (APC):

1 antigen in the form of peptide bound to major histocompatibility (MHC) molecules (reviewed by Banchereau *et al.* (2000));
2 co-stimulation, especially provided by molecules of the B7 and Tumour necrosis factor(TNF)-receptor families (Carreno and Collins, 2002; Rothstein and Sayegh, 2003).

Virtually all cells express on their surface MHC class I molecules in which peptides of cytoplasmic, endogenous molecules are incorporated. In contrast, MHC class II molecules primarily contain peptides from exogenous antigens. To enable activation of naïve MHC class I-restricted cytotoxic T cells, DC are specialized in the so-called cross-presentation of exogenous antigens on MHC class I molecules (reviewed by Melief (2003)). CD1 family members, expressed by Langerhans cells (LC) and some other leukocyte types, may be considered alternative antigen-presentation molecules as they present (glyco-)lipids to natural killer (NK)T cells with a restricted T-cell receptor repertoire (Brigl and Brenner, 2004). Activation of T cells that have made a productive interaction with antigen-presenting and co-stimulatory molecules is supported by cellular adhesion molecules and cytokines. For instance, DC produce interleukin (IL)-2 upon microbial stimulation, thought to play an important role in activation of naïve T cells (Granucci et al., 2002).

In addition to well-characterized antigenic and co-stimulation signals, APC convey less appreciated signals that imprint developing T cells. A third signal relates to the skewing of T cells into a polarized phenotype, such as T-helper-1 or -2. Especially mediators produced by APC, such as IL-12 or -10, mediate this effect (Kalinski et al., 1999). Furthermore, depending on the tissue of origin of the APC, stimulated T cells may be endowed with corresponding tissue-specific homing capacities (Campbell and Butcher, 2002; Dudda et al., 2004). This can be considered a fourth signal delivered by APC to T cells.

Together, the quantity and quality of the distinct signals delivered by APC determine the ensuing T-cell response (Lanzavecchia and Sallusto, 2002). This may lead to a strong effector cell response, activating T-helper or cytotoxic T-cell subsets that are polarized in certain directions. Alternatively, APC are also crucial in the downregulation and tolerization of the adaptive immune system. It is now appreciated that the default function of APC appears to be the induction and maintenance of immune tolerance (Steinman et al., 2003). This is performed either by the induction of anergy or the activation-induced cell death of effector lymphocytes or by stimulation of regulatory T cells. Only in conditions where APC experience danger, primarily by triggering of pathogen-associated molecular pattern receptors such as the TLRs, are they activated to stimulate effector T-cell responses (Matzinger, 1998). Thus, modulation of APC provides a means for tight regulation of the functional T-cell differentiation and therefore regulation of the immune response.

Regulatory functions

Presentation of antigens and subsequent activation of the adaptive immune system may be regarded as a specific example in which DC and macrophages regulate the function of other cells. In fact, mononuclear phagocytes interact with many cell types and effect multiple regulatory tasks, enabled by their ubiquity in most tissues.

Production of a variety of mediators is essential for this function. The immense production potential of mononuclear phagocytes is reflected in their morphology. Although they are morphologically diverse, most mononuclear phagocytes possess a large nucleus with much euchromatin, an extensive endoplasmatic reticulum and Golgi apparatus, many ribosomes, mitochondria and secretory vacuoles in the cytoplasm (Papadimitriou and Ashman, 1989). Secretory products of mono-nuclear phagocytes can be of very distinct molecular nature: proteins such as cytokines, chemokines, or enzymes, as well as low-molecular mass mediators including bioactive peptides such as substance P, regulatory nucleic acid derivatives such as adenosine or cyclic adenosine monophosphate (AMP), steroid hormones such as 1,25-dihydroxyvitamin D3 and lipid mediators such as prostaglandins and leukotrienes (extensive overview by Leenen and Campbell (1993)). Of course, not all phagocytes produce all the molecules mentioned. Which of the productive machineries will be engaged depends on their particular stage of development, acti-vation or cellular subtype. Obviously, most of these products are not specific for macrophages or DC and can be produced by other cells. However, mononuclear phagocytes are often major producers due to their ability to accumulate at sites in large numbers and their impressive production capacity per cell.

Delineating in detail the different regulatory functions of mononuclear phago-cytes listed in Table 3.1 is impossible due to space constraints. Therefore, we will restrict ourselves to their main functions and illustrate their regulatory diversity through a few examples.

As prime cells of the innate immune system, mononuclear phagocytes take part in all phases of the acute and chronic inflammatory responses. Resident macrophages and DC act as sentinel cells in peripheral tissues on the basis of their versatile receptor expression (see above) and become activated upon encountering danger. They quickly produce and release large amounts of proinflammatory cytokines, such as TNF-α and IL-1, and chemokines such as IL-8 and CCL2/MCP-1, and other mediators that attract inflammatory cells of the innate immune system (Aderem, 2001; Malyshev and Shnyra, 2003). Neutrophilic granulocytes often represent the first wave of recruited cells, followed by monocytes. Interestingly, recent investiga-tions by a number of laboratories, including our own, suggest that only a specific sub-set of blood monocytes is recruited to peripheral inflammation (Geissmann et al., 2003; Drevets et al., 2004; Sunderkotter et al., 2004). These inflammatory mono-cytes appear to have recently immigrated from bone marrow and can be distin-guished from more mature monocytes, which have resided longer in circulation, on the basis of their chemokine receptor profile and other markers. These studies have primarily utilized mouse models, but comparable human monocyte subtypes have been identified, suggesting a similar functional dichotomy in man (Grage-Griebenow et al., 2001; Geissmann et al., 2003). These recruited monocytes will probably develop into exudate macrophages and DC. However, depending on the tissue site of inflammation and the eliciting agent, the type of infiltrating mononuclear phagocyte may differ significantly. For instance, at mucosal sites, myeloid DC are rapidly recruited in response to bacterial challenge (McWilliam *et al.*, 1994). In viral infection a specific role has been identified for plasmacytoid DC (PDC), as these cells are major producers of IFN-α upon activation (Cella *et al.*, 1999; Asselin-Paturel *et al.*, 2001). Finally, at a certain point in the inflammatory process, mononuclear phagocytes that develop at the site of inflammation will start producing more IL-10 and suppressor molecules that induce apoptosis of cells in the inflammatory infiltrate (Goerdt *et al.*, 1999; Malyshev and Shnyra, 2003). Thus, these cells initiate the resolution of inflammation before too much damage occurs at the affected site.

As inflammation takes place primarily in connective tissues, it is not surprising that mononuclear phagocytes have a close relationship to connective tissue components. Remarkably, we recently observed that approximately 60% of mouse dermal connective tissue cells are mononuclear phagocytes (Dupasquier *et al.*, 2004). Preliminary data from human skin suggest that a similar predominance of mononuclear phagocytes may exist there. These cells are involved in maintaining homeostasis by their sentinel function, and production and degradation of extracellular matrix components. Together with their impressive ability to recognize and engulf apoptotic cells, this makes mononuclear phagocytes, such as connective tissue histiocytes, lung macrophages and osteoclasts, prime cells in tissue remodeling in steady state, during wound healing and in embryonic development (Peck *et al.*, 1986; Bousquet *et al.*, 1995; Lichanska and Hume, 2000; O'Kane, 2002).

Tissue regulation by mononuclear phagocytes is most prominently illustrated by their interaction with the endocrine and hematopoietic systems. Both male and female gametogenesis are crucially dependent on proper function of macrophages and DC (Hoek *et al.*, 1997; Hales, 2002; Wu *et al.*, 2004), which have a role in clearance and endocrine tissue remodeling, but also modulate hormonal secretion by endocrine cells, primarily by production of cytokines such as IL-1 and -6. In essence, all endocrine organs contain populations of mononuclear phagocytes which appear intimately involved with regulation of endocrine function (Allaerts *et al.*, 1997; Hoek *et al.*, 1997; Simons *et al.*, 1998). Also in hemato- and lymphopoiesis, mononuclear phagocytes play important roles as integral constituents of the hematopoietic stroma in bone marrow and thymus. They are central to erythro- and myelopoiesis in bone marrow as well as selection of developing T cells in the thymus (Brocker, 1999; Sadahira and Mori, 1999).

Together, this minimal overview of mononuclear phagocyte functions shows a kaleidoscopic picture of physiologic processes that are essential to the maintenance of homeostasis. Thus, malfunction of mononuclear phagocytes is thought to be fundamental to many diseases. Given their complexity and diversity, it will become a challenge to exploit our increasing knowledge of the MPS for clinical use.

Phenotypic heterogeneity of the MPS: a static view

The functional diversity of mononuclear phagocytes is clearly reflected in their phenotypic appearances in different tissues. This relates to the morphology of the cells at light microscopic and electron microscopic level, as well as to molecular features of the cells visualized by cytochemical and immunocytochemical methods. Nonetheless, a number of morphologic generalizations at the subcellular level can be made for mononuclear phagocytes, as described earlier. In addition, subtypes may show distinctive morphologic features, such as the racket-shaped Birbeck granules that characterize the LC (Romani *et al.*, 2003). In the last decades, the hybridoma technology provided a wealth of monoclonal antibodies (MAB) against molecules on cell surface or in cytoplasm. Tagging these antibodies with fluorescent dyes in conjunction with advanced flow cytometric technology made immuno-phenotypic labeling of mononuclear phagocytes the most commonly used method for identification. However, these methods revealed no more than a static view of the MPS, allowing only a snap-shot in time and preventing follow-up during cell development, migration or activation. Therefore, it is important to realize that our notion of the developmental and functional relationship between the different mononuclear phagocytes is still limited. Despite this restriction, we feel that morphologic and (immuno)phenotypic identification have brought important insights into the heterogeneity of mononuclear phagocytes, depicted in the following sections.

Phenotypic heterogeneity of macrophages

The extensive diversity of macrophages is illustrated by the lack of a universal, common macrophage marker, despite the vast number of MAB that have been generated against these cells. In the mouse, F4/80 was introduced as a prototypical macrophage marker (Lee *et al.*, 1985; McKnight *et al.*, 1996) but this MAB fails to recognize some populations such as macrophages of the lung and lymphoid organs. Similarly, CD14 and CD68 are widely expressed on human macrophages, but cannot be considered as truly universal markers. Expression of the receptor for macrophage colony-stimulating factor (M-CSF), the essential growth factor for macrophages recognized by CD115 antibodies, has been proposed as a common marker for the MPS (Hume *et al.*, 2002; Sasmono *et al.*, 2003). Indeed, mice deficient in CSF-1 or the CSF-1R show a deficit in several macrophage populations including monocytes, peritoneal macrophages and osteoclasts (Wiktor-Jedrzejczak *et al.*, 1982;

Dai *et al.*, 2002). However, the macrophage deficiency is not complete in these mice, implying that CD115 is also not a universal marker for all macrophages.

The array of markers that has become available for phenotypic labeling allowed a detailed analysis of macrophages in steady-state and in inflammatory conditions. For instance, the study of macrophages in the steady-state spleen in human and mouse, has revealed a significant number of subpopulations differing in phenotype and anatomical location (Buckley *et al.*, 1987; Leenen and Campbell, 1993). Such preliminary studies have increased our consciousness of macrophage heterogeneity, but left many questions about the functional implications. Responding to these questions has resulted in a better understanding of the phenotype-function-link of macrophages. Multiple ways of activation have been identified that are all characterized by a distinct marker profile (Goerdt *et al.*, 1999; Gordon, 2003; Mosser, 2003). However, much remains to be learned. Current developments in molecular profiling by micro-array technology will undoubtedly soon contribute significantly to this field (Wells *et al.*, 2003).

Phenotypic heterogeneity of DC

The highly increased awareness during the last decade of the role of DC in the steering of the immune system and the possible clinical applications, has resulted in a wealth of information about the phenotypic heterogeneity of DC. However, unequivocal interpretation of these findings in developmental and functional terms has proven to be difficult, especially due to the high turn-over of DC, their significant mobility between peripheral and immune organs, and their phenotypic volatility in response to environmental conditions. Thus, the application of the static phenotypic labeling created confusion by definition of many 'new' DC types in different organs, without a clear view of the possible developmental relationships between these and known DC types. Given these restricting considerations, different classifications can be made of phenotypically defined DC types. Figure 3.1 thus provides a schematic overview of some of the DC populations identified in lymphoid and non-lymphoid tissues.

To illustrate the complexity of the DC field, in human thymus three distinct DC populations were found (Bendriss-Vermare *et al.*, 2001), up to five populations in lymph nodes (Takahashi *et al.*, 1998) and tonsils (Summers *et al.*, 2001), and at least three populations in blood (MacDonald *et al.*, 2002). The situation is similarly complicated in mice, since up to six different DC types were found in mouse lymph nodes and spleen (Wilson and Villadangos, 2004). The generation of an overview of lymph node DC is complicated by the fact that, apart from resident DC, the lymph node hosts varying populations of DC that migrate from the periphery. Depending on the tissue drained, different subtypes of DC have been observed in

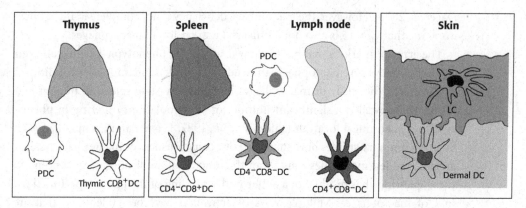

Figure 3.1   Schematic classification of main DC subtypes in lymphoid and non-lymphoid organs.
The phenotypic distinction of DC according to their expression of CD4 and CD8 markers is
based on mouse studies. Depending on the marker combinations used, different, and
often more, subtypes can be distinguished in both mouse and human tissues (see text
for details). PDC: Plasmacytoid DC; LC: Langerhans cell

different lymph nodes (Henri *et al.*, 2001). This points to tissue-specific differences
between DC in peripheral organs, as has been observed earlier for macrophages.

DC in non-lymphoid organs represent a sizeable population of immature cells.
For example, in the skin, LC are located in the epidermis in close proximity to
the basal membrane. Upon stimulation by antigenic or irritant triggering, they
migrate to skin-draining lymph nodes and present accumulated antigens to T cells.
A unique feature of LC is the possession of cytoplasmic Birbeck granules that
makes them distinguishable from other cells at the subcellular level. Related to this,
LC can be uniquely identified by their expression of Langerin, a C-type lectin that
is functionally involved with the induction of Birbeck granules (Valladeau *et al.*,
2000). Next to the LC, a distinct population of skin DC has been identified in the
adjacent dermis. In human, these cells are characterized by the expression of factor
XIIIa and DC-SIGN (Cerio *et al.*, 1989; Turville *et al.*, 2003). Likewise, virtually all
other non-lymphoid tissues contain at least one DC population in the steady state,
with the exception of brain parenchyma (Pashenkov *et al.*, 2003).

Recent studies on phenotypic variability of DC have revealed considerable
promiscuity of DC in expressing molecules previously considered characteristic of
other hematopoietic lineages. Typical examples are the expression of CD4, CD8 and
B220 (CD45R) molecules by particular mouse DC subpopulations. Conversely,
phenotypic features thought to characterize DC uniformly had to be reconsidered.
While classic DC in the mouse all have high-level expression of CD11c, the recently
discovered PDC express only low levels, in combination with the previous B-cell
marker B220 (Nakano *et al.*, 2001; Nikolic *et al.*, 2002) and, in some mouse strains,

Table 3.2 Phenotypic and functional criteria used to distinguish between prototypical macrophages and DC, based on early characterization of the cell types

	Macrophages	DC
Phagocytosis	++	−/±
Adhesion	+	−/±
Acid phosphatase expression	++	± (spot)
Non-specific esterase expression	+	−
Killing of microbes	++	−
MHC class II expression	Inducible	Constitutive
Co-stimulation	±	++
APC for primary response	−	++
APC for secondary response	+	++

the granulocyte marker Gr-1 (Gilliet *et al.*, 2002). Realization of this phenotypic promiscuity and flexibility led to identification of additional DC subtypes, such as the new 'tolerogenic' DC (Wakkach *et al.*, 2003). These cells could be generated *in vitro* by using granulocyte–macrophage colony-stimulating factor (GM-CSF) with IL-10 and were also found in spleen expressing a CD11b$^+$, CD11c$^+$, CD45RB$^+$ phenotype. Time will tell whether this is yet another new DC type or an unrecognized developmental stage of already known DC or macrophages.

Criteria to distinguish DC from macrophages: is this distinction real?

The vast majority of studies published on DC and macrophages might leave the impression that both cell types are separate entities that can be well distinguished on phenotypic and functional criteria. This partition primarily stems from the early characterization of DC as the professional APC, restricted to thymus and secondary lymphoid organs. Such DC are indeed easily distinguished from the macrophages located in peripheral tissues, and defined as professional phagocytes that eliminate debris and micro-organisms. A more extensive list of criteria that separate these prototypical macrophages and DC is provided in Table 3.2.

Before DC were better understood, all phagocytic cells in the periphery were designated macrophages, possibly incorrectly. We know now that immature DC reside as phagocytic cells in the periphery that would be characterized as macrophages by many accepted criteria (Steinman and Inaba, 1999; Mellman and Steinman, 2001). Thus, in many instances the distinction between macrophages and DC appears to become a matter of definition and semantics, rather than biologic reality.

Multiple surface markers are shared between DC and macrophages, and even a combination of several markers does not provide sufficient indication for a clear separation. Both macrophages and myeloid DC in the mouse may express CD11b, both can express CD11c, F4/80, MHC class II, co-stimulatory molecules, among others. It was thought especially that markers related to antigen presentation are expressed constitutively on DC and only upon activation on macrophages. However, this difference was mostly based on a restricted definition of DC as resident cells in secondary lymphoid organs. Furthermore, this criterion is difficult to use in practice, applying mostly non-dynamic phenotypic characterization. The notion that both cell types are very sensitive to environmental conditions and change their phenotype extensively during maturation and activation, makes a general phenotypic distinction between DC and macrophages a treacherous enterprise.

At the level of function, DC can phagocytose significantly *in vitro* as well as *in vivo* (Leenen *et al.*, 1998). They also share with macrophages the potential to produce several cytokines and other soluble factors, which provides them with the potential to perform similar regulatory functions. Conversely, as argued before, some macrophages may activate naïve T cells, at least *in vitro*. Thus, even in these prime functions, no clear-cut difference between DC and macrophages exist.

The *in vitro* generation of DC and macrophages has been a similar source of confusion. For example, the same cytokine, GM-CSF has been used for generation of cells that were either designated DC or macrophages, depending on the definition and characterization (Hamburger *et al.*, 1985; Sallusto and Lanzavecchia, 1994; Godard and Chermann, 1999; Lutz *et al.*, 1999). In general, GM-CSF has now been accepted as a growth factor of choice to generate myeloid DC in both mouse and human, but this may be related to a wider appreciation of the DC-entity.

Taken together, there appear to be no solid criteria to distinguish DC from macrophages in general. Nevertheless, multiple subtypes of cells can be recognized as either DC or macrophage, based on the expression of prototypical features and historic conventions. Given the resulting Babylonic confusion, it is no surprise that a number of studies have reported the conversion from macrophages into DC and vice versa, depending on experimental conditions (Palucka *et al.*, 1998; Rezzani *et al.*, 1999; Ichikawa *et al.*, 2003). We do not expect that unequivocal features separating DC and macrophages will be found in the future, based on the extensive phenotypic and functional overlap between the cells. Developmental origin could have been an alternative way of distinguishing between cell types. However, in the next section, we will elaborate on the comparably heterogeneous and confusing developmental origin of DC and macrophages.

Heterogeneity in the origins of DC and macrophages

In the original concept of the MPS, the members were all considered to be myeloid in nature and to originate from a common progenitor in bone marrow (van Furth *et al.*, 1972). According to this view, the shared direct precursor of macrophages in the periphery is a circulating monocyte that, upon passage through the endothelium of the blood vessel, undergoes final differentiation into a macrophage (Volkman and Gowans, 1965; van Furth and Cohn, 1968; van Furth *et al.*, 1972). A wealth of more recent studies have shown that monocytes can also develop into DC (Sallusto and Lanzavecchia, 1994; Randolph *et al.*, 1999; Geissmann *et al.*, 2003; Nikolic *et al.*, 2003) supporting inclusion of DC in the MPS. Moreover, several studies have demonstrated that DC originate from the bone marrow and can be derived from marrow precursors *in vitro* using different myeloid-related growth factors (Blom *et al.*, 2000; Brasel *et al.*, 2000; Liu, 2001; Gilliet *et al.*, 2002; Baumeister *et al.*, 2003). However, in the following we will argue that the view that all macrophages and DC are myeloid in origin and continuously depend on replenishment by marrow precursors, may be too simplistic.

Studies on early development of DC in mouse and humans suggest that subsets of DC may be developmentally more closely related to lymphocytes than to myeloid cells (Ardavin *et al.*, 1993; Galy *et al.*, 1995). In particular, thymus-derived common T/NK/DC precursors appear to mature into distinctive DC, independent of myeloid development. Human lymphoid-related DC were found to be identical to the enigmatic plasmacytoid cells, the major interferon (IFN)-α producers, upon viral stimulation (Grouard *et al.*, 1997; Cella *et al.*, 1999). Identification of a mouse equivalent PDC underlined the evolutionary importance of this cell type (Bjorck, 2001; Nakano *et al.*, 2001; Nikolic *et al.*, 2002). The lack of the myeloid marker CD11b on their surface, their morphology and other features resembling human PDC point towards their lymphoid origin. However, mouse PDC, unlike human PDC, can develop independently of T cells (Ferrero *et al.*, 2002). This study did not exclude the possibility that, in the mouse, PDC are more related to B cells, and recently a lymphoid heritage for PDC has been demonstrated by the presence of immunoglobulin heavy chain gene rearrangements, CD3 chain messenger RNA (mRNA) expression, and pre-Tα mRNA expression (Corcoran *et al.*, 2003).

Interestingly, similar lymphoid-related molecular markers were observed in thymic CD8α[+] DC, but not in DC from peripheral organs, indicating a closer lymphoid relationship of thymic DC (Corcoran *et al.*, 2003). Previously, CD8α expression was proposed as a marker for lymphoid-related DC (Wu *et al.*, 1996), but this concept was abandoned after finding induction of CD8α on myeloid-related DC under different conditions (Anjuere *et al.*, 2000b; Brasel *et al.*, 2000; Merad *et al.*, 2000; Traver *et al.*, 2000). These findings, together with specific localization of CD8α[+] DC in the T-cell zone of the spleen or lymph nodes, imply that the expression of CD8α on DC probably marks their functional state, rather than origin.

The recent characterization of DC precursors has indicated an impressive plasticity of hematopoietic progenitors in generation of different DC types. For example, both lymphoid- and myeloid-committed progenitors isolated from mice have the ability to generate similar DC types: both develop into $CD8\alpha^+$ and $CD8\alpha^-$ DC *in vitro* or *in vivo* (Manz *et al.*, 2001; Mebius *et al.*, 2001). The frequency of DC originating from myeloid or lymphoid progenitors varies per organ, with general predominance of myeloid derivation.

In contrast to a proposed dual lymphoid and myeloid origin of DC, a separate, distinct lineage derivation for DC has been proposed by Ardavin and collaborators (del Hoyo *et al.*, 2002). They have isolated a precursor population that can give rise to $CD8\alpha^+$ DC, $CD8\alpha^-$ DC as well as PDC. Similarly, it has been shown that the $CD31^+Ly-6C^+$ population in mouse bone marrow can develop into all three types of DC (Bruno *et al.*, 2001). Both studies, however, lack the formal proof that this is possible at the single cell level, and further analyses of the respective DC precursor populations revealed heterogeneity and, thus, possible contamination with other progenitors (de Bruijn *et al.*, 1994; del Hoyo *et al.*, 2004).

An alternative explanation for the confusing lineage derivation of DC has been offered (Canque and Gluckman, 2001). According to this model, hematopoietic progenitors might retain the potential to develop into DC for an extended period during their development, depending on environmental signals. Thus, DC might be generated by a lineage-independent developmental program that has evolved relatively recently and, once switched on, elicits the rapid transformation of distinct leukocytes into professional APC. Recent studies lend support to this view as they suggest that common lymphoid progenitors are flexible cells that can be reprogrammed to develop into myeloid cells, including DC, depending on specific cytokine signals (Prohaska *et al.*, 2002; Iwasaki-Arai *et al.*, 2003). Even pro-B cells might develop into DC, when triggered appropriately (Bjorck and Kincade, 1998).

In a similar manner, macrophages might arise from progenitors that have a lymphoid past, in contrast to their usual myeloid origin. Reprogramming of developing B cells into macrophages was shown by the lack of Pax-5 or enforced expression of transcription factors of the C/EBP family (Rolink and Melchers, 2000; Xie *et al.*, 2004). It could be argued that such genetically manipulated systems bear little resemblance to normal *in vivo* situations. However, bipotential cells capable of developing into B cells and macrophages have also been demonstrated in unmanipulated mice (Borrello *et al.*, 2001; Montecino-Rodriguez *et al.*, 2001). In fact, human Hodgkin's lymphoma cells might represent similar transitional stages, as they derive from germinal center B cells and carry immunoglobulin gene rearrangements, but lack most classic B-cell markers, expressing instead some myeloid features (Thomas *et al.*, 2004).

In addition to a fixed myeloid origin of macrophages and DC, the obligatory replacement of mature cells by precursors derived from bone marrow has also been under scrutiny. During embryonic development, the first CSF-1R expressing cells appear in the yolk sac and spread through the developing embryo (Hume *et al.*, 1995; Lichanska *et al.*, 1999). These are primitive macrophages that play an important role in phagocytosis of dying cells, and therefore in tissue remodeling and organogenesis. Embryonic macrophages do not originate from hematopoietic islands, they do not pass through the monocyte stage, lack F4/80 expression and seem to be independent of PU.1, a key transcriptional regulator in adult macrophage development (Lichanska *et al.*, 1999; Lichanska and Hume, 2000). It has been argued before that they might remain in the adult as bone marrow-independent populations, but this has not been definitively resolved (discussed by Leenen and Campbell (1993)). A problem in these studies is that adequate monitoring of the fate of transplanted, genetically marked bone marrow cells requires conditioning of the host, and thus disturbance of the steady state, including putative local precursors. However, even in this potentially biased setting, lung and liver macrophages remained mostly of host origin, even after a year, and microglia were even less likely to be donor derived (Kennedy and Abkowitz, 1997; Kennedy and Abkowitz, 1998).

Taken together, the ground plan of the MPS has been profoundly completed and confirmed since its establishment. However, a large number of studies have urged revision of the concept of a single lineage of cells that is continuously replenished from bone marrow precursors. The view is emerging that plasticity at the precursor level may allow immature cells from different origins to adopt a developmental program that leads to the generation of mononuclear phagocytes with indistinguishable phenotypes and functions. A good example of this putative multiple origin is provided by the development of LC, residing in epithelial tissue (Figure 3.2).

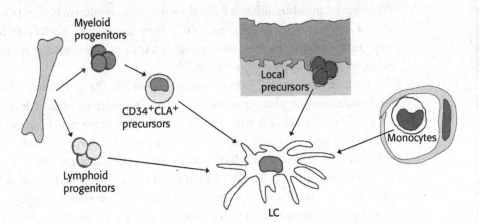

Figure 3.2   Proposed origins for epithelium-residing LC. In different experimental settings, LC were shown to derive from a subset of myeloid progenitors, lymphoid progenitors, circulating monocytes or local precursors (see text for details). CLA: cutaneous lymphocyte antigen

LC have been derived *in vitro* from a distinct human myeloid CD34$^+$ precursor population characterized by expression of the skin-homing molecule cutaneous lymphocyte antigen (CLA) (Caux *et al.*, 1997; Strunk *et al.*, 1997). Alternatively, LC may develop from monocytes under the influence of GM-CSF and transforming growth factor (TGF)-β (Geissmann *et al.*, 1998). *In vivo* studies in mice have suggested that LC may have a lymphoid rather than a myeloid origin (Anjuere *et al.*, 2000a). Last but not least, experiments using parabiotic mice have shown that LC in steady state are maintained independently from the bone marrow (Merad *et al.*, 2002), possibly by local precursors residing in the skin (Larregina *et al.*, 2001). Only when they are collectively depleted by an inflammatory trigger, such as UV irradiation, will marrow-derived cells reoccupy the niche and develop into LC. Thus, while former studies show the potential of different precursor cells to develop into LC, the latter experiments represent the best indication that LC are essentially a bone marrow-independent population of mononuclear phagocytes.

Concluding remarks

Mononuclear phagocytes are characterized by their functional and phenotypic heterogeneity. As outlined above, macrophages and DC have crucial functions in multiple homeostatic processes. This is reflected in their phenotypic characteristics, which are so diverse that no clear-cut phenotypic definition of mononuclear phagocytes can be given. This heterogeneity may originate from different developmental processes.

First, mononuclear phagocytes can have different precursors. The vast majority of mononuclear phagocytes probably stem from the myeloid hematopoietic lineage, but lymphoid progenitors may also give rise to mature DC and macrophages that may either be indistinguishable from their myeloid counterparts (e.g. LC) or constitute a specific subset of cells (e.g. PDC). Even mesenchymal cells may be direct progenitors of adult mononuclear phagocytes, if, as some studies suggest, fetal macrophages persist throughout adult life.

Second, environmental factors crucially influence the generation of diversity among mononuclear phagocytes throughout different phases of their development. At the precursor level, cells will commit to a certain lineage under the influence of local developmental factors. Subsequently, numerous exogenous factors influence the maturation of precursor cells to peripheral macrophages and DC, with obvious functional consequences. Finally, the nature of macrophages and DC as peripheral sentinel cells makes them sensitive par excellence to their environment. These cells carry peripheral messages not only to the immune system, but also to other systems, such as the hematopoietic and neuroendocrine systems.

As the adaptive immune system is vital to host defense and strongly depends on the proper functioning of the MPS, it is no wonder that the observed heterogeneity and redundancy exists. Complete absence of macrophages and DC has, to our knowledge, never been reported in humans or in experimental settings, and would probably be incompatible with life.

Thus, we propose the MPS as a large continuum of cell types of different functions, different phenotypes and even different origins. The flexibility and limits in developmental heterogeneity of the MPS are just now starting to be explored. This research is boosted by the awareness that modulation of the function of the MPS, in either a stimulatory or inhibitory manner, may have great clinical potential in a wide variety of diseases. However, various functions of mononuclear phagocytes have remained poorly investigated, primarily because of the presumption of viewing DC as cells specialized only in immune interaction, and macrophages only as scavengers and destroyers of invaders. Given the recent interest in the mononuclear phagocytes, and DC especially, it may be anticipated that before too long more light will be shed on these 'dark spots' of the MPS.

Acknowledgement

This work was supported by a grant from the Dutch Diabetes Research Foundation (96.606).

REFERENCES

Aderem, A. (2001). Role of Toll-like receptors in inflammatory response in macrophages. *Crit Care Med*, **29**, S16–S18.

Aderem, A. and Underhill, D.M. (1999). Mechanisms of phagocytosis in macrophages. *Annu Rev Immunol*, **17**, 593–623.

Akira, S. and Hemmi, H. (2003). Recognition of pathogen-associated molecular patterns by TLR family. *Immunol Lett*, **85**, 85–95.

Allaerts, W., Salomon, B., Leenen, P.J., *et al.* (1997). A population of interstitial cells in the anterior pituitary with a hematopoietic origin and a rapid turnover: a relationship with folliculo-stellate cells? *J Neuroimmunol*, **78**, 184–197.

Anjuere, F., Martinez del Hoyo, G., Martin, P., *et al.* (2000a). Langerhans cells develop from a lymphoid-committed precursor. *Blood*, **96**, 1633–1637.

Anjuere, F., Martinez del Hoyo, G., Martin, P., *et al.* (2000b). Langerhans cells acquire a CD8+ dendritic cell phenotype on maturation by CD40 ligation. *J Leukoc Biol*, **67**, 206–209.

Ardavin, C., Wu, L., Li, C.L., *et al.* (1993). Thymic dendritic cells and T cells develop simultaneously in the thymus from a common precursor population. *Nature*, **362**, 761–763.

Askew, D., Gatewood, J., Olivas, E., *et al.* (1995). A subset of splenic macrophages process and present native antigen to naive antigen-specific CD4+ T-cells from mice transgenic for an alpha beta T-cell receptor. *Cell Immunol*, **166**, 62–70.

Asselin-Paturel, C., Boonstra, A., Dalod, M., *et al.* (2001). Mouse type I IFN-producing cells are immature APCs with plasmacytoid morphology. *Nat Immunol*, **2**, 1144–1150.

Banchereau, J. and Steinman, R.M. (1998). Dendritic cells and the control of immunity. *Nature*, **392**, 245–252.

Banchereau, J., Briere, F., Caux, C., *et al.* (2000). Immunobiology of dendritic cells. *Annu Rev Immunol*, **18**, 767–811.

Barrington, R., Zhang, M., Fischer, M., *et al.* (2001). The role of complement in inflammation and adaptive immunity. *Immunol Rev*, **180**, 5–15.

Baumeister, T., Rossner, S., Pech, G., *et al.* (2003). Interleukin-3Ralpha+ myeloid dendritic cells and mast cells develop simultaneously from different bone marrow precursors in cultures with interleukin-3. *J Invest Dermatol*, **121**, 280–288.

Bendriss-Vermare, N., Barthelemy, C., Durand, I., *et al.* (2001). Human thymus contains IFN-alpha-producing CD11c(−), myeloid CD11c(+), and mature interdigitating dendritic cells. *J Clin Invest*, **107**, 835–844.

Bjorck, P. (2001). Isolation and characterization of plasmacytoid dendritic cells from Flt3 ligand and granulocyte-macrophage colony-stimulating factor-treated mice. *Blood*, **98**, 3520–3526.

Bjorck, P. and Kincade, P.W. (1998). CD19+ pro-B cells can give rise to dendritic cells *in vitro*. *J Immunol*, **161**, 5795–5799.

Blom, B., Ho, S., Antonenko, S., *et al.* (2000). Generation of interferon alpha-producing pre-dendritic cell (Pre-DC)2 from human CD34(+) hematopoietic stem cells. *J Exp Med*, **192**, 1785–1796.

Borrello, M.A., Palis, J. and Phipps, R.P. (2001). The relationship of CD5+ B lymphocytes to macrophages: insights from normal biphenotypic B/macrophage cells. *Int Rev Immunol*, **20**, 137–155.

Bousquet, J., Vignola, A.M., Chanez, P., *et al.* (1995). Airways remodelling in asthma: no doubt, no more? *Int Arch Allergy Immunol*, **107**, 211–214.

Brasel, K., De Smedt, T., Smith, J.L., *et al.* (2000). Generation of murine dendritic cells from flt3-ligand-supplemented bone marrow cultures. *Blood*, **96**, 3029–3039.

Brigl, M. and Brenner, M.B. (2004). CD1: antigen presentation and T cell function. *Annu Rev Immunol*, **22**, 817–890.

Brocker, T. (1999). The role of dendritic cells in T cell selection and survival. *J Leukoc Biol*, **66**, 331–335.

Bruno, L., Seidl, T. and Lanzavecchia, A. (2001). Mouse pre-immunocytes as non-proliferating multipotent precursors of macrophages, interferon-producing cells, CD8alpha+ and CD8 alpha− dendritic cells. *Eur J Immunol*, **31**, 3403–3412.

Buckley, P.J., Smith, M.R., Braverman, M.F., *et al.* (1987). Human spleen contains phenotypic subsets of macrophages and dendritic cells that occupy discrete micro-anatomic locations. *Amer J Pathol*, **128**, 505–520.

Campbell, D.J. and Butcher, E.C. (2002). Rapid acquisition of tissue-specific homing phenotypes by CD4(+) T cells activated in cutaneous or mucosal lymphoid tissues. *J Exp Med*, **195**, 135–141.

Canque, B. and Gluckman, J.C. (2001). Toward a unified theory of dendritic-cell diversity. *Trends Immunol*, **22**, 664.

Cappello, P., Caorsi, C., Bosticardo, M., *et al.* (2004). CCL16/LEC powerfully triggers effector and antigen-presenting functions of macrophages and enhances T cell cytotoxicity. *J Leukoc Biol*, **75**, 135–142.

Carreno, B.M. and Collins, M. (2002). The B7 family of ligands and its receptors: new pathways for costimulation and inhibition of immune responses. *Annu Rev Immunol*, **20**, 29–53.

Caux, C., Massacrier, C., Vanbervliet, B., *et al.* (1997). CD34+ hematopoietic progenitors from human cord blood differentiate along two independent dendritic cell pathways in response to granulocyte-macrophage colony-stimulating factor plus tumor necrosis factor alpha: II. Functional analysis. *Blood*, **90**, 1458–1470.

Cella, M., Jarrossay, D., Facchetti, F., *et al.* (1999). Plasmacytoid monocytes migrate to inflamed lymph nodes and produce large amounts of type I interferon. *Nat Med*, **5**, 919–923.

Cerio, R., Griffiths, C.E., Cooper, K.D., *et al.* (1989). Characterization of factor XIIIa positive dermal dendritic cells in normal and inflamed skin. *Br J Dermatol*, **121**, 421–431.

Conner, S.D. and Schmid, S.L. (2003). Regulated portals of entry into the cell. *Nature*, **422**, 37–44.

Corcoran, L., Ferrero, I., Vremec, D., *et al.* (2003). The lymphoid past of mouse plasmacytoid cells and thymic dendritic cells. *J Immunol*, **170**, 4926–4932.

Dai, X.M., Ryan, G.R., Hapel, A.J., *et al.* (2002). Targeted disruption of the mouse colony-stimulating factor 1 receptor gene results in osteopetrosis, mononuclear phagocyte deficiency, increased primitive progenitor cell frequencies, and reproductive defects. *Blood*, **99**, 111–120.

de Bruijn, M.F.T.R., Slieker, W.A.T., van der Loo, J.C.M., *et al.* (1994). Distinct mouse bone marrow macrophage precursors identified by differential expression of ER-MP12 and ER-MP20 antigens. *Eur J Immunol*, **24**, 2279–2284.

del Hoyo, G.M., Martin, P., Vargas, H.H., *et al.* (2002). Characterization of a common precursor population for dendritic cells. *Nature*, **415**, 1043–1047.

del Hoyo, G.M., Martin, P., Hernandez Vargas, H., *et al.* (2004). corrigendum: characterization of a common precursor population for dendritic cells. *Nature*, **429**, 205.

Diebold, J. (1986). Mononuclear phagocyte system. Morphology and function of the principal constituting cells. *Ann Pathol*, **6**, 3–12.

Drevets, D.A., Dillon, M.J., Schawang, J.S., *et al.* (2004). The Ly-6C(high) monocyte subpopulation transports listeria monocytogenes into the brain during systemic infection of mice. *J Immunol*, **172**, 4418–4424.

Dudda, J.C., Simon, J.C. and Martin, S. (2004). Dendritic cell immunization route determines CD8+ T cell trafficking to inflamed skin: role for tissue microenvironment and dendritic cells in establishment of T cell-homing subsets. *J Immunol*, **172**, 857–863.

Dupasquier, M., Stoitzner, P., van Oudenaren, A., *et al.* (2004). Macrophages and dendritic cells constitute a major subpopulation of cells in the mouse dermis. *J Invest Dermatol*, **123**, 876–879.

Fanger, N.A., Wardwell, K., Shen, L., *et al.* (1996). Type I (CD64) and type II (CD32) Fc gamma receptor-mediated phagocytosis by human blood dendritic cells. *J Immunol*, **157**, 541–548.

Ferrero, I., Held, W., Wilson, A., *et al.* (2002). Mouse CD11c(+) B220(+) Gr1(+) plasmacytoid dendritic cells develop independently of the T-cell lineage. *Blood*, **100**, 2852–2857.

Figdor, C.G., van Kooyk, Y. and Adema, G.J. (2002). C-type lectin receptors on dendritic cells and Langerhans cells. *Nat Rev Immunol*, **2**, 77–84.

Galy, A., Travis, M., Cen, D., *et al.* (1995). Human T, B, natural killer, and dendritic cells arise from a common bone marrow progenitor cell subset. *Immunity*, **3**, 459–473.

Geijtenbeek, T.B., Engering, A. and Van Kooyk, Y. (2002). DC-SIGN, a C-type lectin on dendritic cells that unveils many aspects of dendritic cell biology. *J Leukoc Biol*, **71**, 921–931.

Geissmann, F., Prost, C., Monnet, J.P., et al. (1998). Transforming growth factor beta1, in the presence of granulocyte/macrophage colony-stimulating factor and interleukin 4, induces differentiation of human peripheral blood monocytes into dendritic Langerhans cells. *J Exp Med*, **187**, 961–966.

Geissmann, F., Jung, S. and Littman, D.R. (2003). Blood monocytes consist of two principal subsets with distinct migratory properties. *Immunity*, **19**, 71–82.

Geske, F.J., Monks, J., Lehman, L., et al. (2002). The role of the macrophage in apoptosis: hunter, gatherer, and regulator. *Int J Hematol*, **76**, 16–26.

Gilliet, M., Boonstra, A., Paturel, C., et al. (2002). The development of murine plasmacytoid dendritic cell precursors is differentially regulated by FLT3-ligand and granulocyte/macrophage colony-stimulating factor. *J Exp Med*, **195**, 953–958.

Godard, C.M. and Chermann, J.C. (1999). Experimental conditions that increase the production of HIV-1 by monocyte-derived macrophages: use of collagen matrix. *Microbes Infect*, **1**, 765–770.

Goerdt, S., Kodelja, V., Schmuth, M., et al. (1996). The mononuclear phagocyte-dendritic cell dichotomy: myths, facts, and a revised concept. *Clin Exp Immunol*, **105**, 1–9.

Goerdt, S., Politz, O., Schledzewski, K., et al. (1999). Alternative versus classical activation of macrophages. *Pathobiology*, **67**, 222–226.

Gordon, S. (2003). Alternative activation of macrophages. *Nat Rev Immunol*, **3**, 23–35.

Grage-Griebenow, E., Flad, H.D. and Ernst, M. (2001). Heterogeneity of human peripheral blood monocyte subsets. *J Leukoc Biol*, **69**, 11–20.

Granucci, F., Andrews, D.M., Degli-Esposti, M.A., et al. (2002). IL-2 mediates adjuvant effect of dendritic cells. *Trends Immunol*, **23**, 169–171.

Grouard, G., Rissoan, M.C., Filgueira, L., et al. (1997). The enigmatic plasmacytoid T cells develop into dendritic cells with interleukin (IL)-3 and CD40-ligand. *J Exp Med*, **185**, 1101–1111.

Hales, D.B. (2002). Testicular macrophage modulation of Leydig cell steroidogenesis. *J Reprod Immunol*, **57**, 3–18.

Hamburger, A.W., White, C.P. and Dunn, F.E. (1985). Cultivation of macrophages derived from human malignant effusions. *Exp Hematol*, **13**, 776–781.

Henri, S., Vremec, D., Kamath, A., et al. (2001). The dendritic cell populations of mouse lymph nodes. *J Immunol*, **167**, 741–748.

Hoek, A., Allaerts, W., Leenen, P.J.M., et al. (1997). Dendritic cells and macrophages in the pituitary and the gonads. Evidence for their role in the fine regulation of the reproductive endocrine response. *Eur J Endocrinol*, **136**, 8–24.

Hume, D.A., Monkley, S.J. and Wainwright, B.J. (1995). Detection of c-fms protooncogene in early mouse embryos by whole mount *in situ* hybridization indicates roles for macrophages in tissue remodelling. *Br J Haematol*, **90**, 939–942.

Hume, D.A., Ross, I.L., Himes, S.R., et al. (2002). The mononuclear phagocyte system revisited. *J Leukoc Biol*, **72**, 621–627.

Ichikawa, M., Sugita, M., Takahashi, M., et al. (2003). Breast milk macrophages spontaneously produce granulocyte-macrophage colony-stimulating factor and differentiate into dendritic cells in the presence of exogenous interleukin-4 alone. *Immunology*, **108**, 189–195.

Iwasaki-Arai, J., Iwasaki, H., Miyamoto, T., *et al.* (2003). Enforced granulocyte/macrophage colony-stimulating factor signals do not support lymphopoiesis, but instruct lymphoid to myelomonocytic lineage conversion. *J Exp Med*, **197**, 1311–1322.

Jung, S., Unutmaz, D., Wong, P., *et al.* (2002). *In vivo* depletion of CD11c(+) dendritic cells abrogates priming of CD8(+) T cells by exogenous cell-associated antigens. *Immunity*, **17**, 211–220.

Kabel, P.J., de Haan-Meulman, M., Voorbij, H.A., *et al.* (1989). Accessory cells with a morphology and marker pattern of dendritic cells can be obtained from elutriator-purified blood monocyte fractions. An enhancing effect of metrizamide in this differentiation. *Immunobiology*, **179**, 395–441.

Kalinski, P., Hilkens, C.M., Wierenga, E.A., *et al.* (1999). T-cell priming by type-1 and type-2 polarized dendritic cells: the concept of a third signal. *Immunol Today*, **20**, 561–567.

Kennedy, D.W. and Abkowitz, J.L. (1997). Kinetics of central nervous system microglial and macrophage engraftment: analysis using a transgenic bone marrow transplantation model. *Blood*, **90**, 986–993.

Kennedy, D.W. and Abkowitz, J.L. (1998). Mature monocytic cells enter tissues and engraft. *Proc Natl Acad Sci USA*, **95**, 14944–14949.

Lanzavecchia, A. and Sallusto, F. (2002). Progressive differentiation and selection of the fittest in the immune response. *Nat Rev Immunol*, **2**, 982–987.

Larregina, A.T., Morelli, A.E., Spencer, L.A., *et al.* (2001). Dermal-resident CD14+ cells differentiate into Langerhans cells. *Nat Immunol*, **2**, 1151–1158.

Lee, S.H., Starkey, P.M. and Gordon, S. (1985). Quantitative analysis of total macrophage content in adult mouse tissues. Immunochemical studies with monoclonal antibody F4/80. *J Exp Med*, **161**, 475–489.

Leenen, P.J.M. and Campbell, P.A. (1993). In: Horton, M.A., ed. *Blood Cell Biochemistry*, Vol. 5. Kluwer Academic/Plenum Publishers, New York, pp. 29–85.

Leenen, P.J.M., Radosevic, K., Voerman, J.S.A., *et al.* (1998). Heterogeneity of mouse spleen dendritic cells: *in vivo* phagocytic activity, expression of macrophage markers, and subpopulation turnover. *J Immunol*, **160**, 2166–2173.

Lichanska, A.M. and Hume, D.A. (2000). Origins and functions of phagocytes in the embryo. *Exp Hematol*, **28**, 601–611.

Lichanska, A.M., Browne, C.M., Henkel, G.W., *et al.* (1999). Differentiation of the mononuclear phagocyte system during mouse embryogenesis: the role of transcription factor PU.1. *Blood*, **94**, 127–138.

Linehan, S.A., Martinez-Pomares, L. and Gordon, S. (2000). Macrophage lectins in host defence. *Microbes Infect*, **2**, 279–288.

Liu, Y.J. (2001). Dendritic cell subsets and lineages, and their functions in innate and adaptive immunity. *Cell*, **106**, 259–262.

Lutz, M.B., Kukutsch, N., Ogilvie, A.L., *et al.* (1999). An advanced culture method for generating large quantities of highly pure dendritic cells from mouse bone marrow. *J Immunol Methods*, **223**, 77–92.

MacDonald, K.P., Munster, D.J., Clark, G.J., *et al.* (2002). Characterization of human blood dendritic cell subsets. *Blood*, **100**, 4512–4520.

Malyshev, I.Y. and Shnyra, A. (2003). Controlled modulation of inflammatory, stress and apoptotic responses in macrophages. *Curr Drug Targets Immune Endocr Metabol Disord*, **3**, 1–22.

Manz, M.G., Traver, D., Miyamoto, T., *et al.* (2001). Dendritic cell potentials of early lymphoid and myeloid progenitors. *Blood*, **97**, 3333–3341.

Marshall, A.S. and Gordon, S. (2004). Commentary: C-type lectins on the macrophage cell surface – recent findings. *Eur J Immunol*, **34**, 18–24.

Matzinger, P. (1998). An innate sense of danger. *Semin Immunol*, **10**, 399–415.

McKnight, A.J., Macfarlane, A.J., Dri, P., *et al.* (1996). Molecular cloning of F4/80, a murine macrophage-restricted cell surface glycoprotein with homology to the G-protein-linked transmembrane 7 hormone receptor family. *J Biol Chem*, **271**, 486–489.

McWilliam, A.S., Nelson, D., Thomas, J.A., *et al.* (1994). Rapid dendritic cell recruitment is a hallmark of the acute inflammatory response at mucosal surfaces. *J Exp Med*, **179**, 1331–1336.

Mebius, R.E., Miyamoto, T., Christensen, J., *et al.* (2001). The fetal liver counterpart of adult common lymphoid progenitors gives rise to all lymphoid lineages, CD45+ CD4+ CD3− cells, as well as macrophages. *J Immunol*, **166**, 6593–6601.

Melief, C.J. (2003). Mini-review: regulation of cytotoxic T lymphocyte responses by dendritic cells: peaceful coexistence of cross-priming and direct priming? *Eur J Immunol*, **33**, 2645–2654.

Mellman, I. and Steinman, R.M. (2001). Dendritic cells: specialized and regulated antigen processing machines. *Cell*, **106**, 255–258.

Merad, M., Fong, L., Bogenberger, J., *et al.* (2000). Differentiation of myeloid dendritic cells into CD8alpha-positive dendritic cells *in vivo*. *Blood*, **96**, 1865–1872.

Merad, M., Manz, M.G., Karsunky, H., *et al.* (2002). Langerhans cells renew in the skin throughout life under steady-state conditions. *Nat Immunol*, **3**, 1135–1141.

Montecino-Rodriguez, E., Leathers, H. and Dorshkind, K. (2001). Bipotential B-macrophage progenitors are present in adult bone marrow. *Nat Immunol*, **2**, 83–88.

Mosser, D.M. (2003). The many faces of macrophage activation. *J Leukoc Biol*, **73**, 209–212.

Muzio, M. and Mantovani, A. (2000). Toll-like receptors. *Microbes Infect*, **2**, 251–255.

Nakano, H., Yanagita, M. and Gunn, M.D. (2001). CD11c(+) B220(+) Gr-1(+) cells in mouse lymph nodes and spleen display characteristics of plasmacytoid dendritic cells. *J Exp Med*, **194**, 1171–1178.

Nikolic, T., Dingjan, G.M., Leenen, P.J., *et al.* (2002). A subfraction of B220(+) cells in murine bone marrow and spleen does not belong to the B cell lineage but has dendritic cell characteristics. *Eur J Immunol*, **32**, 686–692.

Nikolic, T., de Bruijn, M.F., Lutz, M.B., *et al.* (2003). Developmental stages of myeloid dendritic cells in mouse bone marrow. *Int Immunol*, **15**, 515–524.

O'Kane, S. (2002). Wound remodelling and scarring. *J Wound Care*, **11**, 296–299.

Palucka, K.A., Taquet, N., Sanchez-Chapuis, F., *et al.* (1998). Dendritic cells as the terminal stage of monocyte differentiation. *J Immunol*, **160**, 4587–4595.

Papadimitriou, J.M. and Ashman, R.B. (1989). Macrophages: current views on their differentiation, structure, and function. *Ultrastruct Pathol*, **13**, 343–372.

Pashenkov, M., Teleshova, N. and Link, H. (2003). Inflammation in the central nervous system: the role for dendritic cells. *Brain Pathol*, **13**, 23–33.

Peck, W.A., Rifas, L., Cheng, S.L., et al. (1986). The local regulation of bone remodeling. Adv Exp Med Biol, 208, 255–259.

Peiser, L., Mukhopadhyay, S. and Gordon, S. (2002). Scavenger receptors in innate immunity. Curr Opin Immunol, 14, 123–128.

Peters, J.H., Ruppert, J., Gieseler, R.K.H., et al. (1991). Differentiation of human monocytes into CD14 negative accessory cells: do dendritic cells derive from the monocytic lineage? Pathobiology, 59, 122–126.

Prohaska, S.S., Scherer, D.C., Weissman, I.L., et al. (2002). Developmental plasticity of lymphoid progenitors. Semin Immunol, 14, 377–384.

Randolph, G.J., Inaba, K., Robbiani, D.F., et al. (1999). Differentiation of phagocytic monocytes into lymph node dendritic cells in vivo. Immunity, 11, 753–761.

Ravetch, J.V. and Bolland, S. (2001). IgG Fc receptors. Annu Rev Immunol, 19, 275–290.

Rezzani, R., Rodella, L., Zauli, G., et al. (1999). Mouse peritoneal cells as a reservoir of late dendritic cell progenitors. Br J Haematol, 104, 111–118.

Rolink, A.G. and Melchers, F. (2000). Precursor B cells from Pax-5-deficient mice–stem cells for macrophages, granulocytes, osteoclasts, dendritic cells, natural killer cells, thymocytes and T cells. Curr Top Microbiol Immunol, 251, 21–26.

Romani, N., Holzmann, S., Tripp, C.H., et al. (2003). Langerhans cells – dendritic cells of the epidermis. Apmis, 111, 725–740.

Rothstein, D.M. and Sayegh, M.H. (2003). T-cell costimulatory pathways in allograft rejection and tolerance. Immunol Rev, 196, 85–108.

Sadahira, Y. and Mori, M. (1999). Role of the macrophage in erythropoiesis. Pathol Int, 49, 841–848.

Sallusto, F. and Lanzavecchia, A. (1994). Efficient presentation of soluble antigen by cultured human dendritic cells is maintained by granulocyte/macrophage colony-stimulating factor plus interleukin 4 and downregulated by tumor necrosis factor alpha. J Exp Med, 179, 1109–1118.

Salomon, B., Leenen, P.J.M. and Klatzmann, D. (1997). Immune response in dendritic cell depleted mice. Adv Exp Med Biol, 417, 547–550.

Sasmono, R.T., Oceandy, D., Pollard, J.W., et al. (2003). A macrophage colony-stimulating factor receptor-green fluorescent protein transgene is expressed throughout the mononuclear phagocyte system of the mouse. Blood, 101, 1155–1163.

Shortman, K. and Liu, Y.J. (2002). Mouse and human dendritic cell subtypes. Nat Rev Immunol, 2, 151–161.

Simons, P.J., Delemarre, F.G. and Drexhage, H.A. (1998). Antigen-presenting dendritic cells as regulators of the growth of thyrocytes: a role of interleukin-1beta and interleukin-6. Endocrinology, 139, 3148–3156.

Steinman, R.M. and Cohn, Z.A. (1973). Identification of a novel cell type in peripheral lymphoid organs of mice. I. Morphology, quantitation, tissue distribution. J Exp Med, 137, 1142–1162.

Steinman, R.M. and Inaba, K. (1999). Myeloid dendritic cells. J Leukoc Biol, 66, 205–208.

Steinman, R.M., Hawiger, D. and Nussenzweig, M.C. (2003). Tolerogenic dendritic cells. Annu Rev Immunol, 21, 685–711.

Strunk, D., Egger, C., Leitner, G., et al. (1997). A skin homing molecule defines the Langerhans cell progenitor in human peripheral blood. J Exp Med, 185, 1131–1136.

Summers, K.L., Hock, B.D., McKenzie, J.L., *et al.* (2001). Phenotypic characterization of five dendritic cell subsets in human tonsils. *Am J Pathol*, **159**, 285–295.

Sunderkotter, C., Nikolic, T., Dillon, M.J., *et al.* (2004). Subpopulations of mouse blood monocytes differ in maturation stage and inflammatory response. *J Immunol*, **172**, 4410–4417.

Tailleux, L., Neyrolles, O., Honore-Bouakline, S., *et al.* (2003). Constrained intracellular survival of Mycobacterium tuberculosis in human dendritic cells. *J Immunol*, **170**, 1939–1948.

Takahashi, K., Asagoe, K., Zaishun, J., *et al.* (1998). Heterogeneity of dendritic cells in human superficial lymph node: *in vitro* maturation of immature dendritic cells into mature or activated interdigitating reticulum cells. *Am J Pathol*, **153**, 745–755.

Tew, J.G., Thorbecke, G.J. and Steinman, R.M. (1982). Dendritic cells in the immune response: characteristics and recommended nomenclature (A report from the Reticuloendothelial Society Committee on Nomenclature). *J Reticuloendothel Soc*, **31**, 371–380.

Thomas, R.K., Re, D., Wolf, J., *et al.* (2004). Part I: Hodgkin's lymphoma – molecular biology of Hodgkin and Reed-Sternberg cells. *Lancet Oncol*, **5**, 11–18.

Traver, D., Akashi, K., Manz, M., *et al.* (2000). Development of CD8alpha-positive dendritic cells from a common myeloid progenitor. *Science*, **290**, 2152–2154.

Turk, J.L. and Narayanan, R.B. (1982). The origin, morphology, and function of epitheloid cells. *Immunobiology*, **161**, 274–282.

Turville, S., Wilkinson, J., Cameron, P., *et al.* (2003). The role of dendritic cell C-type lectin receptors in HIV pathogenesis. *J Leukoc Biol*, **74**, 710–718.

Valladeau, J., Ravel, O., Dezutter-Dambuyant, C., *et al.* (2000). Langerin, a novel C-type lectin specific to Langerhans cells, is an endocytic receptor that induces the formation of Birbeck granules. *Immunity*, **12**, 71–81.

van Furth, R. (1980). In: van Furth, R. ed. *Mononuclear Phagocytes: Functional Aspects*. Martinus Nijhoff, Dordrecht, pp. 1–30.

van Furth, R. (1985). Monocyte production during inflammation. *Comp Immunol Microbiol Infect Dis*, **8**, 205–211.

van Furth, R. and Cohn, Z.A. (1968). The origin and kinetics of mononuclear phagocytes. *J Exp Med*, **128**, 415–435.

van Furth, R., Cohn, Z.A., Hirsch, J.G., *et al.* (1972). The mononuclear phagocyte system: a new classification of macrophages, monocytes, and their precursor cells. *Bull World Health Organ*, **46**, 845–852.

Volkman, A. and Gowans, J.L. (1965). The origin of macrophages from bone marrow in the rat. *Br J Exp Pathol*, **46**, 62–70.

Wakkach, A., Fournier, N., Brun, V., *et al.* (2003). Characterization of dendritic cells that induce tolerance and T regulatory 1 cell differentiation *in vivo*. *Immunity*, **18**, 605–617.

Wells, C.A., Ravasi, T., Sultana, R., *et al.* (2003). Continued discovery of transcriptional units expressed in cells of the mouse mononuclear phagocyte lineage. *Genome Res*, **13**, 1360–1365.

Wiktor-Jedrzejczak, W.W., Ahmed, A., Szczylik, C., *et al.* (1982). Hematological characterization of congenital osteopetrosis in op/op mouse. Possible mechanism for abnormal macrophage differentiation. *J Exp Med*, **156**, 1516–1527.

Williams, G.T. and Williams, W.J. (1983). Granulomatous inflammation – a review. *J Clin Pathol*, **36**, 723–733.

Wilson, N.S. and Villadangos, J.A. (2004). Lymphoid organ dendritic cells: beyond the Langerhans cells paradigm. *Immunol Cell Biol*, **82**, 91–98.

Wu, L., Li, C.L. and Shortman, K. (1996). Thymic dendritic cell precursors: relationship to the T lymphocyte lineage and phenotype of the dendritic cell progeny. *J Exp Med*, **184**, 903–911.

Wu, R., Van der Hoek, K.H., Ryan, N.K., *et al.* (2004). Macrophage contributions to ovarian function. *Hum Reprod Update*, **10**, 119–133.

Xie, H., Ye, M., Feng, R., *et al.* (2004). Stepwise reprogramming of B cells into macrophages. *Cell*, **117**, 663–676.

4

The immunological basis of Langerhans cell histiocytosis

Cristiana E.T. da Costa, Nicola E. Annels and R. Maarten Egeler

Although Langerhans cell histiocytosis (LCH) was first described a century ago, the aetiology is still not understood. Recent studies on the role of cytokines, chemokines, immunological dysfunction, cell surface antigen expression, clonality and cell-cycle regulation have provided new insights into the pathogenesis of LCH. Much of the data from these studies points to the Langerhans cell (LC) being intrinsically abnormal in LCH. Studies have shown that there is a proliferation of clonal LCs in the lesions of LCH. Furthermore, these LCH cells not only have differences in cytoplasmic and surface markers compared to the normal LC but also show abnormalities in cytokine production and antigen presentation. The recent progress in LCH research has provoked much discussion on whether LCH is a reactive disease resulting from environmental triggers, or a neoplastic process (Arceci et al., 2002; Egeler et al., 2004; Nezelof and Basset, 2004). Unfortunately, there is as yet no clear answer.

Continuing progress in the field of dendritic cell (DC) biology has allowed us to gain an increased understanding of the phenotype and function of LCH cells and their interaction with their microenvironment and hence the pathophysiology of this disease. Conversely, LCH, as an in vivo example of a DC abnormality, may serve as a 'lesson' to DC biologists (Laman et al., 2003). This chapter summarises some of the most recent studies investigating the immunological basis of LCH.

Phenotypic characterisation of LCH cells

Typically, the LCH cell phenotype corresponds to the early-activated stage of DC maturation, combining an immature phenotype with high-level cytokine expression. LCH cells have many features in common with early-activated DCs that develop from the immature DC on contact with bacterial products (Ricciardi-Castagnoli and Granucci, 2002). However, in contrast to early-activated DC, LCH cells have rounded morphology, and show high expression of some co-stimulatory molecules that drive interactions with T-cells. One such co-stimulatory molecule,

CD40, is highly expressed by LCH cells in lesional sites (Egeler *et al.*, 2000). There is also prominent expression of CD40L by T-cells in LCH lesions suggesting potential interactions between these cell types. The CD40–CD40L interaction leads to upregulation of two other co-stimulatory molecules involved in antigen presentation, CD80 and CD86 (B7-2), also expressed by LCH cells (Emile *et al.*, 1994; Egeler *et al.*, 2000). However, another study showed frequent detection of CD80 expression but no CD86 on the majority of LCH cells in most bone and some skin lesions (Geissmann *et al.*, 2001). This suggests that functional ability of LCH cells may differ between restricted skin lesions and disseminated ostotic lesions. Whether productive antigen presentation to T-cells is occurring at all, is questionable, as major histocompatability complex (MHC) class II expression is only moderate (Geissmann *et al.*, 2001).

Although LCH cells have been described as undergoing a 'maturation block' (Annels *et al.*, 2003; Laman *et al.*, 2003), several reports have observed expression of more mature DC markers by LCH cells. In one such study, DC-LAMP and CD83, markers of mature DCs, were found to be expressed by scattered LCH cells in LCH lesions. Interestingly, cases of skin-only LCH showed higher expression of CD83 and DC-LAMP than bone lesions. Moreover, the highest DC-LAMP positivity was evident in spontaneously regressive disease, suggesting that these cells had overcome any potential blockade in their maturation resulting in resolution of the disease (Geissmann *et al.*, 2001). Another marker of LC activation is fascin, a highly selective marker for DCs of lymphoid tissues and peripheral blood, and completely absent from normal epidermal LCs. This actin bundling protein is involved in the formation of dendritic processes in maturing epidermal LCs. Fascin expression has been shown to correlate with dendritic morphology, cell differentiation and antigen-presenting activity of normal DCs (Ross *et al.*, 2000; Al-Alwan *et al.*, 2001). In contrast, despite being positive for fascin, LCH cells have been shown to be functionally defective in antigen-presentation *in vitro* (Geissmann *et al.*, 2001). Thus, the fascin positivity of LCH cells represents another aberration in their phenotype (Pinkus *et al.*, 2002).

One of the abnormal features of LCH cells is their occurrence at sites where normal LCs are not found (e.g. bone). Aberrant migration and homing of LCs resulting from the expression of cellular adhesion molecules may play a role in the pathogenesis of LCH. Recent investigations have shown that LCH cells indeed express different adhesion molecules from normal LCs (Ruco *et al.*, 1993; De Graaf *et al.*, 1994, 1995). CD54 (ICAM-1), CD58 (LFA-3), and the β1 integrin α4, adhesion molecules that are expressed during activation of normal LCs, were shown to be upregulated in LCH lesions. In addition, adhesion molecules not found on normal LCs, such as CD2, CD11a, and CD11b, could be demonstrated on LCH cells in a number of cases (De Graaf *et al.*, 1995). The aberrant expression of these molecules may result in homotypic adhesion of LCH cells through ligand binding of CD2 to CD58 or CD11a to CD54. Another molecule aberrantly expressed by LCH cells was CD62L. CD62L is only found in LCs in normal skin and is shed from monocytes after activation (Stibenz and Buhrer, 1994). Thus, the expression of CD62L by LCH cells is peculiar, as these cells are thought to be in an early-activated state. One can speculate that the aberrant activation of LCH cells results in failure to shed CD62L (De Graaf *et al.*, 1995).

Normal LCs express high levels of the homophilic adhesion molecule E-cadherin and undergo E-cadherin-dependent adhesion with epidermal keratinocytes (Tang *et al.*, 1993). E-cadherin expression is markedly downregulated upon the migration and maturation of epidermal LCs (Borkowski *et al.*, 1994). A study carried out to investigate whether or not E-cadherin expression correlates with clinical outcome, showed that LCH cells of seven children with skin-only involvement were positive for E-cadherin, whereas seven children who developed disseminated LCH displayed negative or low expression (Geissmann *et al.*, 1997). It has already been observed that E-cadherin downregulation in many carcinomas correlates with tumour cell metastasis. Thus, one can speculate that downregulation of E-cadherin surface expression by LCH cells similarly correlates with the occurrence of dissemination of the disease.

Based on the phenotypic studies to date, it is clear that LCH cells display an abnormal phenotype that includes characteristics of both normal epidermal LCs and activated LCs. This phenotype is indicative of LCH cells being in an arrested state of activation and/or differentiation. Whether this phenotype is due to a dysregulated immune response to an antigenic stimulus, or is a reflection of an intrinsic defect of LCH cells, remains unknown.

The immune function of LCH cells

Since LCH cells display an abnormal phenotype in which immature markers coexist with adhesion molecules and antigen-presentation markers, it seems logical that these cells also display defective functional capabilities. The presence of many T-cells within LCH lesions raises the question of whether there is an immune interaction between T- and LCH cells. To date only a few studies have assessed the functional activity of LCH cells, due to the paucity of fresh material.

Normal LCs are potent antigen-presenting cells (APCs) and activators of T-cells (Banchereau and Steinman, 1998). In order to determine whether LCH cells function as APCs, an early study used highly purified LCH cells as stimulator cells in an allogeneic mixed cell reaction (Yu *et al.*, 1995). This study, of three LCH patients, showed that the antigen-presenting capacity of LCH cells, derived from four different organs affected by LCH namely skin, lymph node, bone and gum, was greatly reduced when compared to normal epidermal LCs. This result correlated with an earlier study from the same group, in which lesional LCH cells from a fatal case of LCH also displayed poor alloantigen-presenting activity *in vitro* (Yu *et al.*, 1992).

Several receptors and their ligands are involved in DC/T-cell interaction. The CD40–CD40L pathway is an integral part of this bi-directional communication. The ligation of CD40 expressed by DCs, is an early and pivotal signal for the upregulation of antigen-presenting functions by these cells (Laman *et al.*, 1996). In addition, ligation of CD40L expressed by activated CD4+ T-cells is crucial to T-cell priming and cytokine production (Peng *et al.*, 1996). In a more recent study, LCH cells stimulated by CD40L, were shown to be able to mature *in vitro* and acquire potent immunostimulatory characteristics (Geissmann *et al.*, 2001). In this study, sorted CD1a+ LCH cells and control immature DCs, were cultured with CD40L or CD32-transfected fibroblasts for two days before being added to allogeneic lymphocytes. Although LCH cells and immature DCs cultured with CD32-transfected cells retained an immature phenotype and stimulated lymphocyte proliferation equally poorly, both LCH cells and the control cells stimulated with CD40L, expressed high membrane MHC class II and CD86, and showed strong capacity to stimulate lymphocytes. Interestingly, in spontaneously regressive disease, including self-healing cutaneous lesions, LCH cells frequently exhibit the expression of mature markers, such as CD86 and DC-LAMP *in situ*, suggesting that they represent more mature DCs (Geissmann *et al.*, 2001).

It is still unclear why LCH cells *in vivo* appear to have reduced functional activity. The fact that this defect appears to be confined to LCH cells and does not affect all cells of DC lineage in LCH patients (Holter *et al.*, 2002), plus the ability of LCH cells to mature *in vitro*, suggests that the lesional microenvironment may be having a suppressive effect on the LCH cells. The detection of interleukin (IL)-10, a cytokine capable of downregulating the expression of B7 molecules and class II antigens by DCs, in bone and lymph node lesions, but not in skin lesions from patients with limited or self-healing disease (Geissmann *et al.*, 2001), perhaps gives further evidence that the cytokine environment is the extrinsic factor affecting the differentiation and functional capabilities of LCH cells *in vivo*.

The role of cytokines in LCH

A central feature of normal immunological regulation involves the production and local action of cytokines. However this action is normally short lived. In cases of immunological dysregulation, as is thought to occur in LCH, the over-production of cytokines can lead to pathological consequences. Indeed, LCH is characterized by a lesional 'cytokine storm', a term referring to both the high level and diversity of cytokines produced locally (Egeler *et al.*, 1999).

In LCH lesions, the predominant sources of the 'cytokine storm' are T-cells and LCH cells. LCH cells produce high levels of a range of cytokines, including pro-inflammatory (IL-1α) and interferon-γ (IFN-γ), anti-inflammatory (IL-10), and growth factors (e.g. granulocyte/macrophage colony stimulating factor, GM-CSF).

The pro-inflammatory cytokine IFN-γ is known to be produced by activated natural killer (NK) cells and in larger amounts by effector T-cells, and thus appears mainly after induction of an adaptive immune response. Elevated levels of IFN-γ are also expressed by T- and LCH cells in LCH lesions. Indeed, IFN-γ has been reported to be a marker of LCH cells in the skin (Neumann *et al.*, 1988). However, IFN-γ+ LCH cells were also found in bone and lymph node lesions, suggesting that IFN-γ is not a specific marker of skin LCH cells (De Graaf *et al.*, 1996). The fact that IFN-γ is highly expressed in LCH lesions suggests that it possibly plays a stimulatory role on LCH cells, such as enhancing their IL-1 secretory capacity (Arenzana-Seisdedos *et al.*, 1986).

Indeed, IL-1α, IL-1β and another pro-inflammatory cytokine, tumour necrosis factor alpha (TNF-α), were shown to be present in high amounts in LCH lesions (De Graaf *et al.*, 1996; Egeler *et al.*, 1999). This finding may help explain the osteolytic capacity of LCH cells, as these cytokines are known to activate osteoclastic bone resorption (Kudo *et al.*, 2002). Multinucleated giant cells resembling osteoclasts, found in LCH bone lesions, may originate from macrophage activation under such IL-1 and TNF-α influence. Besides the expression of IL-1 in LCH lesions, a study showed elevated levels of IL-1 receptor antagonist (IL-1Ra), a naturally occurring IL-1 antagonist, in LCH patients. Whereas the IL-1/IL-1R complex triggers several inflammatory events, such as cyclo-oxygenase-2 induction and the production of prostaglandin E2 (Arend *et al.*, 1998), the IL-1Ra/IL-R complex on the cell membrane does not induce any response. The role of IL-1Ra in the pathophysiology of LCH is however unknown. Two main hypotheses have been proposed: IL-1Ra is a primary product of abnormal DCs, or it is produced by normal cells in an attempt to cope with LCH and its manifestations (Rosso *et al.*, 2003).

Another pro-inflammatory cytokine highly expressed in LCH lesions is IL-2. IL-2 is involved in the interaction of antigen-presenting LCs with T-cells, being involved in T-cell activation as well as programmed cell death. A study has shown that the IL-2 receptor (IL-2R) is expressed by LCH cells, suggesting that LCs are activated and induced to proliferate in LCH lesions (Barbey *et al.*, 1987). Furthermore, elevated amounts of soluble IL-2R (sIL-2R) were found in the sera of seven children with various forms of LCH (Schultz *et al.*, 1998). sIL-2R is capable of binding to IL-2, potentially inhibiting the normal immune response by occupying the binding region of this T-cell derived cytokine.

In contrast to the pro-inflammatory cytokines, anti-inflammatory cytokines, such as transforming growth factor (TGF)-β or IL-10, may prevent LC maturation. In particular, IL-10 is capable of downregulating the expression of B7 molecules and class II antigens by DCs *in vitro* (Ozawa *et al.*, 1996). Two recent studies report conflicting results regarding the expression of IL-10 in LCH. In one study, both LCH cells and macrophages appeared to be the source of the IL-10 in 9 of 11 bone and lymph node biopsies (Egeler *et al.*, 1999). However, in a second study, IL-10-expressing cells in eosinophilic granuloma were predominantly large-sized CD3-, Langerin-, CD68+ cells, and therefore were neither LCH cells nor T-cells, but macrophages (Geissmann *et al.*, 2001). In another study of adult lung patients, IL-10 was not detected in five of five LCH lesions in which the LCH cells expressed CD86 (Tazi *et al.*, 1999). This difference between pulmonary and bone LCH lesions, suggests that the different clinical picture characteristic of pulmonary LCH, where LCH cells present a more mature phenotype, may be a consequence of the absence of this anti-inflammatory cytokine. Further evidence to support this hypothesis comes from the observation that macrophages are very rare in skin lesions from patients with limited or self-healing disease, and there are consistently no IL-10+ cells (Geissmann *et al.*, 2001). Another anti-inflammatory cytokine, TGF-β, is also present in LCH lesions. TGF-β is known to be involved in LC differentiation (Jaksits *et al.*, 1999), and has been identified as the major player producing tissue fibrosis (Border and Noble, 1994), thus explaining this outcome in LCH lesions.

Cytokines are also known to induce proliferation, differentiation and activation of normal LCs. One such cytokine is the growth factor GM-CSF. In three studies (Emile *et al.*, 1993, 1994, 1995) GM-CSF was detected within the cytoplasm of all the LCH cells but not other cell types within the lesions. Children with disseminated active LCH, but not localized (e.g. bone) LCH, had an elevated serum GM-CSF level. Additionally, LCH cells from all samples stained positively with granulocyte/macrophage colony stimulating factor receptor (GM-CSFR)-antibody. This suggests that GM-CSF may be a growth factor for LCH cells and that the GM-CSF level is related to the extent and activity of LCH.

The presence of this 'cytokine storm' probably explains the abnormal phenotype and function of LCH cells and may provide these cells with an optimal microenvironment to prolong their viability, possibly by creating autocrine loops. Thus it is highly likely that cytokines play a prominent role in the pathogenesis of LCH and may explain common phenomena, such as osteolysis and fibrosis, and the recruitment of typical inflammatory infiltrates.

The role of chemokines in LCH

Chemokines are chemo-attractant molecules that determine the tissue distribution of many cell types. LCH lesions may be present in skin or lymph nodes where one expects LCs, but also in many other sites. This inappropriate accumulation of LCs at various sites in LCH suggests an abnormality of cell trafficking. Several studies have demonstrated that the movement of LCs from the site of antigen capture to the draining lymphoid organs involves selective chemokines which act on maturing LCs through particular chemokine receptors (Dieu *et al.*, 1998; Sozzani *et al.*, 1998).

Immature DCs respond to many chemokines, in particular CCL20, which appears to be the most powerful chemokine to induce migration of CD34+-derived immature DCs (Dieu *et al.*, 1998). CCL20 mRNA expression seems to be restricted to epithelium and is upregulated by inflammation (Hromas *et al.*, 1997). Thus it is thought that during pathogen invasion, immature LCs expressing CCR6, the major functional CCL20 receptor, would be attracted to the site of inflammation through the local production of chemokines, such as CCL20. After antigen uptake, the maturation of DC results in a complete reprogramming of the cell, with downregulation of endocytic activity (Sallusto *et al.*, 1995), upregulation of MHC, adhesion and co-stimulatory molecules (Cella *et al.*, 1997) as well as a striking switch in chemokine receptor usage (Sozzani *et al.*, 1998). The response to a set of chemokines, in particular CCL20, is rapidly lost due to downregulation of CCR6 expression, enabling LCs to escape the local gradient of CCL20. At the same time, maturing LCs start to express CCR7, resulting in attraction of these cells to CCL19 and CCL21 which are expressed in the T-cell zones of lymph nodes (Gunn *et al.*, 1998). As these two chemokines can attract mature DC and lymphocytes, they are likely to play a key role in helping antigen-loaded DC to encounter specific naive T-cells.

Through our own work on LCH, we have demonstrated that lesional LCs are indeed in an immature state as defined by their expression of the chemokine receptor CCR6. Conversely, CCR7 expression appears to be absent on these cells, in keeping with the fact that LCH cells are hardly ever found in lymph nodes draining the lesional sites. Thus, despite various inflammatory stimuli, such as TNF-α, which should induce LC maturation, the lesional CD1a+ cells do not lose their expression of CCR6 and do not upregulate CCR7 (Annels *et al.*, 2003). Other work has shown that the lesional CD1a+ cells have the intrinsic capability to fully differentiate and mature once removed from the lesion (Geissmann *et al.*, 2001), indicating that a factor/factors in LCH lesions prevents full differentiation. This, together with the high expression of the CCR6 ligand CCL20 in LCH lesions, probably prevents lesional CD1a+ cells from leaving their peripheral tissue sites and instead enhances their accumulation.

In contrast to our findings, Fleming recently reported coincident expression of the chemokine receptors CCR6 and CCR7 by pathological LCH cells (Fleming *et al.*, 2003). One possibility for the discrepancy could be the type of lesion that was studied. In some LCH cases *in vivo*, most notably in self-healing cutaneous lesions, a more mature phenotype can be observed and LCH cells appear to downregulate CD14 and upregulate CD86 and DC-LAMP (Geissmann *et al.*, 2001). It may be that in these lesions, the LCH cells have partially overcome the maturation blockade and are able to downregulate CCR6 and upregulate CCR7 as they mature. This would in turn release these cells from the local control of CCL20, and allow them to follow the normal lymphoid drainage pathways, thus explaining the spontaneous resolution which may be seen.

In our study of chemokine/chemokine receptor interactions involved in LCH (Annels *et al.*, 2003), we showed that lesional CD1a+ cells express not only CCL20 but other inflammatory chemokines, such as CCL5 and CXCL11. These chemokines are likely responsible for the recruitment of other inflammatory cell types, characteristic of LCH lesions. Indeed, as well as expressing CXCR3, the receptor for CXCL11, the infiltrating T-cells in LCH lesions also expressed CCR6. This finding along with the finding that CCL20 specifically attracts the memory subset of T-cells *in vitro* (Liao *et al.*, 1999), strongly implicates CCL20 as an important chemo-attractant responsible for T-cell recruitment in LCH lesions. In another study, CCL22-positive DCs were shown to be present in LCH lesions (Vulcano *et al.*, 2001). CCL22 is a constitutively produced DC chemokine known to be chemotactic for DCs, IL-2-activated NK-cells and chronically activated T-lymphocytes (Godiska *et al.*, 1997). This finding suggests a role for CCL22 in co-localization and interaction of lesional CD1a+ cells and T-cells in LCH lesions. Thus, lesional CD1a+ cells, through their production of various chemokines, may not only be causing their own recruitment and retention, but that of other inflammatory cells as well.

In future studies, it will be interesting to see if the same spectrum of chemokines/chemokine receptors are expressed in spontaneously resolving lesions and in adult pulmonary LCH lesions.

Cell-cycle regulation and proliferation in LCH

It is often assumed that the massive accumulation of LCs in LCH lesions results not only from aberrant chemo-attraction, but also from abnormal local proliferation of these cells. This uncontrolled proliferation could be due to a neoplastic transformation of the LCH cells or to locally secreted cytokines (De Graaf *et al.*, 1996; Egeler *et al.*, 1999), perhaps as part of a dysregulated immune response. In order to address this, genetic and functional alterations, essential for tumorigenic growth (controlling proliferation and apoptosis), have been investigated.

Two recent studies measured the proliferative activity of LCs in LCH by studying the expression of the proliferation marker Ki-67 (Schouten *et al.*, 2002; Bank *et al.*, 2003). In both studies, and in agreement with an earlier study (Hage *et al.*, 1993), Ki-67 nuclear-positive LCs were found in all the lesions examined, ranging from a small number of clusters to the majority of the cells. As Ki-67 is expressed during all active phases of the cell cycle, but not in resting cells, this suggests that the cell cycle is not terminated in LCH cells. In addition, mitotic figures were observed in

34 of 61 evaluated specimens (Bank *et al.*, 2003), in keeping with a number of earlier reports (Shamoto, 1977; Pierard *et al.*, 1982; Risdall *et al.*, 1982; Ruco *et al.*, 1993), giving further support to the interpretation that LCH infiltrates have local proliferative activity.

Another element critically involved in the cellular pathways controlling proliferation, DNA repair, or apoptosis is the transcription factor p53. p53 regulates the normal cell cycle by activating transcription of genes that control progression through the cycle, and of other genes that cause arrest in G1 when the genome is damaged. In some cell types, p53 can also promote apoptosis (Lane, 1992). In normal cells, the p53 gene product is expressed at very low levels, undetectable by immunohistochemical methods because of rapid turnover. In contrast, mutant p53 proteins have a stable conformation, resulting in the accumulation of the protein to detectable levels (Reich *et al.*, 1983). Several groups have investigated the expression of p53 (Bank *et al.*, 2002; Schouten *et al.*, 2002) as well as p53 gene mutations in LCH cells (Weintraub *et al.*, 1998). In all the studies p53 protein was detectable by immunohistochemistry specifically localized to the LCs in LCH lesions. Furthermore, p53 expression occurred in all cases of LCH studied, including patients with localized bone lesions and multisystem disease, thus abnormal p53 expression is not limited to severe forms of LCH, but is also found in the mildest, frequently self-resolving forms. Mutations in the single copy p53 gene are the most frequent genetic changes associated with human cancers. However, by polymerase chain reaction or single-stranded conformational polymorphism (PCR/SSCP), no mutations in exons 4 to 11 of the p53 gene in LCH cells were found (Weintraub *et al.*, 1998). Another mechanism that can cause abnormal expression of the p53 protein is stabilization of the protein as a result of binding of p53 to other proteins. One such protein is mdm2, an oncogene product, which binds to the transactivation domain of p53 and downregulates its ability to activate transcription. Following DNA damage, the p53 protein induces the transcription of the mdm2 oncogene that in turn inhibits p53-dependent transcriptional activation, creating a feedback loop resulting in downregulation of p53 activity. The study by Schouten *et al.* found heterogeneous over-expression of mdm2 by lesional LCs, probably induced by p53, and reflecting the existence of the auto-regulatory feedback loop between p53 and mdm2 (Schouten *et al.*, 2002).

Only one study so far has investigated the expression of a number of other key factors that control proliferation and apoptosis, namely p21, p16 and Rb. p53 activates p21 in response to DNA damage; p21 inhibits cell cycle progression at both G1 and G2 checkpoints (El Deiry *et al.*, 1994). Another important pathway for detecting DNA damage and inducing cell-cycle arrest is the p16–Rb pathway. Both the p21 and p16–Rb pathways were found to be active in virtually all LCH cases studied (Schouten *et al.*, 2002).

As well as abnormal proliferation, the accumulation of LCH cells may also be due to disturbances in normal apoptosis (programmed cell death). The product of the Bcl-2 gene is an important regulator of apoptosis (Bomer, 2003), now recognized as a survival factor for many cell types. In LCH, over-expression of the Bcl-2 protein has been found (Savell et al., 1998; Schouten et al., 2002), possibly playing a role in the activation of p53 and p16 and subsequent arrest of apoptosis.

Correlating the results of these studies leaves a fairly conflicting picture of the cell proliferation and apoptotic pathways that may be involved in LCH. Indeed, both stimulatory and inhibitory pathways of cell proliferation and apoptosis appear to be upregulated. Survival and proliferation are probably supported by several mechanisms in LCH. Firstly, proliferation of LCH cells is probably due to various cytokines present in LCH lesions. Secondly, the high level of expression of Bcl-2 will inhibit apoptosis and thirdly, the observed mdm2 expression will inhibit p53 suppressive activity. Despite the fact that these stimulation pathways result in a high level of cellular proliferation, there are also several counter-regulatory pathways active in LCH. The suppressive cytokine TGF-β is present, as are the TGF-β receptors (Schouten et al., 2002) and downstream, the inhibitory p53–p21 and p16–Rb pathways are also activated. As the outcome is enhanced LCH cell proliferation and survival despite the presence of negative regulators, it appears that the counter-regulatory pathways are unable or insufficient to keep the cells in check.

LCH: A clonal proliferative disease

Several studies showing that LCH cells are intrinsically proliferative (Hage et al., 1993; Schouten et al., 2002; Bank et al., 2003), led to the question of whether LCH is a reactive polyclonal disorder or is due to proliferation of a single LCH cell resulting in a clonal histiocytic disease. Studies that can detect clonal or polyclonal X chromosome inactivation patterns in female tissues have been performed in LCH. These studies have unequivocally shown that the LCs from single system and multisystem LCH lesions are clonal (Willman et al., 1994b). In a further study, clonality was shown in CD1a-positive cells, fluorescence-activated cell sorter (FACS) sorted from lesions of females with multisystem disease (Yu et al., 1994). The fact that clonal histiocytes were found in all forms of LCH, including clinically benign disease, led to the opinion that LCH is most likely a clonal neoplastic disease with highly variable biological behaviour (Willman 1994a). The number of patients studied is small however, and it remains a controversial point. In future studies, it would be interesting to determine whether multiple samples from different sites or from a single patient over-time, show identical clonality.

When clonality was assessed in adult pulmonary LCH, a unique form of the disease commonly affecting smokers in the third to fifth decades, the disease was found to be non-clonal (Yousem *et al.*, 2001). Thus, adult pulmonary LCH appears to be primarily a reactive process, possibly due to tobacco smoke-driven hyperplasia of LCH cells in which occasional clones may arise.

LCH: A role for viruses?

Regardless of whether the disease is monoclonal or polyclonal, the proliferation of LCH cells may be induced by some intrinsic mutation or by external factors, such as a virus. Immature DCs typically respond to pathogen exposure by undergoing a maturation process that facilitates induction of further innate and adaptive immune responses (Banchereau *et al.*, 2000). Maturation is induced when immature DCs are exposed to pathogens, such as *Escherichia coli*, *Candida*, and influenza virus or to inflammatory cytokines (Banchereau *et al.*, 2000; Huang *et al.*, 2001). However, some viruses, such as HIV, vaccinia, measles and dengue viruses, interfere with DC function and maturation in order to evade immune surveillance (Grosjean *et al.*, 1997; Engelmayer *et al.*, 1999; Tortorella *et al.*, 2000; Izmailova *et al.*, 2003). In addition, viral infection of DCs can induce aberrant or uncontrolled cytokine production, a major feature of LCH (Moss, 1996; Braun *et al.*, 1997; Smith *et al.*, 1997). Thus, it is highly plausible that a viral infection may be a pathogenic factor causing the immunological abnormality in LCH.

In an early study nucleic acid extracts of biopsy specimens from LCH patients were injected into mice. Cell suspensions were subsequently made from the lungs of these animals and assayed for cytopathic effects on primary human embryo cultures. The presence of syncytia and nuclear changes were interpreted as evidence of a transmissible agent (Nastac *et al.*, 1970). Since then studies have detected the presence of human herpesvirus (HHV) 6 (Leahy *et al.*, 1993) and cytomegalovirus (CMV) (Kawakubo *et al.*, 1999) in LCH cells. However, just as many published studies refute these findings (McClain *et al.*, 1994; McClain and Weiss, 1994; Jenson *et al.*, 2000). In one study, the presence of nine different viruses which commonly infect children, namely adenovirus, CMV, Epstein–Barr virus (EBV), herpes simplex virus, HHV6, parvovirus, human T-cell viruses type I and II and HIV, was investigated. *In situ* hybridisation (ISH) and PCR performed on 56 cases of LCH did not result in consistent evidence of any viral genome and the study concluded that none of the viruses tested was responsible for LCH (McClain *et al.*, 1994).

In a recent publication, the presence of viral particles as well as DNA from the HHV-6B variant that is associated with disease in humans, was detected by immunohistochemistry and ISH in a large number of patients with LCH, again raising the possibility of a viral trigger (Glotzbecker *et al.*, 2004). However, in the same study a high prevalence of HHV-6 was found in control tissues, thus the presence of a virus does not establish a causal role in LCH. However, even if a virus is not the causative factor in LCH, this does not preclude the involvement of other microbial agents.

LCH: A reactive or neoplastic disease?

For decades it has been thought that LCH is a reactive rather than a neoplastic process. This was based on the absence of aneuploidy (Rabkin *et al.*, 1988), the failure to identify consistent cytogenetic alterations, and the occurrence of spontaneous clinical regression. However, the finding of proliferation of LCs in LCH lesions, and the clonality studies quoted above, has renewed the arguments that LCH may indeed be a neoplasm. Despite the fact that clonality is widely considered to be characteristic of neoplastic disease, there are several circumstances in which clonal populations may be detected over several years without the development of a malignancy (Weiss *et al.*, 1986; Kurahashi *et al.*, 1991). Furthermore, adaptive immune responses are associated with clonal expansions that may be detected over many years and are certainly not malignant (Maini *et al.*, 1999). The fact that LCH cells are clonal, however, raises the possibility that these cells may acquire somatic mutations in a gene or genes that regulate cell growth, survival, or proliferation. Indeed, there is now evidence of increased chromosomal breakage in patients with LCH, from investigations using comparative genomic hybridization (CGH) and other molecular methods (Betts *et al.*, 1998; Scappaticci *et al.*, 2000; Murakami *et al.*, 2002). Besides chromosomal instability, abnormal clones showing a t(7;12) (q11.2;p13) translocation have been observed (Betts *et al.*, 1998). These data strongly suggest that there is a component of genetic instability in LCH, as observed in some types of neoplasms and myelodysplastic disorders. Furthermore, as described, the cell-cycle regulation of LCH cells is severely disrupted (Bank *et al.*, 2002; Schouten *et al.*, 2002), probably as a result of a combination of external signals (growth factors and cytokines), and intrinsic factors from as yet unidentified DNA changes. To test the hypothesis of malignancy, more rigorous studies are needed into the expression of oncogenes and anti-oncogenes by LCH cells. To date, only one such study has been carried out in which it was reported that the c-myc and H-ras proto-oncogenes were expressed in the active terminal phases of the disease, but not in the quiescent phase (Abdelatif *et al.*, 1990). However, now that the pathways and molecules involved in oncogenesis are much better defined, it is known that the expression of these oncogenes is associated with proliferative activity of any kind of cell.

Once the role and expression of oncogenes and their pathways in LCH has been fully assessed, the argument about a reactive *versus* a neoplastic disorder can finally be laid to rest.

REFERENCES

Abdelatif, O.M., Chandler, F.W, Pantazis, C.G., *et al.* (1990). Enhanced expression of c-myc and H-ras oncogenes in Letterer–Siwe disease. *Arch Pathol Lab Med*, **114**, 1254–1260.

Al-Alwan, M.M., Rowden, G., Lee, T.D., *et al.* (2001). Fascin is involved in the antigen presentation activity of mature dendritic cells. *J Immunol*, **166**, 338–345.

Annels, N.E., da Costa, C.E.T., Prins, F.A., *et al.* (2003). Aberrant chemokine receptor expression and chemokine production by Langerhans cells underlies the pathogenesis of Langerhans cell histiocytosis. *J Exp Med*, **197**, 1385–1390.

Arceci, R.J., Longley, J. and Emanuel, P.D. (2002). Atypical cellular disorders. *Hematology*, 297–314.

Arend, W.P., Malyak, M., Guthridge, C.J., *et al.* (1998). Interleukin-1 receptor antagonist: role in biology. *Ann Rev Immunol*, **16**, 27–55.

Arenzana-Seisdedos, F., Marbey, S., Virelizier, J.L., *et al.* (1986). Histiocytosis X. Purified (T6+) cells from bone granuloma produce interleukin 1 and prostaglandin E2 in culture. *J Clin Invest*, **77**, 326–329.

Banchereau, J. and Steinman, R. (1998). Dendritic cells and the control of immunity. *Nature*, **392**, 245–252.

Banchereau, J., Briere, F., Caux, C., *et al.* (2000). Immunobiology of dendritic cells. *Ann Rev Immunol*, **18**, 767–811.

Bank, M.I., Rengtved, P., Carstensen, H., *et al.* (2002). p53 expression in biopsies from children with Langerhans cell histiocytosis. *J Pediatr Hematol Oncol*, **24**, 733–738.

Bank, M.I., Rengtved, P., Carstensen, H., *et al.* (2003). An evaluation of histopathological parameters, demonstration of proliferation by Ki-67 and mitotic bodies. *Acta Pathol, Microbiol Immunol Scand*, **111**, 300–308.

Barbey, S., Gane, P., Pelletier, O.L., *et al.* (1987). Histiocytosis X Langerhans cells react with antiinterleukin-2 receptor monoclonal antibody. *Pediatr Pathol*, **7**, 569–574.

Betts, D.R., Leibundgut, K.E., Feldges, A., *et al.* (1998). Cytogenetic abnormalities in Langerhans cell histiocytosis. *Br J Cancer*, **77**, 552–555.

Bomer, C. (2003). The bcl-2 protein family: sensors and checkpoints for life-or-death decisions. *Mol Immunol*, **39**, 615–647.

Border, W.A. and Noble, N.A. (1994). Transforming growth factor β in tissue fibrosis. *New Engl J Med*, **331**, 1286–1292.

Borkowski, T.A., Van Dyke, B.J., Schwarzenberger, K., *et al.* (1994). Expression of E-cadherin by murine dendritic cells: E-cadherin as a dendritic cell differentiation antigen characteristic of epidermal Langerhans cells and related cells. *Eur J Immunol*, **24**, 2767–2774.

Braun, D.K., Dominiquez, G.D. and Pellett, P.E. (1997). Human herpes virus 6. *Clin Microbiol Rev*, **10**, 521–567.

Cella, M., Engering, A., Pinet, V., *et al.* (1997). Inflammatory stimuli induce accumulation of MHC class II complexes on dendritic cells. *Nature*, **388**, 782–787.

De Graaf, J.H., Tamminga, R.Y.J., Kamps, W.A., *et al.* (1994). Langerhans cell histiocytosis: expression of leukocyte cellular adhesion molecules suggests abnormal homing and differentiation. *Am J Pathol*, **144**, 466–472.

De Graaf, J.H., Tamminga, R.Y.J., Kamps, W.A., *et al.* (1995). Expression of cellular adhesion molecules in Langerhans cell histiocytosis and normal Langerhans cells. *Am J Pathology*, **147**, 1161–1171.

De Graaf, J.H., Tamminga, R.Y.J., Dam-Meiring, A., *et al.* (1996). The presence of cytokines in Langerhans cell histiocytosis. *J Pathol*, **180**, 400–406.

Dieu, M.C., Vanbervliet, B., Vicari, A., *et al.* (1998). Selective recruitment of immature and mature dendritic cells by distinct chemokines expressed in different anatomic sites. *J Exp Med*, **188**, 373–386.

Egeler, R.M., Annels, N.E. and Hogendoorn, P.C. (2004). Langerhans cell histiocytosis: a pathologic combination of oncogenesis and immune dysregulation. *Pediatr Blood Cancer*, **42**, 401–403.

Egeler, R.M., Favara, B.E., van Meurs, M., *et al.* (1999). Differential *in situ* cytokine profiles of Langerhans-like cells and T cells in Langerhans cell histiocytosis: abundant expression of cytokines relevant to disease and treatment. *Blood*, **94**, 4195–4201.

Egeler, R.M., Favara, B.E., Laman, J.D., *et al.* (2000). Abundant expression of CD40 and CD40-ligand (CD154) in paediatric Langerhans cell histiocytosis lesions. *Eur J Cancer*, **36**, 2105–2110.

El Deiry, W.S., Harper, J.W., O'Connor, P.M., *et al.* (1994). WAF1/CIP1 is induced in p53-mediated G1 arrest and apoptosis. *Cancer Res*, **54**, 1169–1174.

Emile, J.F., Fraitag, S., Pascale, A., *et al.* (1995). Expression of GM-CSF receptor by Langerhans cell histiocytosis cells. *Virchows Arch*, **427**, 125–129.

Emile, J.F., Peuchmaur, M., Fraitag, S., *et al.* (1993). Immunohistochemical detection of granulocyte/macrophage colony-stimulating factor in Langerhans cell histiocytosis. *Histopathology*, **23**, 327–332.

Emile, J.F., Tartour, E., Brugieres, L., *et al.* (1994). Detection of GM-CSF in the sera of children with Langerhans cell histiocytosis. *Pediatr Allergy Immunol*, **5**, 162–163.

Engelmayer, J., Larsson, M., Subklewe, M., *et al.* (1999). Vaccinia virus inhibits the maturation of human dendritic cells: a novel mechanism of immune evasion. *J Immunol*, **163**, 6762–6768.

Fleming, M.D., Pinkus, J.L., Alexander, S.W., *et al.* (2003). Coincident expression of the chemokine receptors CCR6 and CCR7 by pathologic Langerhans cells in Langerhans cell histiocytosis. *Blood*, **101**, 2473–2475.

Geissmann, F., Emile, J.F., Andry, P., *et al.* (1997). Lack of expression of E-cadherin is associated with dissemination of Langerhans cell histiocytosis and poor outcome. *J Pathol*, **181**, 301–304.

Geissmann, F., Lepelletier, Y., Fraitag, S., *et al.* (2001). Differentiation of Langerhans cells in Langerhans cell histiocytosis. *Blood*, **97**, 1241–1248.

Glotzbecker, M.P., Carpentieri, D.F. and Dormans, J.P. (2004). Langerhans cell histiocytosis: a primary viral infection of bone? Human herpesvirus 6 protein detected in lymphocytes from tissue of children. *J Pediatr Orthop*, **24**, 123–129.

Godiska, R., Chantry, D., Raport, C.J., *et al.* (1997). Human macrophage derived chemokine (MDC) a novel chemoattractant for monocytes, monocyte derived dendritic cells, and natural killer cells. *J Exp Med*, **185**, 1595–1604.

Grosjean, I., Caux, C., Bella, C., *et al.* (1997). Measles virus infects human dendritic cells and blocks their allostimulatory properties for CD4+ T cells. *J Exp Med*, **186**, 801–812.

Gunn, M.D., Tangemann, K., Tam, C., *et al.* (1998). A chemokine expressed in lymphoid high endothelial venules promotes the adhesion and chemotaxis of naïve T lymphocytes. *Proc Natl Acad Sci USA*, **95**, 258–263.

Hage, C., Willman, C.L., Favara, B.E., *et al.* (1993). Langerhans cell histiocytosis (histiocytosis X): immunophenotype and growth fraction. *Hum Pathol*, **24**, 840–845.

Holter, W., Ressmann, G., Grois, N., *et al.* (2002). Normal monocyte-derived dendritic cell function in patients with Langerhans-cell-histiocytosis. *Med Pediatr Oncol*, **39**, 181–186.

Hromas, R., Gray, P.W., Chantry, D., *et al.* (1997). Cloning and characterization of exodus, a novel beta-chemokine. *Blood*, **89**, 3315–3322.

Huang, Q., Liu, D., Majewski, P., *et al.* (2001). The plasticity of dendritic cell responses to pathogens and their components. *Science*, **294**, 870–875.

Izmailova, E., Bertley, F.M.N., Huang, Q., *et al.* (2003). HIV-1 Tat reprograms immature dendritic cells to express chemoattractants for activated T cells and macrophages. *Nat Med*, **9**, 191–197.

Jaksits, S., Kriehuber, E., Charbonnier, A.S., *et al.* (1999). CD34+ cell-derived CD14+ precursor cells develop into Langerhans cells in a TGF-beta 1-dependent manner. *J Immunol*, **163**, 4869–4877.

Jenson, H.B., McClain, K.L., Leach, C.T., *et al.* (2000). Evaluation of human herpesvirus type 8 infection in childhood Langerhans cell histiocytosis. *Am J Hematol*, **64**, 237–241.

Kawakubo, Y., Kishimoto, H., Sato, Y., *et al.* (1999). Human cytomegalovirus infection in foci of Langerhans cell histiocytosis. *Virchows Arch*, **434**, 109–115.

Kudo, O., Fujikawa, Y., Itonaga, I., *et al.* (2002). Proinflammatory cytokine (TNF alpha/ IL-1 alpha) induction of human osteoclast formation. *J Pathol*, **198**, 220–227.

Kurahashi, H., Hara, J. and Yumura-Yagi, K. (1991). Monoclonal nature of transient abnormal myelopoiesis in Down's syndrome. *Blood*, **77**, 1161–1163.

Laman, J.D., Claassen, E. and Noelle, R.J. (1996). Functions of CD40 and its ligand, gp39 (CD40L). *Crit Rev Immunol*, **16**, 59–108.

Laman, J.D., Leenen, P.J., Annels, N.E., *et al.* (2003). Langerhans-cell histiocytosis 'insight into DC biology'. *Trends Immunol*, **24**, 190–196.

Lane, D.P. (1992). Cancer: p53, guardian of the genome. *Nature*, **358**, 15–16.

Leahy, M.A., Krejci, S.M., Friednash, M., *et al.* (1993). Human herpesvirus 6 is present in lesions of Langerhans cell histiocytosis. *J Invest Dermatol*, **101**, 642–645.

Liao, F., Rabin, R.L., Smith, C.S., *et al.* (1999). CC-chemokine receptor 6 is expressed on diverse memory subsets of T cells and determines responsiveness to macrophage inflammatory protein 3 alpha. *J Immunol*, **162**, 186–194.

Maini, M.K., Casorati, G., Dellabona, P., *et al.* (1999). T cell clonality in immune responses. *Immunol Today*, **20**, 262–266.

McClain, K. and Weiss, R.A. (1994). Viruses and Langerhans cell histiocytosis: is there a link? *Br J Cancer*, **70**, S34–S36.

McClain, K., Jin, H., Gresik, V., *et al.* (1994). Langerhans cell histiocytosis: lack of a viral etiology. *Am J Hematol*, **47**, 16–20.

Moss, B. (1996). Poxviridae: the viruses and their replication. In: Fields B.N., Knipe, D.M. and Howley, P.M., eds. *Fields Virology*, 3rd edn. Lipincott-Raven, Philadelphia, pp. 26–37.

Murakami, I., Gogusev, J., Fournet, J.C., *et al.* (2002). Detection of molecular cytogenetic aberrations in Langerhans cell histiocytosis of bone. *Hum Pathol*, **33**, 555–560.

Nastac, E., Athanasiu, P., Lungu, M., *et al.* (1970). Experimental investigations in human eosinophilic granuloma. *Rev Roumaine Inframicrobiol*, **7**, 125–149.

Neumann, C., Schaumberg-Lever, G., Dopfer, R., *et al.* (1988). Interferon gamma is a marker for histiocytosis X cells in the skin. *J Invest Dermatol*, **91**, 280–282.

Nezelof, C. and Basset, F. (2004). An hypothesis. Langerhans cell histiocytosis: the failure of the immune system to switch from an adaptive mode. *Pediatr Blood Cancer*, **42**, 398–400.

Ozawa, H., Aiba, S., Nakagawa, S., *et al.* (1996). Interferon-γ and interleukin-10 inhibit antigen presentation by Langerhans cells for T helper type 1 cells by suppressing their CD80 (B7-1) expression. *Eur J Immunol*, **26**, 648–652.

Peng, X., Kasran, A., Warmerdam, P.A., *et al.* (1996). Accessory signalling by CD40 for T cell activation: induction of Th1 and Th2 cytokines and synergy with interleukin-12 for interferon-gamma production. *Eur J Immunol*, **26**, 1621–1627.

Pierard, G.E., Franchimont, C. and Lapiere, C.M. (1982). Proliferation of the characteristic histiocyte of histiocytosis X in the skin. *Am J Dermatopathol*, **4**, 215–221.

Pinkus, G.S., Lones, M.A., Matsumura, F., *et al.* (2002). Immunohistochemical expression of fascin, a dendritic cell marker. *Hematopathol*, **118**, 335–343.

Rabkin, M.S., Wittwer, C.T., Kjeldsberg, C.R., *et al.* (1988). Flow-cytometric DNA content of histiocytosis X (Langerhans cell histiocytosis). *Am J Pathol*, **131**, 283–289.

Reich, N.C., Oren, M. and Levine, A.J. (1983). Two distinct mechanisms regulate the levels of a cellular tumour antigen, p53. *Mol Cell Biol*, **3**, 2143–2150.

Ricciardi-Castagnoli, P. and Granucci, F. (2002). Interpretation of the complexity of innate immune responses by functional genomics. *Nat Rev Immunol*, **2**, 881–888.

Risdall, R.J., Dehner, L.P., Duray, P., *et al.* (1982). Histiocytosis X (Langerhans cell histiocytosis): prognostic role of histopathology. *Arch Pathol Lab Med*, **107**, 59–63.

Ross, R., Jonileit, H., Bros, M., *et al.* (2000). Expression of the actin-bundling protein fascin in cultured human dendritic cells correlates with dendritic morphology and cell differentiation. *J Invest Dermatol*, **115**, 658–663.

Rosso, D.A., Ripoli, M.F., Roy, A., *et al.* (2003). Serum levels of interleukin-1 receptor antagonist and tumor necrosis factor-alpha are elevated in children with Langerhans cell histiocytosis. *J Pediatr Hematol Oncol*, **25**, 480–483.

Ruco, L.P., Stoppacciaro, A., Vitolo, D., *et al.* (1993). Expression of adhesion molecules in Langerhans cell histiocytosis. *Histopathol*, **23**, 29–37.

Sallusto, F., Cella, M., Danieli, C., *et al.* (1995). Dendritic cells use macropinocytosis and the mannose receptor to concentrate macromolecules in the major histocompatibility complex II compartment: downregulation by cytokines and bacterial products. *J Exp Med*, **182**, 389–400.

Savell Jr, V.H., Sherman, T., Scheuermann, R.H., *et al.* (1998). Bcl-2 expression in Langerhans cell histiocytosis. *Pediatr Develop Pathol*, **1**, 210–215.

Scappaticci, S., Danesino, C., Rossi, E., *et al.* (2000). Cytogenetic abnormalities in PHA-stimulated lymphocytes from patients with Langerhans cell histiocytosis. *Br J Hematol*, **111**, 258–262.

Schouten, B., Egeler, R.M., Leenen, P.J.M., *et al.* (2002). Expression of cell cycle-related gene products in Langerhans cell histiocytosis. *J Pediatr Hematol Oncol*, **24**, 727–732.

Schultz, C., Klouche, M., Friedrichsdorf, S., *et al.* (1998). Langerhans cell histiocytosis in children: does soluble interleukin-2-receptor correlate with both the disease extent and activity? *Med Pediatr Oncol*, **31**, 61–65.

Shamoto, M. (1977). Mitotic histiocytes and intranuclear Langerhans cell granules in histiocytosis X. *Virchows Arch B: Cell Pathol* **24**, 87–90.

Smith, G.L., Symons, J.A., Khanna, A., *et al.* (1997). Vaccinia virus immune evasion. *Immunol Rev*, **159**, 137–154.

Sozzani, S., Allavena, P., D'Amico, G., *et al.* (1998). Differential regulation of chemokine receptors during dendritic cell maturation: A model for their trafficking properties. *J Immunol*, **161**, 1083–1086.

Stibenz, D. and Buhrer, C. (1994). Down-regulation of L-selectin surface expression by various leukocyte isolation procedures. *Scand J Immunol*, **39**, 59–63.

Tang, A., Amagai, M., Granger, L.G., *et al.* (1993). Adhesion of epidermal Langerhans cells to keratinocytes mediated by e-cadherin. *Nature*, **361**, 82–85.

Tazi, A., Moreau, J., Bergeron, A., *et al.* (1999). Evidence that Langerhans cells in adult pulmonary Langerhans cell histiocytosis are mature dendritic cells: importance of the cytokine microenvironment. *J Immunol* **163**, 3511–3515.

Tortorella, D., Gewurz, B.E., Furman, M.H., *et al.* (2000). Viral subversion of the immune system. *Ann Rev Immunol*, **18**, 861–926.

Vulcano, M., Albanesi, C., Stoppacciaro, A., *et al.* (2001). Dendritic cells as a major source of macrophage-derived chemokine/CCL22 *in vitro* and *in vivo*. *Eur J Immunol*, **31**, 812–822.

Weintraub, M., Bhatia, K.G., Chandra, R.S., *et al.* (1998). p53 expression in Langerhans cell histiocytosis. *J Pediatr Hematol Oncol*, **20**, 12–17.

Weiss, L.M., Wood, G.S. and Trela, M. (1986). Clonal T cell populations in lymphomatoid papulosis: evidence of a lymphoproliferative origin for a clinically benign disease. *New Engl J Med*, **315**, 475–479.

Willman, C.L. (1994a). Detection of clonal histiocytes in Langerhans cell histiocytosis: biology and clinical significance. *Br J Cancer*, **23**, 29–33.

Willman, C.L., Busque, L., Griffith, B.B., *et al.* (1994b). Langerhans'-cell histiocytosis (histiocytosis X): a clonal proliferative disease. *New Engl J Med*, **331**, 154–160.

Yousem, S.A., Colby, T.V., Chen, Y-Y., *et al.* (2001). Pulmonary Langerhans'cell histiocytosis. Molecular analysis of clonality. *Am J Surg Pathol*, **25**, 630–636.

Yu, R.C., Alaibac, M. and Chu, A.C. (1995). Functional defect in cells involved in Langerhans cell histiocytosis. *Arch Dermatol Res*, **287**, 627–631.

Yu, R.C., Morris, J.F., Pritchard, J., *et al.* (1992). Defective alloantigen-presenting capacity of 'Langerhans cell histiocytosis cells'. *Arch Dis Child*, **67**, 1370–1372.

Yu, R.C., Chu, C., Buluwela, L., *et al.* (1994). Clonal proliferation of Langerhans cells in Langerhans cell histiocytosis. *Lancet*, **343**, 767–768.

5

The genetics of Langerhans cell histiocytosis

Maurizio Aricò, Susi Scappaticci and Cesare Danesino

Langerhans cell histiocytosis (LCH) is a rare disorder with heterogeneous clinical manifestations (Aricò and Egeler, 1998). A continuous effort by the clinical investigators, especially in the pediatric field, has led to improved, standardized definitions of the clinical and pathologic diagnostic criteria (Chu *et al.*, 1987; Broadbent *et al.*, 1989; Favara *et al.*, 1997). On this basis, better comparison of pathological and clinical data, including retrospective evaluation of large series of patients, has improved our clinical knowledge of LCH, including the isolated or uncommon manifestations (The French LCH Study Group, 1996; Willis *et al.*, 1996). Moreover, this has been the basis for development of multicenter, international prospective clinical trials, producing definition of standard treatment for LCH in children (Gadner *et al.*, 2001).

Over a century after the first reports, despite these recent advances in clinical management and some very interesting findings from basic research, LCH remains an intriguing disease with many unanswered questions. The etiology and pathogenesis remain largely undefined, and we still are unable to understand why it has such heterogeneous clinical behavior in the absence of identifiable differences in pathology of involved tissues. Although localized skin or bone disease is usually regarded as a benign, self-healing disease, there is a continuing debate as to the possible neoplastic origin of the disseminated form of LCH, which can be associated with a severe course and a high mortality rate (Gadner *et al.*, 2001). On the basis of the evidence of clonality obtained by HUMARA assay in the lesions of nine patients, Willman suggested that LCH is a clonal neoplastic disorder with highly variable biologic behavior and that gene mutations might be identified (Willman *et al.*, 1994). These findings have not been widely reproduced however, and thus clonality of LCH cannot yet be taken for granted (Nezelof and Basset, 2004).

Recent work has raised interest in the possibility of genetic mechanisms playing a role in LCH. Genetic mechanisms may be involved with the pathogenesis of LCH in several different ways. One of these is through an aberrant immune response to a common infectious agent. Extensive laboratory and clinical work over two decades has been unable so far to definitively associate LCH and viral infections (Kawakubo *et al.*, 1999; Jenson *et al.*, 2000; Slacmeulder *et al.*, 2002). Recently however human herpes virus (HHV)-6 has been found in a high percentage of LCH lesional tissue by immunohistochemistry and *in situ* hybridization (ISH) by investigators from the Children's Hospital of Philadelphia, who suggest that all the manifestations of LCH could be secondary to a viral infection of lymphocytes (Glotzbecker *et al.*, 2002, 2004). Further studies to clarify the role of HHV-6 and other viruses is necessary.

Despite this however, there is as yet no definite evidence at present to consider LCH as a virally induced disease. Yet, common pathogens do represent a daily challenge for humans. Increasing evidence support the concept that variants in the immune system may lead to altered immune responses. These in turn trigger mechanisms which result in pathogenic reactive disorders. Thus, inherited variants of genes involved in the anti-infective immune response might well result in inherited constitutional phenotypes that are prone to have persistence of more severe infections. These persistent infections and the resulting hyperimmune state may in turn be associated with overproduction of inflammatory cytokines and the clinical manifestations of LCH.

Changes in regulatory gene(s) might alter control of immune responses at several levels with the hyperimmune state potentially resulting from exuberant cell proliferation and/or defective apoptotic mechanisms. The large number of genes potentially involved in such mechanisms however, prevents their routine screening in patients with LCH.

LCH has always been considered as a sporadic disorder affecting both sexes at any age. Epidemiological studies have failed to identify predisposing factors (Bhatia *et al.*, 1997), but an increased risk of hematologic and solid tumors has been clearly identified in LCH patients (Egeler *et al.*, 1998), giving credence to the possibility of underlying germ-line genetic aberrations.

Taken together, all of the above has been sufficient to stimulate the interest of investigators in the evaluation of the genetics of LCH. As a result several studies were carried out during the last few years, including a search for familial cases among large patient series, as well as an evaluation of chromosomal aberrations occurring at different stages of the disease.

Family studies in LCH

The occurrence of familial clustering of a rare disorder is considered to be evidence in favor of a genetic component in the pathogenesis of the disease. For this reason in our search for a genetic link to LCH, we first undertook an evaluation of familial clustering of this disease.

Table 5.1 LCH in monozygotic twins: summary of published cases

Source	Sex	Age at onset (months)	Zygosity indicators	Disease extent (sites)
Lightwood (1954)	M	6	Blood groups, fingerprint	Disseminated (skin, bone, lymph nodes)
	M	–		None; asymptomatic at 7+ years
Bierman (1966)	M	8	Not defined	Disseminated (including bone)
	M	8		Disseminated (including bone)
Caldarini (1966)	M	6	Blood groups, fingerprint	Disseminated (skin, hepatosplenomegaly)
	M	6		Disseminated (skin, hepatosplenomegaly)
Juberg (1970)	M	12	Blood group	Disseminated (skin, ear)
	M	12		Disseminated (including bone, diabetes insipidus)
Jacobson (1987)	M	18	Not defined	Disseminated (bone, proptosis)
	M	11		Disseminated (skin, bone)
Kuwabara (1990)	NS	NS	Not defined	Localized (bone)
Katz (1991)	M	11	Not defined	Disseminated (with skin + ear)
	M	11		Disseminated (with skin + ear)
Enjolras (1992)	M	Birth	Not defined	Localized (skin)
	M	Birth		Localized (skin)
Kanold (1994)	F	4	HLA type, DNA analysis	Disseminated (with bone)
	F	4		Disseminated (with bone)

NS: non-significant. Reproduced with permission from Aricò, M., Nichols, K., Whitlock, J.A., *et al.* (1999a). Familial clustering of Langerhans cell histiocytosis. *Br J Haematol*, **107**, 883–888.

Twin study

Studying twins is an old but still reliable method of assessing if a genetic component is present in a disease. The initial study was a comparison of the rate of concordance of LCH in monozygotic and dizygotic twins. The study was conducted using published data as well as specific data collection.

Looking at the reported cases of 'familial LCH', five of five reported monozygotic twin pairs were found to be concordant for LCH (Table 5.1), while in contrast, only one of three reported dizygotic pairs was concordant for the disease (Lightwood and Tizard, 1954; Bierman, 1966; Caldarini, 1966; Juberg *et al.*, 1970; Jakobson *et al.*, 1987; Kuwabara and Takahashi, 1990; Katz *et al.*, 1991; Enjolras *et al.*, 1992; Kanold *et al.*, 1994; Aricò *et al.*, 1999a, 2000).

In addition, we performed a survey of the presence of twins among patients with LCH in Italy. Of the 590 families identified with one member diagnosed with LCH, we found five families in which the propositus had a twin and all were dizygotic. Among the five, four pairs were discordant for the disease while only one pair of girls, who were also HLA discordant, simultaneously developed multisystem LCH.

Further to this study, an international survey was performed, with the aim of collecting a larger number of cases, although we are aware that such studies are limited by both the voluntary participation and the lack of a solid denominator. Overall, we have identified 21 patients with a twin sibling in whom we have evaluated the rate of concordance for LCH. Eight of the twin pairs were assumed to be monozygotic based on their concordance for sex, blood groups or HLA. Seven of the eight monozygotic pairs were concordant for LCH with similar clinical features, pattern of dissemination and age of onset which was simultaneous in five while the age difference at diagnosis in the remaining two was up to 40 months (Table 5.2). The median age at the disease onset was 4 months. All but three had multisystem disease.

By contrast, of 10 patients with a dizygotic twin, only one companion twin was also affected by LCH. Their median age at disease onset was 21 months; five of nine had multisystem disease (Table 5.3).

Of the remaining five twin pairs who were concordant for sex, but in whom the zygosity could not be clearly assessed, none were concordant for the disease (Table 5.4). The data thus shows a higher rate of concordance for LCH (92.3%) in presumed monozygotic twins, versus dizygotic ones (10%) and strongly suggests that a genetic component is relevant in the pathogenesis of LCH.

Familial clustering of LCH

If a genetic component is in fact present in LCH, we might expect to observe families in which more than one subject, other than twins, develops the disease. Indeed, we have recently reported three families with more than one affected sibling or cousin (Aricò *et al.*, 2000); the fourth case (Family M) described in the same report is now excluded because of unconfirmed paternity. Overall, there is at present evidence of six families in which two siblings developed LCH. Only in one case were the parents consanguineous. In three of the six families LCH was limited to a single system (bone or skin), while in the remaining three it was multisystem in at least one of the siblings. The age at diagnosis was often very similar, but very large differences (up to 25 years) were also observed. LCH was also observed in two first-cousin pairs with multifocal bone or multisystem disease.

Familial occurrence of LCH is not restricted to the same generation: overall we have identified seven families in which LCH occurred in a child or adult (up to 42 years) and in one parent (or aunt in one case) (Aricò *et al.*, 2000).

Overall on the basis of available data, it appears that around 1% of children with LCH have an affected relative; a similar finding has been found in the preliminary data-set obtained by the Histiocyte Society Adult Study Group on adult patients (Aricò *et al.*, 2003).

Table 5.2 Major features of eight presumed monozygotic twins with LCH

Family	Sex	Age at diagnosis (months)	Zygosity indicators	Clinical manifestations	Course and outcome
1	M	8	Sex, blood groups	Intrauterine growth retardation; skin (since birth); subsequently bone, spleen, LN, cytopenia, CNS, mouth	Reactivation; CR at 7+ years
	M	8		Intrauterine growth retardation; skin (since birth); subsequently bone, ear, liver, spleen, LN	Reactivation; CR at 7+ years
2	M	4	Sex, blood groups, HLA	Bone, ear, thymus; subsequently LN	Reactivation; CR at 7+ years
	M	4		Bone, ear, LN, thymus	Reactivation; AWD (otitis) at age 7 years
3	M	11	Sex, blood groups, HLA	Skin, ear, lung, bone, BM, HSM	No follow-up
	M	11		Skin, ear, lung, HSM	No follow-up
4	M	11	Sex, HLA	Skin, spleen, thrombocytopenia, lung	CR at age 6 years
	F	1		None	Asymptomatic at age 6 years
5	F	NA	Sex, blood groups, placental examination	Skin, soft tissues, bone, HM	Reactivation; APL at age 8.9, died at age 11 years
	M	3		Skin, soft tissues, bone, HM	Alive and well at age 13.5 years
6	M	3	Sex, HLA	Bone, skin, LN, liver, BM, lung	Reactivation, CR at an age of 2.9 years
	F	4		Lymphnodes, lung, bone	Reactivation; CR at age of 2.9 years
7	F	2	Phenotype	Ear, maybe bone	CR
	M	42		lymph nodes	CR
8	M	22	Sex, HLA	Bone multifocal	AWD
	M	22		Bone multifocal	AWD

LN: lymph node(s); CNS: central nervous system; CR: complete response; AWD: alive with disease; BM: bone marrow; H(S)M: hepato(spleno)megaly; APL: acute

neumoblastic leukaemia; NA: not applicable; HLA: human leukocyte antigen.

Table 5.3 Major features of 10 dizygotic twins with LCH

Family	Sex	Age at diagnosis	Zygosity indicators	Clinical manifestations	Course and outcome
1	F	21 months	Discordant for HLA	Skin, bone, HSM, BM, LN, ear, proptosis	Reactivation; APL at age 5 years
	F	21 months		Skin, bone, HSM, LN, ear	CR at age 6 years
2	M	32 months	Sex	Bone, skin	Reactivation; CR age 9.5 years
	F	NA		None	Asymptomatic at age 9.5 years
3	F	14 months	Discordant for HLA	Skin, LN, liver	DOD at age 22 months
	F	NA		None	Asymptomatic at age 3.5 years
4	M	12 years	Bi-amniotic	Bone, skin, LN, ear	Asymptomatic at age 18 years
	M	NA		None	Asymptomatic at age 18 years
5	M	38 months	Sex	Bone	CR at age 4 years
	F	NA		None	Asymptomatic at age 4 years
6	M	17 months	Sex	Skin, liver, BM	DOD (early progression?)
	F	NA		None	No follow-up
7	F	4 months	Sex	Bone	Reactivation; CR at age 2.2 years
	M	NA		None	No follow-up
8	M	11.5 years	Sex	Bone multifocal	CR at age 26 years
	F	NA		None	Asymptomatic at age 26 years
9	M	35 months	Sex	Multifocal	Asymptomatic
	F	NA		None	Asymptomatic
10	M	48 months	HLA	Skin (prepuce)	Asymptomatic, 12 years
	M	NA		None	Asymptomatic, 12 years

DOD: dead of disease.

Table 5.4 LCH in twins with unknown zygosity

Family	Sex	Age at diagnosis	Clinical manifestations	Course and outcome
1	F	1 month	Skin	Asymptomatic at age 3 years
	F	NA	None	Asymptomatic at age 3 years
2	F	24 days	Skin, bone, lung	Asymptomatic at age 3 years and 5.5 years
	F	NA	None	No follow-up
3	M	13 years	Bone	CR at age 19 years
	M	NA	None	No follow-up
4	F	4 months	Lymph nodes	No follow-up
	F	NA	None	No follow-up
5	M	25 years	Bone multifocal	Asymptomatic at age 27 years
	M	NA	None	Asymptomatic at age 27 years

Genetic models to explain 'familial LCH'

The occurrence of LCH in a minority of families may be explained by several models. LCH might occur as a consequence of the expression of a combination of specific alleles of a group of genes conferring susceptibility to the disease. All members of the family who share such alleles, would also share a propensity to developing the disease. The non-random association between LCH and a specific mannose-binding lectin (MBL) allele constitutes preliminary evidence for such a model (Carstensen, 1999; de Filippi et al., submitted). Additional genetic or acquired conditions which may substantially affect the immune response could play a role in the propensity to develop LCH. The observation of histiocytosis in children with associated conditions should be carefully considered. The identification of mutations in the perforin gene as the cause of the cellular cytotoxicity defect in some patients with hemophagocytic lymphohistiocytosis (HLH), suggests that histiocytoses may occur as a result of uncontrolled proliferation of lymphocytes and histiocytes in subjects unable to effect a normal immune response against viruses or other infectious agents (Stepp et al., 1999; Clementi et al., in press). Therefore, the association of HLH or LCH with DiGeorge syndrome (Levendoglu-Tugal et al., 1996; Aricò et al., 1999b; Touraine et al., 1999; Cesaro et al., 2003) is not casual.

An alternative model is the presence of mutations in an 'LCH-gene'. In most cases mutation of this putative gene would be somatic mutations; in a minority of cases germinal mutations may occur and explain the familial cases. Genetic heterogeneity and the relationship between simple and complex inheritance are further issues that need to be investigated.

Chromosome studies in LCH

As a genetic component has long been suspected to play a role in the pathogenesis of the disease, extensive chromosomal studies in LCH patients may provide additional insights. Normal karyotypes from peripheral blood lymphocytes are usually observed in LCH patients. Betts *et al.* documented a t(7;12)(q11.2;p13) translocation in unsorted cells cultured from an eosinophilic granuloma (Betts *et al.*, 1998). This report prompted many investigators to try to verify whether the reported breakpoints contained a potential 'LCH gene', but as yet without success.

We have analyzed the karyotypes of 16 patients with LCH at diagnosis or during the disease course, using phytohemagglutinin-stimulated peripheral blood lymphocytes. An increased number of chromatid and chromosomal breaks were observed in 13 patients. These were seen more often in cases with disseminated disease. Polyploid cells or cells with chromosomal pulverization (Figure 5.1) were also observed in some cases (Scappaticci *et al.*, 2000). Our data demonstrate that chromosomal instability is frequent in LCH, in keeping with data reported by Betts, although at that time instability was considered less relevant than the reported translocation (Betts *et al.*, 1998).

Several human conditions share constitutional chromosomal instability and a propensity to develop neoplasia (Cohen and Levy, 1989). These diseases are however, characterized by a specific phenotype that is not present in our patients, nor has it ever been reported in LCH. Interestingly, we have observed chromosomal

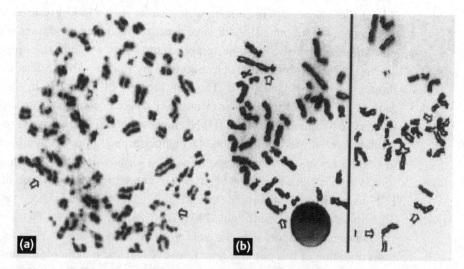

Figure 5.1   Case 1: (a) chromosome pulverization, (b) chromosome and chromatid breaks and chromosome interchanges (reproduced with permission from Scappaticci, *et al.* (2000). *Br J Haematol*, **111**, 258–262, Blackwell Publishing, Oxford)

instability at any stage of the disease, including untreated subjects or asymptomatic ones at the time of long-term follow-up. This may suggest that it is not dependent on the acute phase of the disease nor on its treatment. Nevertheless no evidence is yet available to suggest that instability results from a genetic defect of the DNA-handling mechanisms, and that LCH may represent a new chromosomal instability syndrome.

The association between chromosomal instability and exposure to viral agents has been known for over 25 years (Watt *et al.*, 1977; Neel *et al.*, 1996; Shimura *et al.*, 1999). Evidence of chromosomal pulverization in association with herpes virus and respiratory syncythial virus in children (Scappaticci *et al.*, unpublished data), provides further support to the hypothesis that viruses represent a possible trigger of LCH. The presence of different types of chromosomal alterations together with the variability in the number of chromosomal breaks, are in keeping with the hypothesis that the abnormalities may be virus driven. Even in patients in whom clinical viral infections are not reported, a preclinical infection may be difficult to rule out. If chromosomal aberrations are virus related, this would fit with the hypothesis that a defect in some step of anti-infective immune mechanisms may underlie LCH.

Association between LCH and genetic polymorphism

Recently an indication of a possible link between the HLA system and LCH has been found. McClain *et al.* showed that patients presenting with single bone disease had an especially high frequency of the DR4 type and in this patient group, every Caucasian patient had either Cw7 or DR4 (McClain *et al.*, 2003). Additionally, in a study of Nordic patients, patients with single-system disease more often had the phenotype HLA-DRB1*03, compared with patients with multisystem disease, suggesting an immunogenetic heterogeneity between these two clinical entities of LCH (Bernstrand *et al.*, 2003).

Few candidate genes have been investigated in patients with LCH. In one study, McClain *et al.* found fewer mutations in the promoter region of the tumour necrosis factor (TNF)-alpha gene in the patients with LCH than in the general population (McClain *et al.*, 2003).

We have recently studied the association between LCH and polymorphism of the MBL gene. We have shown that variant alleles causing low levels of MBL may be associated with severe forms of LCH in patients with early onset of the disease, but it does not appear to be associated with LCH in general. Thus, the mbl2 gene may be a disease modifier in LCH. The biological mechanisms behind this finding has not yet been elucidated, but if the association is confirmed in independent studies, MBL defective patients might require a more aggressive surveillance and treatment than MBL sufficient ones (de Filippi *et al.*, submitted).

Conclusion

Although the pathogenesis of LCH is far from being clarified, recently available data strongly suggest a relevant genetic component in the development of the disease. Since familial cases are likely to be under-reported, we suggest that a careful family history is taken for every patient with LCH, with special attention paid to the possibility of localized or oligo-symptomatic diseases in relatives. A joint effort between paediatricians and adult specialists could be the means of determining the real incidence of the disease, and of identifying the true genetic component of LCH. Future studies should address the issue of whether a single rare mutation of an 'LCH-gene' may account for the disease or alternatively whether several predisposing genetic factors may collectively result in the development and expression of LCH. Whenever possible, constitutional and lesional DNA samples from the patient and affected relatives in familial cases should be collected and stored for further investigation. The results of such studies will allow more specific counselling for the families and provide tools to refine treatment programs.

REFERENCES

Aricò, M. and Egeler, R.M. (1998). Clinical aspects of Langerhans cell histiocytosis. *Hematol Oncol Clin North Am*, **12**, 247–258.

Aricò, M., Nichols, K., Whitlock, J.A., *et al.* (1999a). Familial clustering of Langerhans cell histiocytosis. *Br J Haematol*, **107**, 883–888.

Aricò, M., Bettinelli, A., Maccario, R., *et al.* (1999b). Hemophagocytic lymphohistiocytosis in a patient with deletion of 22q11.2. *Am J Med Genet*, **87**, 329–330.

Aricò, M., Haupt, R., Spica Russotto, V., *et al.* (2000). Langerhans' cell histiocytosis in two generations: a new family and review of the literature. *Med Pediatr Oncol*, **36**, 314–316.

Aricò, M., Girschikofsky, M., Genereau, T., *et al.* (2003). Langerhans cell histiocytosis in adults. Report from the International Registry of the Histiocyte Society. *Eur J Cancer*, **39**, 2341–2348.

Bernstrand, C., Carstensen, H., Jakobsen, B., *et al.* (2003). Immunogenetic heterogeneity in single- and multisystem Langerhans cell histiocytosis. *Pediatr Res*, **54**, 30–36.

Betts, D.R., Leibundgut, K.E., Feldges, A., *et al.* (1998). Cytogenetic abnormalities in Langerhans cell histiocytosis. *Br J Cancer*, **77**, 552–555.

Bhatia, S., Nesbit, M.E., Egeler, R.M., *et al.* (1997). Epidemiologic study of Langerhans cell histiocytosis in children. *J Pediatr*, **130**, 774–784.

Bierman, H.R. (1966). Apparent cure of Letterer-Siwe disease. Seventeen-year survival of identical twins with nonlipoid reticuloendotheliosis. *J Am Med Assoc*, **196**, 156–158.

Broadbent, V., Gadner, H., Komp, D.M., *et al.* (1989). Histiocytosis syndromes in children: II. Approach to the clinical and laboratory evaluation of children with Langerhans cell histiocytosis. Clinical Writing Group of the Histiocyte Society. *Med Pediatr Oncol*, **17**, 492–495.

Caldarini, G. (1966). Remarks on a case of Letterer-Siwe disease in a pair of twins. *Clin Pediatr* (Bologna) **48**, 315–332.

Carstensen, H. (1999). Plasma levels of mannose-binding lectin in children with Langerhans cell histiocytosis. *Proceedings of the 15th Annual Meeting of the Histiocyte Society*, Toronto, p. 55.

Cesaro, S., Messina, C., Sainati, L., *et al.* (2003). Del 22Q11.2 and hemophagocytic lymphohisti-ocytosis: a non-random association. *Am J Med Genet*, **116A**, 208–209.

Chu, T., D'Angio, G.J., Favara, B.E., *et al.* (1987). Histiocytosis syndromes in children. *Lancet*, **2**, 41–42.

Cohen, M.M. and Levy, H.P. (1989). Chromosome instability syndromes. *Adv Hum Genet*, **18**, 43–149.

Egeler, R.M., Neglia, J.P., Aricò, M., *et al.* (1998). The relation of Langerhans cell histiocytosis to acute leukemia, lymphomas, and other solid tumors. The LCH-Malignancy Study Group of the Histiocyte Society. *Hematol Oncol Clin North Am*, **12**, 369–378.

Enjolras, O., Leibowitch, M., Bonacini, F., Vacher Lavenu, M.C. and Escande, J.P. (1992). Histio-cytoses Langerhansiennes congenitales cutanees. Apropos of 7 cases. *Ann Dermatol Venereol*, **119**, 111–117.

Favara, B., Feller, A., Paulli, M., *et al.*, for the Reclassification Working Group of the Histiocyte Society (1997). Contemporary classification of histiocytic disorders. *Med Pediatr Oncol*, **29**, 157–166.

Gadner, H., Grois, N., Aricò, M., *et al.*, for the Histiocyte Society (2001). A randomized trial of treatment for multisystem Langerhans' cell histiocytosis. *J Pediatr*, **138**, 728–734.

Glotzbecker, M.P., Carpentieri, D.F. and Dormans, J.P. (2002). Langerhans cell histiocytosis: clin-ical presentation, pathogenesis, and treatment from the LCH etiology research group at the Children's Hospital of Phildelphia. *UPOJ*, **15**, 67–73.

Glotzbecker, M.P., Carpentieri, D.F. and Dormans, J.P. (2004). Langerhans cell histiocytosis: a primary viral infection of bone? Human herpes virus-6 latent protein detected in lympho-cytes from tissue of children. *J Pediatr Orthop*, **24**, 123–129.

Jakobson, A.M., Kreuger, A., Hagberg, H. and Sundstrom, C. (1987). Treatment of Langerhans cell histiocytosis with alpha-interferon [letter] *Lancet*, **2**, 1520–1521.

Jenson, H.B., McClain, K.L., Leach, C.T., *et al.* (2000). Evaluation of human herpesvirus type 8 infection in childhood Langerhans cell histiocytosis. *Am J Hematol*, **64**, 237–241.

Juberg, R.C., Kloepfer, H.W. and Oberman, H.A. (1970). Genetic determination of acute disseminated histiocytosis X (Letterer-Siwe syndrome). *Pediatrics*, **45**, 753–765.

Kanold, J., Vannier J.P., Fusade, T., Drouin, V., Thomine, E., Prudent, M. and Tron, P. (1994). Langerhans-cell histiocytosis in twin sisters. *Arch Pediatr*, **1**, 49–53.

Katz, A.M., Rosenthal, D., Jakubovic, H.R., Pai, R.K., Quinonez, G.E. and Sauder, D.N. (1991). Langerhans cell histiocytosis in monozygotic twins. *J Am Acad Dermatol*, **24**, 32–37.

Kawakubo, Y., Kishimoto, H., Sato, Y., *et al.* (1999). Human cytomegalovirus infection in foci of Langerhans cell histiocytosis. *Virch Arch*, **434**, 109–115.

Kuwabara, S. and Takahashi, M. (1990). Eosinophilic granuloma of the skull in identical twins – case report. *Neurol Med Chir*, Tokyo, **30**, 1043–1046.

Levendoglu-Tugal, O., Noto, R., Juster, F., *et al.* (1996). Langerhans cell histiocytosis associated with partial DiGeorge syndrome in a newborn. *J Pediatr Hematol Oncol*, **18**, 401–404.

Lightwood, R. and Tizard, J.P.M. (1954). Recovery from infantile non lipoid reticulo-endotheliosis (?Letterer-Siwe disease). *Acta Paediatr*, **43** (suppl 100), 453–468.

McClain, K.L., Laud, P., Wu, W.S., *et al.* (2003). Langerhans cell histiocytosis patients have HLA Cw7 and DR4 types associated with specific clinical presentations and no increased frequency in polymorphisms of the tumor necrosis factor alpha promoter. *Med Pediatr Oncol*, **41**, 502–507.

Neel, J.V., Major, E.O., Awa, A.A., *et al.* (1996). Hypothesis: 'Rogue cell' type chromosomal damage in lymphocytes is associated with infection with the JC human polyoma virus and has implications for oncogenesis. *Proc Natl Acad Sci*, **93**, 2690–2695.

Nezelof, C. and Basset, F. (2004). An hypothesis Langerhans cell histiocytosis: the failure of the immune system to switch from an innate to an adaptive mode. *Pediatr Blood Cancer*, **42**, 398–400.

Scappaticci, S., Danesino, C., Rossi, E., *et al.*, for the AIEOP-Istiocitosi Group (2000). Cytogenetic abnormalities in PHA-stimulated lymphocytes from patients with Langerhans cell histiocytosis. *Br J Haematol*, **111**, 258–262.

Shimura, M., Onozuka, Y., Yamaguchi, T., *et al.* (1999). Micronuclei formation with chromosome breaks and the amplification caused by Vpr, an accessory gene on human immunodeficiency virus. *Cancer Res*, **59**, 2259–2264.

Slacmeulder, M., Geissmann, F., Lepelletier, Y., *et al.* (2002). No association between Langerhans cell histiocytosis and human herpes virus-8. *Med Pediatr Oncol*, **39**, 187–189.

Stepp, S.E., Dufourcq-Lagelouse, R., Le Deist, F., *et al.* (1999). Perforin gene defects in familial hemophagocytic lymphohistiocytosis. *Science*, **286**, 1957–1959.

The French Langerhans' Cell Histiocytosis Study Group (1996). A multicentre retrospective survey of Langerhans' cell histiocytosis: 348 cases observed between 1983 and 1993. *Arch Dis Child*, **75**, 17–24.

Touraine, R.L., Pondarre, C., Till, M., *et al.* (1999). Hemophagocytic lymphohistiocytosis and del22q11. *Genet Counsel*, **10**, 114–115.

Watt, J.L., Page, B.M. and Davidson, R.J.L. (1977). Cytogenetic study of 10 cases of infectious mononucleosis. *Clin Genet*, **12**, 167–274.

Willis, B., Ablin, A., Weinberg, V., *et al.* (1996). Disease course and late sequelae of Langerhans' cell histiocytosis: 25-year experience at the University of California, San Francisco. *J Clin Oncol*, **14**, 2073–2082.

Willman, C.L., Busque, L., Griffith, B.B., *et al.* (1994). Langerhans'-cell histiocytosis (histiocytosis X) – a clonal proliferative disease. *New Engl J Med*, **331**, 154–160.

6

Langerhans cell histiocytosis: a clinical update

Jean Donadieu, R. Maarten Egeler and Jon Pritchard

Introduction

In 1953, Lichtenstein coined the term histiocytosis X for the different forms of Langerhans cell histiocytosis (LCH), the X denoting his uncertainty about the disease and its pathogenesis (Lichtenstein, 1953). Fifty years later some of the uncertainty still exists. The histopathological appearance of the various forms of 'LCH' is identical, yet the intriguing question remains. How is it that patients with such a variable clinical profile, from a single self-healing bone lesion to a generalized disorder resistant to any known therapy, seem to have the same disease? Many more pieces of the 'LCH jigsaw puzzle' are still missing and need to be fitted in. Meanwhile, descriptions of the clinical features, the natural history of the disease and the long-term outcome provide a useful framework for clinicians, for recognition and management of the disease. In describing the clinical picture of LCH, we have focused on those few studies which have included more than 50 patients (Table 6.1). It is noteworthy that until April 2004, only 14 studies, the product of just 10 centres or cooperative groups, have reported on more than 100 patients.

Clinical involvement by specific organs

The frequency of involvement of specific organs or 'organ systems' is described in the following sections in descending order of frequency. Most cooperative studies record specific system involvement at diagnosis; in some cases, events during the course of LCH are also included.

Bone

In most surveys, bone lesions are present in around 80% of patients. The skeletal system is therefore by far the most frequently involved. Symptoms include pain, swelling or a combination of both, and rarely a pathological fracture. Painless swellings occur most often over the skull bones and represent soft tissue extension of lesions arising

Table 6.1 Clinical studies including more than 50 patients with LCH, by publication year

References	Institutions	Years of study	Adult included	Focus of the survey	Multi centre study	Number of patients
Lahey (1975)	CCSG	1966–1975 (?)	–	Therapeutic trial	+	83
Carlson *et al.* (1976)	Mayo Clinic	1962–1973	–	Lung	–	81
Nezelof *et al.* (1979)	Necker, Paris	1952–1979	–	Multivisceral	–	50
Komp *et al.* (1980)	SWOG	1971	–	Long-term sequelae	+	75
Greenberger *et al.* (1979)	Boston	1941–1975	+	–	–	127
Broadbent (1986)	GOS, London	1961–1982	–	–	–	70
Berry *et al.* (1986)	POG	1982	–	–	+	92
Chomette *et al.* (1987)	Pitié, Paris	1966–1986	+	Stomatology	–	61
Rivera-Luna *et al.* (1988)	Mexico	1972–1986	–	–	–	124
Raney and D'Angio (1989)	CHOP, Philadelphia	1970–1984	–	–	–	64
McLelland *et al.* (1990)	GOS, London	1980–1987	–	–	–	58
Dimentberg and Brown (1990)	Montreal	1955–1987	–	Bone	–	52
Bollini *et al.* (1991)	Marseille	1975–1988	–	Bone	–	62
Ha *et al.* (1992)	GOS, London	1981–1987	–	Lung	–	61
Egeler *et al.* (1993)	Amsterdam	1969–1988	–	–	–	50
Ceci *et al.* (1988)	Italian Group	1983–1988	–	Treatment study	+	90
Gadner *et al.* (1994); Grois *et al.* (1995)	DAL HX 83, GPOH	1983–1989	–	Treatment study	+	106 of 199
Kilpatrick *et al.* (1995)	Mayo Clinic	1915–1995	–	Bone	–	263
Rivera-Luna *et al.* (1996)	Mexico	1978–1988	–	Age <2 years	–	55
Willis *et al.* (1996)	UCSF, San Francisco	1969–1994	+	–	–	71
Lieberman *et al.* (1996)	MSKKC, NY	1942–1994	+	Pathological registry	–	298
The French LCH Study Group (1996)	Cooperative French Centers	1983–2002	–	–	+	348
Braier *et al.* (1999)	Garahan Institute	1987–1996	–	–	–	123
Howarth *et al.* (1999)	Mayo Clinic	1946–1996	+	–	–	314
Nanduri *et al.* (2000)	GOS, London	1966–1998	–	Endocrine	–	144

Male (%)	Bone (%)	Skin (%)	DI (%)	Liver (%)	Lung (%)	Hem (%)	Liver or lung or blood (%)	Overall survival (%)
56	5	–	20	–	–	–	40	71
–		–		–	8.6	–	–	–
70	82	80	40	36	60	26	76	52
–	68	–	20	–	–	–	–	80
60	83	63	23	53.5	40	35	72	37.8
60	82	54	NA	15.7	21	13	21 at least	89
54	72	58	29	7.6	5.4	12	15	15
72	100	2	NA	0	26	0	26	97
53	82	55	19	51	23	46	NA	63
57	76	30	3.1	8	3.1	6.3	14	89
69	–	–	36	–	–	–	38	82
48	100	21	17	2	11	19	27	90
64.5	97	–	–	–	–	5	9	98
70	75	78	NA	19.7	29.5	24	73	88
54	86	38	14	10	2	10	16	94
64	80	20	20	7	3.5	10	12.2	93 (at 4 years)
–			15.1				19.8	90
61	100	13	15	5	7	4	NA	95
55	69	76	NA	38	29	63	71	36
–	92	45	26	–	–	–	39	77 at 20 years
65.9	71	4.4	6.7	0	4.7	0	4.7	93.3 (60% of death in adults)
55	81	39	15.8	14	13	11	16	91 (at 5 years)
58	93	24	14	10	11	11	15	86
–	60	24	14	1.6	41	0	43	91.1
–	–	–	44 (18 of overall survey)	–	–	–	–	86.9

(continued)

Table 6.1 (*continued*)

References	Institutions	Years of study	Adult included	Focus of the survey	Multi centre study	Number of patients
Surico *et al.* (2000)	Italian Group	1982–1995	–	Ear involvement	+	220
Minkov *et al.* (2000)	DAL HX 83–90	1983–1991	–	Treatment MS patients	+	63 of 324
Titgemeyer *et al.* (2001)	DAL HX 83–90	1983–1991	–	Therapeutic study Single-system patients	+	178 of 275
Gadner *et al.* (2001)	HS Study	1991–1995	–	Randomized trial	+	143
Donadieu *et al.* (2004b)	Cooperative French Centers	1983–2002	–	Endocrine	+	589

Studies dealing exclusively with adults were not included. The percentage of organs involved was calculated, including documentation of sites of recurrence. DI: diabetes inspidus; Hem: hemotopoietic system; MS: multisystem; NA: not applicable.

in skull. Frequently, a bony defect can be felt deep to the lesion or at their perimeters. Bone disease may also be identified on X-rays ordered because of an intercurrent event, such as trauma. In orthopaedic surveys (Dimentberg and Brown, 1990; Kilpatrick *et al.*, 1995), about half the bone lesions are asymptomatic and only revealed during radiological 'screening'. The typical lesion appears as a 'punched-out' area in a long (Figure 6.1) or flat bone (Figure 6.2). Sometimes, the radiological appearance is worrying, with cortical disruption and a periosteal reaction suggestive of Ewing's sarcoma or bone lymphoma (Figure 6.3). Occasionally lesions involve the metaphyses with lysis of cartilage (Figure 6.4). 'Vertebra plana', due to compression of a vertebral body, is often seen (Figure 6.5). Other complications include spinal instability, spinal cord compression and proptosis. Loss of dental lamina dura may result in loose teeth. Rarely, osteolysis can be complicated by hypercalcaemia requiring specific treatment (McLean and Pritchard, 1996).

The skeletal distribution of LCH lesions has been evaluated in several surveys (Dimentberg and Brown, 1990; Bollini *et al.*, 1991; Kilpatrick *et al.*, 1995) and one large literature review (Slater and Swarm, 1980). The distribution is definitely 'centripetal', possibly because the overall 'bulk' of axial bones are greater than limb bones, or because the cellular environment in axial bones is more hospitable to LCH cells. Around half of all lesions occur in the skull and facial bones, 20% in proximal limbs, about 5% in distal limbs, hardly any in the digits, 12% in pelvis and

Male (%)	Bone (%)	Skin (%)	DI (%)	Liver (%)	Lung (%)	Hem (%)	Liver or lung or blood (%)	Overall survival (%)
55	–	–	15.7 (of survivors)	–	–	–	15.8	91.5
52	–	–	17.5	–	–	–	–	81 (5-year survival)
61	87	10	3	0	0	0	0	100
50	–	–	25	–	–	–	–	80
55	80	45	24% (at 10 years)	17	16	13.4	37	85 (at 15 years)

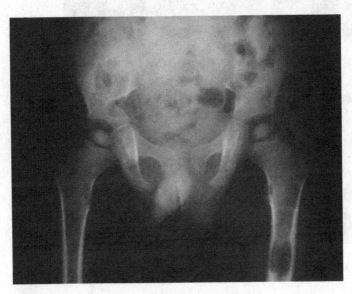

Figure 6.1   Typical LCH lytic lesions in a long bone

scapulae, and 10% in vertebrae. The results differ between surveys, both because of the inevitable variation in patient cohorts, and because there are two ways to do the calculations. The total number of patients with specific localizations is always counted as the 'numerator' but the 'denominator' might be the number of bone lesions or the

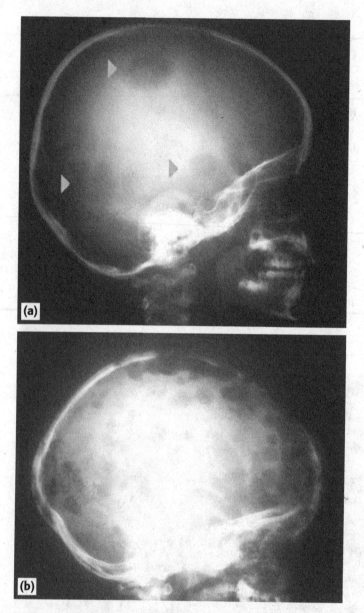

Figure 6.2   Different aspects of skull lesions in LCH

total number of patients. In large surveys, the mean number of bones involved per patient is about 1.5. Single bone ('monostotic') involvement is observed in around half the cases, whilst in the other half more than one bone is involved. In addition, each patient may experience one or more 'reactivations' of disease, which, naturally, increases the 'bone events' per patient.

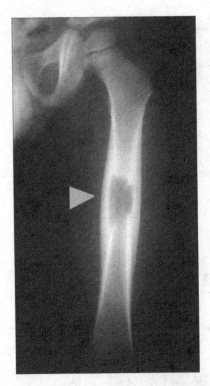

Figure 6.3   'Atypical' LCH with a periosteal reaction

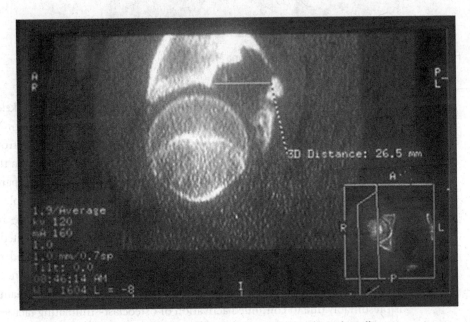

Figure 6.4   Lytic lesion of the head of femur with involvement of metaphyseal cartilage

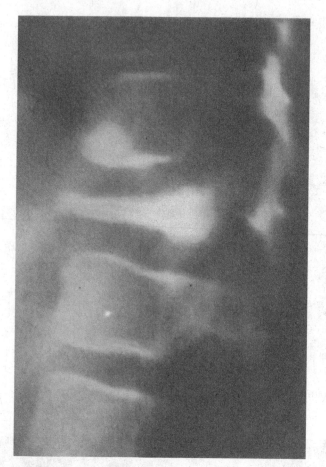

Figure 6.5   Radiograph showing vertebra plana

Extent of bone involvement is usually assessed by plain radiography ('skeletal survey'). 99technetium (^{99}Tc) scintigraphy is a complementary investigation (Dogan *et al.*, 1996; Howarth *et al.*, 1996). Somatostatin scintigraphy and positron emission tomography (PET) scanning measure the 'activity' (metabolism) in the associated granulomas, but there is as yet no hard data on their utility compared with X-rays and ^{99}Tc scanning (Calming *et al.*, 2002), and they are not available in most hospitals. There is also no clear relationship between the number of bones involved and the outcome. The duration of healing of lytic lesions is documented in one study (Sartoris and Parker, 1984). Destructive lesions in the skull and mastoid bones especially, can persist for at least a year after diagnosis and sometimes as long as 10 years or more. This uniquely 'delayed healing' has not been explained, but is presumably due to continued activation of osteoclast-stimulating factors by the disease process or suppression of osteoblast activity by the 'cytokine/chemokine storm' that accompanies it. Radiologically, peripheral sclerosis is often the hallmark of healing. A final point worth noting is that, especially in the case of chronic skull lesions, there may be a necrotic centre to bone lesions, which may erupt as a 'sinus' through the skin. This may occur at the time of diagnosis and be confused with low-grade infection.

Skin

The skin is the second most commonly involved organ. In big surveys of paediatric LCH, skin disease is reported in 30–60% of patients. Skin involvement may be present during the first few months of life, in either of the two forms. The commoner is a rash consisting of papulo-squamous lesions, which can be petechial when the platelet count is reduced, affecting the scalp (Figure 6.6) the seborrhoeic zones (skin folds including gluteal cleft) and the midline of the trunk (Figure 6.7). The distal limbs are usually spared. Unless there are obvious additional signs suggesting LCH (otitis, hepatosplenomagaly, blood cytopaenias), the rash may be mistaken for seborrhoeic eczema. Due to this resemblance, persistent 'seborrhoeic dermatitis' should be biopsied, since otherwise a more invasive biopsy may be needed from a deeper organ. The second and much rarer form is a chickenpox-like rash consisting of small, single or multiple violaceous papulo-nodular and sometimes vesicular lesions, a form usually seen in the condition known as 'Hashimoto–Pritzker' disease, which usually affects only the skin and may disappear spontaneously (see Chapter 7 for discussion). Perianal or genital area involvement is commoner in adults. It can be extremely uncomfortable and disabling, itchy and resistant to treatment.

The 'late effects' of skin disease include scarring, with slightly altered skin pigmentation and rarely evolution to juvenile xanthogranuloma (JXG) (Hoeger et al., 2001).

Soft tissue including muscle

Usually these lesions are extensions of bone, skin or lymph node infiltration. They can be large, with necrosis in some cases. Except for one case of probable extra-ocular muscle involvement causing proptosis and papilloedema (Werner et al., 2003), primary muscle involvement has not been reported to date.

Ear, nose and throat

Recurrent aural discharge is frequent, and sometimes leads to the diagnosis of LCH, especially if combined with a skin rash and other suggestive clinical features. The outer, middle and inner ears can be involved separately or together. Involvement of the external canal (otitis externa) is usually due to the extension of scalp or facial skin rash into the ear canals, and secondary infection often with Pseudomonas

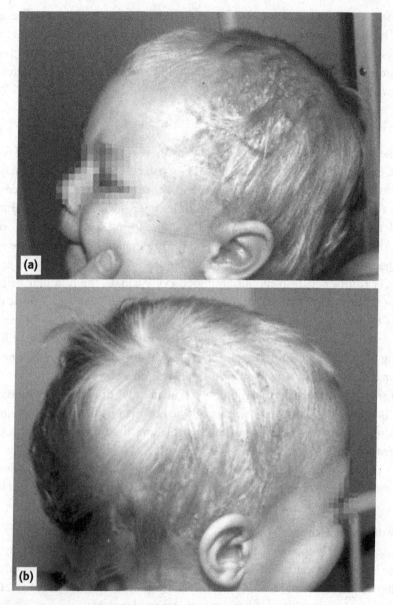

Figure 6.6   Seborrhoeic rash on the scalp of an infant with LCH

aeruginosa. Middle and inner ear involvement are usually secondary to involvement of the petrous temporal bone and/or mastoid. Middle ear involvement is often chronic, with secondary infection and perforation of the tympanic membrane, causing intermittent ear discharge and secondary polyps. Inner ear involvement can present with deafness or behavioural disturbance in younger children because of acute hearing loss (Nanduri *et al.*, 1998). The sinuses and nasal mucosa can also

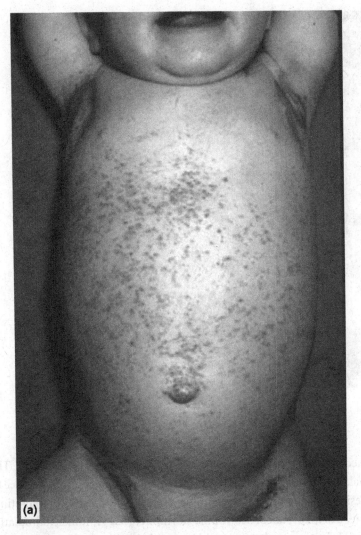

Figure 6.7   An LCH skin rash involving the trunk

be infiltrated. In general, ear, nose and throat (ENT) involvement is present in about 15% of patients. Some have suggested that it is associated with severer forms of the disease and it is considered to be a bad prognostic feature (Cunningham *et al.*, 1989; Surico *et al.*, 2000). As regards 'late effects', hearing is usually preserved, with some conductive loss, unless the inner ear is involved.

Endocrine involvement

'Pituitary involvement' is usually diagnosed following detection of a deficiency of one of the hypophyseal hormones or, rarely, as an incidental finding on magnetic

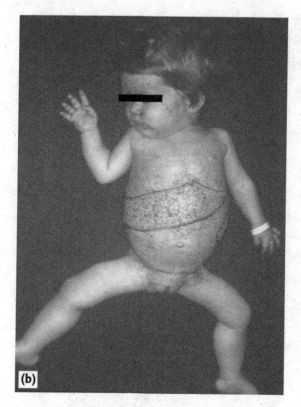

(b)

Figure 6.7   (*contd*)

resonance imaging (MRI) or computed tomography (CT) scanning. The term 'hypothalamic–pituitary axis' (HPA) involvement is more appropriate since the level of the lesion causing diminished pituitary trophic hormone (thyroid-stimulating hormone, TSH; adrenocorticotrophic hormone, ACTH; follicle-stimulating hormone, FSH; leutinizing hormone, LH; growth hormone, GH) secretion is often unknown: the lesion may be in the hypothalamus rather than the pituitary stalk or pituitary gland. MRI is unquestionably the most sensitive way of detecting HPA involvement and has revealed much variation between cases. Characteristic appearances range from subtle thickening of the pituitary stalk with loss of the normal 'bright signal' seen in 90% of normal individuals on T2 sequences, to a mass lesion in the pituitary fossa or hypothalamus. No specific hormone deficiency or pattern of deficiencies is specific for LCH (Dattani, 2001). The differential diagnosis of pituitary failure poses a considerable problem, when it is the presenting feature of the disease (Maghnie *et al.*, 2000).

The association between LCH and diabetes insipidus (DI) has been recognized since the first description in 1893 (Hand, 1893). However, the proportion of

Table 6.2 Endocrine dysfunction in three paediatric LCH studies

	DAL HX 83 Study[a]	Great Ormond Street Survey[b]	French Survey[c]
Number of patients at risk	199	275	589
Median observation time (years)	5.2	Not stated	11.6
DI alone (%)	9.5	17.8	23.9
GH insufficiency (GHI) (%)	3.5	7.6	10.4
DI and GHI combined (%)	(?) or (−)	7.3	5.9
DI and one or more additional endocrinopathies (%)	(?) or (−)	2.5	4.9
Central hypothyroidism (%)	0	1.8	3.9
Primary hypothyroidism (Grave's disease) (%)	0	−	0.2
Gonadotrophin deficiency* (all in association) (%)	1.5	2.5	2.9
Corticotrophin deficiency* (all in association) (%)	(?) or (−)	1.1	1.7
Panhypopituitarism (%)	(?) or (−)	1.1	1.5
Primary hypothyroidism (%)	0	−	0.3

*These figures are 'minimum estimates' since tests of endocrine function, inevitably in retrospective studies, were not standardized.
[a]Grois *et al.* (1995); [b]Nanduri *et al.* (2000); [c]Donadieu *et al.* (2004b).

patients with HPA involvement, including DI, is quite variable in published surveys. The lowest rate of DI, reported by the Austro-German group, was 2% (Titgemeyer *et al.*, 2001). Most other studies have yielded an incidence of 15–35% whilst a few reported over 40% (Broadbent, 1986; Dunger *et al.*, 1989; Nezelof *et al.*, 1979). This variation may be explained by methodological differences, different duration of follow-up and the degree to which endocrinologists are involved. In some centres a diagnosis of DI is based on water-deprivation testing only, but children do not tolerate this procedure well so the results may be misleading. Other centres measure urinary arginine vasopressin (AVP) levels, probably the most sensitive method (Dunger *et al.*, 1989), but this method is not widely available.

The patterns of endocrinopathies observed by the Austro-German Group (Grois *et al.*, 1995), the Great Ormond Street Group (Nanduri *et al.*, 2000) and the French Group (Donadieu *et al.*, 2004a,b) are shown in Table 6.2. GH insufficiency can be demonstrated in around half of all patients with DI, and deficiency of other pituitary hormones also occurs (Nanduri *et al.*, 2000; Donadieu *et al.*, 2004b).

Determinants of DI and anterior pituitary insufficiency are not as easy to analyse as their incidence, but two groups of investigators made the attempt, with concordant results (Donadieu *et al.*, 2004a; Grois *et al.*, 2004). Disease activity, as reflected by the reactivation rate during the first 3 years after LCH diagnosis, was 2–3-fold higher in patients with HPA dysfunction than those with normal function. HPA dysfunction also appears to be related to the anatomical distribution of LCH lesions, especially with involvement of facial bones and skull base, and mucous membranes of the nose and sinuses. In contrast, the 'acute' disseminated form of LCH, often with haematological involvement and interstitial pneumonitis occurring usually in infants, is not associated with an increased risk of pituitary dysfunction. Slowly progressive LCH, typified by lung cysts and/or bullae with or without pneumothorax as well as biliary fibrosis (sclerosing cholangitis), appears to be strongly associated with HPA dysfunction. These two clinical profiles appear, superficially, to be mutually exclusive. If so, and if LCH is just one – albeit a variable – entity, why is this? Perhaps there are clues in the observed 'natural history' of LCH. For example, HPA-related endocrinopathy was already present in almost half the patients prior to the appearance of other organ involvement (Grois *et al.*, 1995; Braier *et al.*, 1999; Gadner *et al.*, 2001; Donadieu *et al.*, 2004b). Thus, the anatomic sites of LCH associated with the DI are not necessarily a risk factor for DI, but may be instead an association. There are two possible explanations for this. The first is that LCH cells infiltrating the nasal mucosa may follow, retrograde, the lymphatic drainage channels from the base of the brain through the cribriform plate; 'reverse flow' in these channels might offer a route for dendritic cells to enter the brain cavity (Perry, personal communication). The alternative explanation is that the appearance of DI depends on one or more intrinsic determinants, and that the persistent lesions in the facial skeleton and adjacent structures (as well as other chronic progressive lesions, such as lung fibrosis and sclerosing cholangitis), similarly reflect the same determinants.

DI is almost always permanent (Broadbent and Pritchard, 1997). There are a few reports of 'recovery', either spontaneously or after specific treatments (Braier *et al.*, 1999; Ottaviano and Finlay, 2003), but it is difficult to know in these cases whether the diagnosis of DI was correct or whether 'resolution' simply involves a reduction in 1-desamino-8-D-arginine vasopressin, DDAVP (a desmopressin, which is a combination of vasopressin and antidiuretic hormone (ADH)) requirement rather than true recovery of ADH secretion. A point from the LCH1 trial of the Histiocyte Society is worth noting. One of the 'questions' in 'LCH1' was whether a drug that crosses the blood–brain barrier (such as etoposide) would reduce the incidence of DI as compared to vinblastine. In the event, the incidence of DI was exactly the same (25%) in each arm of the trial (Gadner *et al.*, 2001). This is in contrast to the finding from two other trials, that more intensive and longer therapy reduced the incidence of DI (Ceci *et al.*, 1988; Grois *et al.*, 1995). Whether DI is preventable with chemotherapy or is an inevitable consequence of a specific form of LCH remains controversial.

Neurological involvement

Central nervous system (CNS) involvement, which affects up to 10% of patients with multisystem disease, is categorized as either 'tumour-like' or 'neurodegenerative'. Rare biopsy data suggests that 'tumour-like' LCH is usually caused by one or more 'active' lesions in the brain, causing elevated intracranial pressure, seizures or focal neurological deficits. In these cases, MRI shows a space-occupying lesion in the cerebral cortex with a mass effect and peri-lesional oedema. 'Neurodegenerative' LCH on the other hand, is characterized by progressive cerebellar dysfunction with nystagmus, dysarthria and hypotonia, which may progress to spastic tetraparesis and pseudobulbar palsy with or without cranial nerve palsies. The natural history of this alarming sequela varies considerably, but in the worst cases there may be progression to severe disability and near-total dependency upon caregivers. MRI typically shows symmetrical non-enhancing changes in the dentate nuclei of the cerebellum with no mass effect. Later, cerebellar atrophy often develops. There may also be imaging abnormalities in the basal ganglia, pons and midbrain (Barthez et al., 2000). A detailed classification of LCH CNS lesions, according to MRI findings, has been proposed (Grois et al., 1998).

An important distinction can be made between the two forms of CNS LCH. Tumour-like LCH is usually part of the acute (active) phase of disease and lesional cells are CD1a positive. Neurodegenerative disease, on the other hand, is a 'late' complication usually recognized 5–15 years after the original diagnosis. 'Functional' imaging techniques, such as PET scans or functional MRI, may help us to understand the progression of this lesion, as will autopsy studies which should be requested as there is 'still a great deal to learn' (Calming et al., 2002; Corry et al., 2004). Interestingly, almost all patients with neurodegenerative disease reported in the literature have had DI. Conversely, in a recent French series, with a mean of 15 years follow-up, the incidence of DI was 10.8% in patients with HPA dysfunction but less than 0.4% in patients without HPA dysfunction.

Blood and bone marrow

Involvement of the haematopoietic system is one of the major features of more severe forms of LCH. Literature review (Berry et al., 1986; Kilpatrick et al., 1995; Willis et al., 1996) reveals that haematopoietic involvement is present in 60–70% of patients who die of LCH. However, many of its features are poorly understood and some definitions are unsatisfactory. An early definition of 'haematopoietic involvement', based on decreased complete blood count (CBC) values, was included in the Lahey criteria (Lahey, 1975). Many patients with isolated anaemia would be judged to have 'anaemia of chronic disease' (reduced serum iron and total iron-binding capacity (TIBC), normal iron saturation), but neutropaenia and thrombocytopaenia usually have serious significance. Bone marrow examination (both aspirates and trephines are recommended) may be difficult to interpret. The percentage of bone marrow 'LCH cells' is often not studied because CD1a immunostaining is not usually performed. Sometimes, marrow aspiration is difficult, and involvement is only assessable via biopsy because of disease-induced myelofibrosis (Pinckney and Parker, 1977; Sartoris and Resnick, 1985). Histopathologists may not do CD1a immunostaining on paraffin block sections or electron microscopy (EM) for Birbeck granules, because the latter is expensive and time consuming. In the few reliable reports available, massive bone marrow infiltration by 'LCH cells' is rare, even in the presence of severe pancytopaenia. More commonly, a few clusters of 'LCH cells' or single 'LCH cells' are seen. There are no reports of 'LCH cells' being reliably identified in peripheral blood, although they must spread through vascular and/or lymphatic routes.

It has become apparent that one likely explanation for cytopaenia is not direct infiltration as occurs in acute leukaemia, but a secondary haemophagocytic syndrome due to macrophage activation by LCH (Sartoris and Resnick, 1985; Favara *et al.*, 2002). Other features supporting this hypothesis include evidence of concurrent acute viral infections, such as cytomegalovirus (CMV) or Epstein–Barr virus (EBV) (Klein *et al.*, 1999), although the infection may simply initiate the process, and specific antiviral therapy is unlikely to be helpful. If the haemophagocytosis is severe, the bone marrow may become quite severely hypoplastic, due to phagocytosis of haematopoietic precursors including, perhaps, multipotent stem cells.

Haematological dysfunction is often associated with dysfunction of other organs, especially the spleen, liver and lungs, and there is often nutritional impairment and myelofibrosis.

Lung and airways

The proportion of patients with lung involvement varies between surveys (Table 6.1), perhaps because of the varying criteria used to define this complication, particularly the question of whether or not 'occult' lung involvement – as judged by lung function tests – should be included (Ha *et al.*, 1992). Probably around 15% of children with LCH have lung involvement at diagnosis. The primary lesion is a peribronchiolar granuloma causing 'interstitial' lung disease. This lesion may regress, or progress causing alveolar destruction, fusion and microcyst formation. Further progression leads to confluence of the cysts, bullous formation and sometimes pneumothorax (Vassallo *et al.*, 2002). Pneumothorax can be bilateral (Figures 6.8 and 6.9). There seem to be two distinct presentations of lung involvement according to age (Carlson *et al.*, 1976; Nondahl *et al.*, 1986; Ha *et al.*, 1992). In infants, lung disease is associated with acute 'generalized' LCH and may not progress beyond the nodular (granulomatous) stage. By contrast, older patients – invariably smokers – often

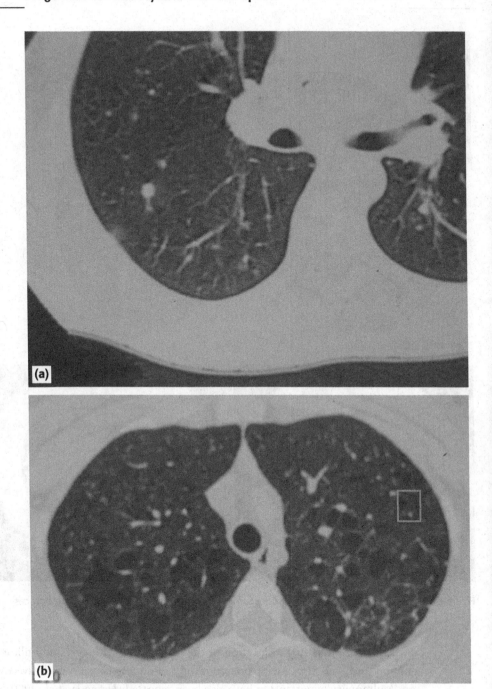

Figure 6.8   Lung LCH (a) CT showing limited lung nodules and (b) CT demonstrating nodules and cysts in lung

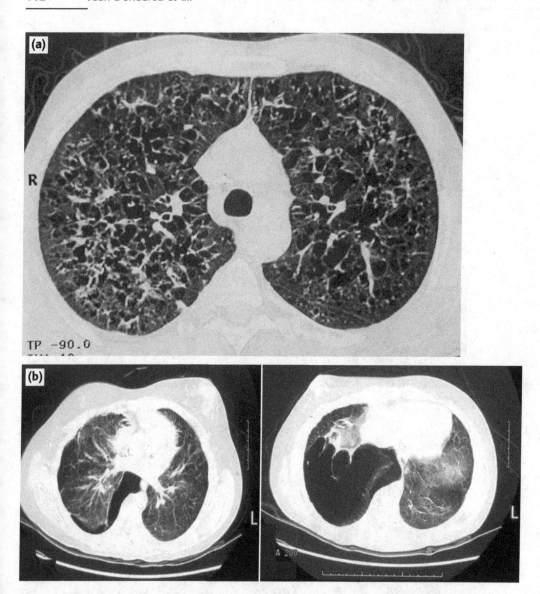

Figure 6.9   Lung LCH (a) CT showing 'honeycomb' lung and (b) CT showing pneumothoraces

present with interstitial infiltration of the lungs, often with cyst and bullous for-mation and sometimes with pneumothorax. Pulmonary veno-occlusive disease and pulmonary hypertension have also been reported (Hamada *et al.*, 2000).

Lung biopsy is the most precise way of confirming the diagnosis but in practise lung involvement is usually inferred from chest X-rays and CT scans, unless it is the sole site of disease, as it may be in adult smokers. Biopsies can either be transthoracic or transbronchial, according to available skills. High-resolution thin-slice CT (hrCT) scans are highly sensitive (Brauner *et al.*, 1997). The earliest lesion is a micronodular change with small cysts progressing to larger cysts, with large areas of parenchymal destruction. Broncho-alveolar lavage (BAL) has some advocates because the percentage of CD1a-positive cells may reflect LCH activity. There are pitfalls to this procedure (Réfabert *et al.*, 1996), but BAL has a useful role in eliminating associated infections, such as *Pneumocystis carinii*.

For monitoring, pulmonary function testing is the most practical, non-invasive and accurate method. Results may show a restrictive abnormality or a combination of restrictive and obstructive changes. Clearly, such tests must be done when there is no intercurrent upper or lower respiratory infection. Infection must also be excluded if function is subnormal. Active and passive smoking should be avoided by all patients who have or have had LCH because of incontrovertible evidence that it worsens lung involvement (Bernstrand *et al.*, 2000; Bernstrand *et al.*, 2001).

The late sequelae of pulmonary involvement range from mild restrictive lung disease, with some exercise intolerance to frank respiratory failure, requiring lung or heart–lung transplantation. In one series, 6% of patients had symptomatic lung involvement at a mean of 15 years off treatment (Nanduri *et al.*, 2003). LCH can re-occur in transplanted lungs (Gabbay *et al.*, 1998).

Liver and bile ducts

It is clinically useful to distinguish between acute liver involvement, invariably a component of multisystem disease, and the chronic form, usually occurring months to years after presentation, although occasionally present at diagnosis. The acute presentation is characterized by soft hepatomegaly, often with splenomegaly (which may represent splenic infiltration by LCH or 'reactive' change) and occasionally also with jaundice. Liver function tests at this stage are characterized by failure of protein synthesis, the coagulation times are prolonged and the serum albumin is low. It is unusual, however, for the 'liver enzymes' (aspartic aminotransferase (AST), alanine aminotransferase, (ALT) and gamma glutamyl transpeptidase, (γGT)) to be elevated. At this stage, liver infiltration with CD1a-positive cells and accompanying inflammatory cells, with a prominent biliary tropism, is characteristically present, but liver biopsy is often too risky because of accompanying coagulopathy, thrombocytopaenia or both.

The chronic liver disease of LCH is typically a sclerosing cholangitis, probably representing direct progression from the CD1a-positive acute phase via fibrosis induced by the chemokine/cytokine 'storm' which is a major component of LCH (Annels *et al.*, 2003). The diagnosis can be confirmed by biopsy or via transhepatic or retrograde cholangiography (Figure 6.10). More recently magnetic resonance cholangiography (MRC) is often used. This technique is less invasive but may not

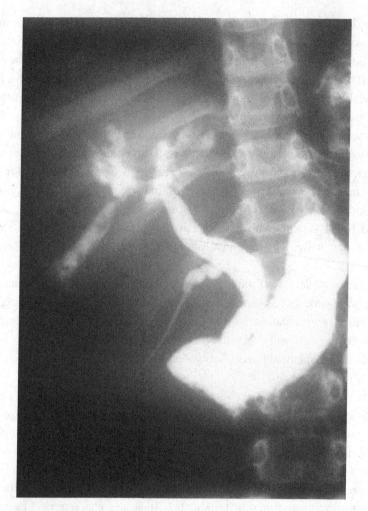

Figure 6.10 Cholangiogram with sclerosing cholangitis

be as sensitive as X-ray cholangiography. Sclerosing cholangitis often progresses to biliary cirrhosis with or without portal hypertension, and in some cases liver failure (Braier *et al.*, 2002; Debray, 2003). Biopsy at this stage shows only fibrosis; CD1a-positive cells are absent. In some cases cholestasis is rapidly progressive and dominates the clinical picture. In such cases, the differential diagnosis includes Caroli disease (Al Asiri *et al.*, 2000) and other causes of sclerosing cholangitis, such as inflammatory bowel disease and inherited or acquired immunodeficiency.

Spleen

Spleen enlargement can be judged clinically or by abdominal ultrasonography. Splenomegaly in LCH patients is often assumed to be due to direct involvement, although biopsy data are few because of the risks of biopsy of such a vascular organ, especially if there is coagulopathy and/or thrombocytopaenia. Splenic size varies from borderline to massive and in rare cases splenic rupture has been observed (Broadbent *et al.*, 1990). When there is haematological dysfunction and especially when there is a massive transfusion requirement, hypersplenism may also be present but splenectomy does not usually reduce the blood product transfusion requirement. The spleen can also be enlarged in biliary cirrhosis complicated by portal hypertension, and is then often associated with thrombocytopaenia.

Lymph nodes and thymus

Lymph node involvement is part of the clinical presentation but is less common than expected, bearing in mind that normal Langerhans cells and T-lymphocytes normally 'converse' in these structures. Node enlargement is usually part of multisystem LCH but sometimes only lymph nodes are involved, sometimes in association with a single bone lesion, an association termed 'osteolymphatic' LCH. Superior vena cava syndrome can result from mediastinal lymph node or thymic enlargement (Mogul *et al.*, 1993). Typically, in thymic involvement, flecks of calcification are seen, especially on CT scanning.

Chronic skin sinuses from underlying LCH-affected nodes may be a late sequela (Figure 6.11).

Mouth and gums

The mucous membranes of the mouth, perianal or genital area can be involved, sometimes extensively. Gingival involvement results in gingivitis with gum hypertrophy, and, in a young child, premature eruption of the milk teeth, an almost pathognomonic sign. Later, the secondary dentition may be affected. Although discrete lytic lesions do occur in both maxilla and mandible, a more common appearance is uniform resorption of the lamina dura and adjacent bone, with loosening of those teeth. This gives rise to speculation that the commonest oral LCH lesion arises in the tooth sockets and the gums, rather than more deeply in bone.

Loss of permanent dentition is a common sequela of oro-dental disease.

Gastrointestinal tract

Gastrointestinal (GI) involvement is rarely reported but is probably commoner than previously believed, and simply not thoroughly investigated because of other clinical priorities. It is usually part of multisystem disease and may present at any age. Symptoms include loose stools with blood and mucous if the colon is involved. Sometimes the enteropathy can be exudative with associated hypoproteinaemia and steatorrhoea. The disease is often focal, macroscopically and microscopically.

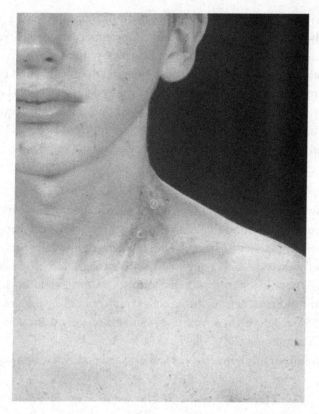

Figure 6.11   Chronic skin sinuses from an underlying LCH-affected nodes

Alpha-4 beta-7 protein is claimed to be expressed on 'LCH cells' in the GI tract. One study suggests that this protein expression pattern is specific for GI involvement (Geissmann *et al.*, 1996). LCH can be identified from almost any part of the GI tract, including small intestine, colon and rectum (Nanduri *et al.*, 1999), but symptoms may be subtle and erroneously attributed to intercurrent illness (Egeler *et al.*, 1990).

Orbits and eyes

Orbital soft tissue involvement, not related to orbital bone lesions, can be observed but, *per se*, rarely cause visual difficulties. Intrinsic eye involvement is exceptional, though it may be found at autopsy. In those cases, the retina, uveal tract and corneas may be involved, with varying visual consequences (Moore *et al.*, 1985; Daras *et al.*, 1995). There has been one recent report of extrinsic ocular muscle involvement (Werner *et al.*, 2003).

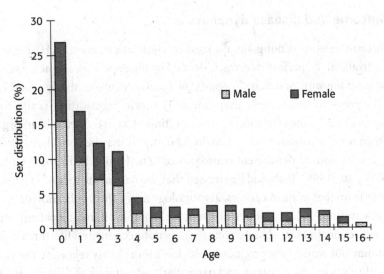

Figure 6.12 Age and sex distribution in a sample of 348 patients

Organs rarely reported

The urological tract, including the bladder, may be involved (Witters *et al.*, 1991). Infiltration of the kidney itself has not been reported but concomitant glomerulonephritis has been reported (Duranay *et al.*, 1996), as have peri-renal and abdominal masses compressing the urological tract and causing hydronephrosis (Tsuchiya *et al.*, 1995); LCH with pancreatic involvement (Yu *et al.*, 1993; Muwakkit *et al.*, 1994), and Langerhans cell histiocytosis presenting with a para-aortic lesion and heart failure (Chen *et al.*, 2001). There is therefore hardly an organ which is not sometimes involved.

Demography and distribution of lesions

LCH patients of 55–65% are male, especially in patients with 'single-system' disease. This gender inequality is so far unexplained. Irrespective of the organs involved, median age for diagnosis is usually around 2 years. Figure 6.12 shows the age and sex distribution in a large French survey (The French LCH Study Group, 1996). The diagnosis may be made at birth, and there is one report of intrauterine death related to multisystem LCH (Yu *et al.*, 1990). On the whole, clinical manifestations relate to age. 'Haematological dysfunction' is usually seen only in children <2 years and usually <1 year of age, whilst the median age of onset of HPA dysfunction is about 4 years. There is also diversity in the symptomatology according to age, for lung involvement. Infants usually have interstitial nodular disease whilst teenagers and adults often develop cysts, bullae and complicating pneumothoraces.

Long-term outcome and disease dynamics

The term 'relapse' is not generally used by clinicians treating LCH. 'Recurrence' or 'reactivation', the preferred terms, is defined by the appearance of new sites of 'active' disease in the same or different organ(s) of a patient in whom the signs and symptoms of the previous episode has disappeared. The term 'reactivation' is also sometimes used to describe the extension or deterioration of 'active' disease in an organ that is known to be involved. DI or sclerosing cholangitis may be considered alternatively as 'reactivation' or permanent consequence (The French LCH Study Group, 1996; Willis *et al.*, 1996). It should be stressed that the natural history of LCH is very different from that of most cancers. Terminology apart, the implication of 'recurrence' or 'reactivation' in LCH is quite different to the implication for a patient with cancer or leukaemia. In LCH, disease recurrence is not necessarily a life-threatening event and may not worsen the prognosis, which is more closely related to the variety and extent of organ involvement, and particularly whether or not the patient has 'vital organ failure' at each episode. Nor is the number of 'reactivations' generally relevant. In different series the 'reactivation' rate varies from 15% to 60%, presumably reflecting differences in the definition of such episodes (The French LCH Study Group, 1996; Willis *et al.*, 1996; Titgemeyer *et al.*, 2001). The 'reactivation' rate varies with the type of initial involvement. It ranges from 10% to 20% for 'single-system' disease to 30–60% for patients with vital organ involvement. The total number of 'reactivations' varies from 0 to as many as 15, with around 5% of patients experiencing more than 3 'reactivations'.

Classification

Many eponyms and classifications have been used to describe the various forms of LCH in different eras: eosinophilic granuloma, Letterer–Siwe, Hashimoto–Pritzker and Hand–Schüller–Christian disease. The terms are sometimes useful because they tend to correspond to distinct clinical profiles of LCH. For instance, the Hashimoto–Pritzker variant of cutaneous LCH is hardly ever seen in patients outside infancy (see Chapter 7). Various classifications of disease severity have also been used. The 'Lahey' classification (Lahey, 1975) was in common use for over 40 years, but a more recent classification devised by the Histiocyte Society, is now coming into use (Table 6.3). These classifications have been developed to assist with therapeutic decision-making, and to clarify the reporting of multicentre studies. However, classifications may have a negative effect because they may ignore some of the intricacies of LCH, which often appears in unexpected combinations and/or degrees of severity. The underlying philosophical point is whether it is better in these circumstances, to be a 'lumper' or a 'splitter' of the various forms of LCH. At present there is no reason

Table 6.3 Classification used in the LCH III Histiocyte Society Protocol

Group	Definition
'High-risk' patients (at least one 'risk organ' involved)	Lung, spleen, liver or haematological dysfunction
Multivisceral risk without 'risk organs'	Any organs involved but no lung, spleen, liver or haematological dysfunction
Single system	One-organ system*

*Usually bone; occasionally skin, lymph nodes or pituitary.

to contest the 'unity' of the disease because the histopathology is the same in all (Cline, 1994). This 'unity' of LCH is a crucial reason to have an open approach to each newly diagnosed patient and not limit investigations to one or a few organs.

Disease activity: clinical assessment scales

Evaluation of disease activity has been one of the most difficult areas in LCH therapy and to date has been very subjective. Bearing in mind the diversity of LCH and the high incidence of late sequelae, clinical scales that could be used to objectively evaluate the patient's condition would be a very useful tool to help physicians formulate treatment plans, and could improve the reliability of reporting of clinical trials. However, scales like these are poorly developed in LCH. Recently one such scale has been proposed to allow objective evaluation of disease activity (Donadieu et al., 2004c).

In addition, a scoring system that may help in the assessment of cerebellar symptoms, such as the International Cooperative Ataxia Rating Scale (Trouillas et al., 1997) and, more generally, the severity of the numerous sequelae which can impair the quality of life of LCH patients (Nanduri et al., 2003), would be useful in long-term follow-up of LCH patients.

The development of objective scores will be a valuable addition to the therapeutic armamentarium in LCH.

LCH associated with other histiocytoses

True histological LCH can be associated with various other histiocytoses, such as Rosai Dorfman disease (Wang et al., 2002) or JXG (Hoeger et al., 2001). These observations, although anecdotal, do suggest plasticity in the pathobiology of dendritic cells and their derivatives.

LCH associated with other non-histiocytic diseases

The observation that LCH can be associated with other truly malignant tumours, especially T-cell non-Hodgkin's lymphoma (NHL), is worrisome and probably not coincidental (see Chapter 14 for discussion). There is a suggestion that other diseases too are commoner in LCH patients than in the general population, but there is very great diversity (e.g. kidney malformations and CNS disorders) and no consistent pattern has been described as yet (Sheils and Dover, 1989; The French LCH Study Group, 1996).

Genetics of LCH

The observation that up to 1% of all patients have a first degree relative with LCH add very considerable weight to the view that LCH patients have an underlying 'genetic predisposition' (Aricò *et al.*, 2001) (see Chapter 5 for discussion).

Diagnosis

Definitive diagnosis should always be made by biopsy (Chu *et al.*, 1987). However, all 'good rules have exceptions'. In patients with 'isolated' DI without a suprasellar mass, the diagnosis of LCH should always be considered, but biopsy of the pituitary stalk may be too risky a procedure. Anti-CD1a antibody scans may be helpful in this regard, but are not widely available (Kelly and Pritchard, 1994) and the murine monoclonal antibody has been reported to result in anaphylactic reactions.

Cytology, as opposed to histology, may be helpful but does not permit morphological examination of tissue. Formal histological criteria (see Chapter 2) require both the 'characteristic' morphological appearance and the expression of either CD1a antigen or langerin. Immunostaining is usually done on frozen samples but techniques are now available for formalin-fixed tissue (Emile *et al.*, 1995). EM is now only used in a few centres or in instances of genuine diagnostic doubt, as it is time consuming, expensive and because the density of Birbeck granules varies from tissue to tissue (for instance, high in the skin and lung, and lower in the liver).

Differential diagnosis

Given the varied presentations described earlier, the differential diagnosis can be quite extensive. Punched-out bone lesions or vertebra plana, commonly due to LCH, may also be seen in leukaemia, bone lymphoma, idiopathic juvenile osteoporosis and atypical mycobacterial infection (Edgar *et al.*, 2001). A simple dermoid cyst can be responsible for a bone defect in the skull. Vertebra plana can be caused by Ewing's sarcoma (Papagelopoulos *et al.*, 2002), lymphoma, infantile myofibromatosis and JXG (Dehner, 2003). The similarity between the surnames of Paul Langerhans and Theodore Langhans may, if the histopathology report is mistyped or read wrongly, cause confusion between atypical tuberculosis and LCH (Pritchard *et al.*, 2003). Gorham disease (vanishing bone disease), a form of bony and soft tissue lymphangiomatosis in which bone defects can be associated with interstitial lung changes, often with a pleural effusion, can also be a source of confusion. Primary hypoparathyroidism, although exceptional in childhood, can be associated with bone pain, bone tumours and sometimes localized osteolysis. If a suprasellar mass is present, germinoma should always be considered, especially since both LCH and germ cell tumours can involve both suprasellar and pineal areas.

The differential diagnosis in other 'organ systems' is also considerable. Suffice to say that 'if in doubt, biopsy it!'

Work-up at diagnosis or at reactivation

The aim of the evaluation is to define disease extent, to acquire key information in order to use appropriate therapy and to decide on the frequency and method of follow-up. At the initial consultation the details, past history and family history, should be taken, not forgetting the specific manifestations of LCH, some of which may have occurred months or years before presentation. In particular enquiry should be made about the possible onset of polyuria and polydypsia, height and weight percentiles should be measured and recorded. Clinical examination requires full ENT and dental/mouth evaluation as well as examination of other muco-cutaneous junctions, including anus and vaginal introitus. The initial panel of 'essential' tests is quite small – CBC, liver function tests and coagulation studies, early morning urine osmolality, skeletal survey, chest X-ray and abdominal ultrasound are all that is needed. Isotope bone scans are probably less sensitive overall, than skeletal surveys, although the latter need not include the hands and the feet, which are rarely involved in LCH. If these 'screening tests' are negative no more need to be done, but specific abnormalities require further follow-up.

Haematological abnormalities require a bone marrow evaluation (aspirate and trephine). Suspected lung involvement by symptomatology or X-ray should be explored by hrCT scan, pulmonary function tests (if the patient is old enough to cooperate) and, if in doubt, by BAL/biopsy. Abnormal liver function tests may require MRC or liver biopsy. HPA dysfunction must be investigated by MRI and appropriate pituitary function tests.

Storing portions of frozen biopsy samples are crucial for present and future biological research.

In follow-up, the frequency and type of repeat studies varies with each patient, depending mostly on the organs deemed to be involved at diagnosis. Most families find frequent follow-up visits helpful initially but can manage with less frequent visits if the disease becomes quiescent. In most cases, however, many years of follow-up are required and facilities should be available locally so that adolescents and adults can continue to be followed in the most appropriate setting.

If possible, HPA dysfunction requires MRI follow-up to allow for detection of early CNS degenerative lesions and correlation of the findings with outcome over time (Donadieu *et al.*, 2004a; Grois *et al.*, 2004).

Survival and prognostic factors

Survival is related to the number and degree of organ involvement, and to the therapy. The treatment era is probably important, too. Thanks to more intensive supportive care and greater knowledge of LCH, crude rates of survival have increased over the last 20 years. The impact of therapy on the disease itself is more difficult to assess. From surveys of newly diagnosed patients, 5-year survival is usually reported at around 90% in childhood (The French LCH Study Group, 1996) (Figure 6.13). Late deaths, after 5 years from diagnosis, are uncommon and mostly related to the late sequelae of LCH in the lungs, liver or CNS. The main prognostic factors in most published series have been young age at diagnosis, the type and number of disease sites, organ dysfunction and response to treatment. Involvement of liver, spleen,

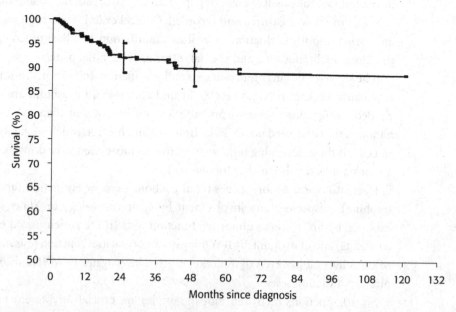

Figure 6.13 Overall survival in a sample of 348 patients

lungs, digestive tract and haematopoietic system are usually associated with a poor outcome. Young age at diagnosis has been a poor prognostic factor in univariate analysis but not as strongly in multivariate analysis, reflecting the association between young age, organ dysfunction and/or initial response to chemotherapy. The prognostic value of response to treatment at 6 weeks is now validated in several studies (The French LCH Study Group, 1996; Gadner *et al.*, 2001). The negative influence of a poor initial response to therapy reflect the fact that until recently there have been few effective alternatives in cases of treatment failure.

Late sequelae (see Chapter 15 for details)

The permanent consequences (late sequelae) of LCH are numerous and have already been briefly described in the sections dedicated to each organ. Their frequency ranges from 0% to 50%, depending on the series and the initial extent of disease, from only 7% for unifocal bone involvement, to about 40% for LCH with organ dysfunction (Komp *et al.*, 1980; The French LCH Study Group, 1996; Titgemeyer *et al.*, 2001). Despite the frequency of bone lesions, orthopaedic sequelae are uncommon, but do include facial and orbital asymmetry, chronic dental problems, kypho-scoliosis and height loss. The aesthetic/cosmetic problems of facial or mandibular lesions can be very distressing. Hearing loss follows involvement of the middle or inner ear. An HPA dysfunction is common, although usually treatable. Neurodegenerative LCH is one of the most serious and worrying problems, because it can be life threatening. The same applies to severe pulmonary destruction and sclerosing cholangitis but at least, in these cases, organ transplantation is a possibility. 'Late deaths' may occur many years (probably up to 20 years at least) after diagnosis, either from end-organ failure or treatment-induced complications including 'second tumours'.

The clinical challenge

The outcome of LCH is very variable indeed. Improvements in therapy have been frustrated because the pathogenesis of the disorder has not yet been defined. However, and as described in other chapters, a great deal of research work is moving us towards that goal. More specific 'targeted treatments' are now on the horizon. Corticosteroids and chemotherapy are, after all, 'blunderbuss' therapies that do help most patients, but also have side-effects which are at least bothersome and at worst life threatening. The clonality of the LCH cell (except in adult lung disease) is a crucial experimental finding (Willman *et al.*, 1994), and the definition of 'cytokine storm' identified in LCH granulomas (Laman *et al.*, 2003) provides the explanation for the severe tissue damage that can occur. However, there are many inexplicable findings, the cerebellar degenerative syndrome being one example, and a great deal more work to do. Another ill-understood phenomenon is the great variability in severity of the disease, in individual patients but also from time to time in the same patient. The more adult patients one sees, the more one suspects that in some patients at least, the disease has been present since infancy but not recognized (Aricò *et al.*, 2003; Aricò, 2004). The publicity that this volume will provide for adult LCH patients – 'the real orphans of this disease', may be one of its most valuable contributions.

REFERENCES

Al Asiri, R., Al Shahed, M. and Wali, S. (2000). Histiocytosis X and Caroli's disease. *Saudi Med J*, 21, 306–307.

Annels, N.E., da Costa, C.E.T., Prins, F.A., *et al.* (2003). Aberrant chemokine receptor expression and chemokine production by Langerhans cells underlies the pathogenesis of Langerhans cell histiocytosis. *J Exp Med*, 197, 1385–1390.

Aricò, M. (2004). Langerhans cell histiocytosis in adults: more questions than answers? *Eur J Cancer*, 40(10), 1467–1473.

Aricò, M., Haupt, R., Russotto, V.S., *et al.* (2001). Langerhans cell histiocytosis in 2 generations: a new family and review of the literature. *Med Pediatr Oncol*, 36, 314–316.

Aricò, M., Girschikofsky, M., Généreau, T., *et al.* (2003). Langerhans cell histiocytosis in adults. Report from the International Registry of the Histiocyte Society. *Eur J Cancer*, 39, 2341–2348.

Barthez, M.A., Araujo, E. and Donadieu, J. (2000). Langerhans cell histiocytosis and the central nervous system in childhood: evolution and prognostic factors. Results of a collaborative study. *J Child Neurol*, 15, 150–156.

Bernstrand, C., Cederlund, K., Åhstrom, L., *et al.* (2000). Smoking preceded pulmonary involvement in adults with Langerhans cell histiocytosis diagnosed in childhood. *Acta Paediatr*, 89, 1389–1392.

Bernstrand, C., Cederlund, K., Sandstedt, B., *et al.* (2001). Pulmonary abnormalities at long-term follow-up of patients with Langerhans cell histiocytosis. *Med Pediatr Oncol*, 36, 459–468.

Berry, D.H., Gresik, M.V., Humphrey, G.B., *et al.* (1986). Natural history of histiocytosis X: a Pediatric Oncology Group Study. *Med Pediatr Oncol*, 14, 1–5.

Bollini, G., Jouve, J.L., Gentet, J.C., *et al.* (1991). Bone lesions in histiocytosis X. *J Pediatr Orthoped*, 11, 469–477.

Braier, J., Chantada, G., Rosso, D., *et al.* (1999). Langerhans cell histiocytosis: retrospective evaluation of 123 patients in a single institution. *Pediatr Hematol Oncol*, 16, 377–385.

Braier, J., Cioccca, M., Latella, A., *et al.* (2002). Cholestasis, sclerosing cholangitis, and liver transplantation in Langerhans cell histiocytosis. *Med Pediatr Oncol*, 38, 178–182.

Brauner, M.W., Grenier, P., Tijani, K., *et al.* (1997). Pulmonary Langerhans cell histiocytosis: evolution of lesions on CT scans. *Radiology*, 204, 497–502.

Broadbent, V. (1986). Favourable prognostic features in histiocytosis X: bone involvement and absence of skin disease. *Arch Dis Child*, 61(12), 1219–1221.

Broadbent, V. and Pritchard, J. (1997). Diabetes insipidus associated with Langerhans celll histiocytosis: is it reversible? *Med Pediatr Oncol*, **28**, 289–293.

Broadbent, V., Williams, M. and Dossetor, J. (1990). Ruptured spleen as a cause of death in an infant with Langerhans cell histiocytosis (histiocytosis X). *Pediatr Hematol Oncol*, **7**, 297–299.

Calming, U., Bernstrand, C., Mosskin, M., *et al.* (2002). Brain 18-FDG PET scan in central nervous system Langerhans cell histiocytosis. *J Pediatr*, **141**, 435–440.

Carlson, R.A., Hattery, R.R., O'Connell, E.J., *et al.* (1976). Pulmonary involvement by histiocytosis X in the pediatric age group. *Mayo Clin Proc*, **51**, 542–547.

Ceci, A., de Terlizzi, M., Colella, R., *et al.* (1988). Etoposide in recurrent childhood Langerhans' cell histiocytosis: an Italian cooperative study. *Cancer*, **62**, 2528–2531.

Chen, C.Y., Wu, M.H., Huang, S.F., *et al.* (2001). Langerhans' cell histiocytosis presenting with a para-aortic lesion and heart failure. *J Formos Med Assoc*, **100**, 127–130.

Chomette, G., Auriol, M., Ragot, J.P., *et al.* (1987). Histiocytosis X of the jaw. I. Anatomico-clinical study apropos of 61 cases. *Rev Stomatol Chir Maxillofac*, **88**, 334–338.

Chu, T., D'Angio, G.J., Favara, B., *et al.* (1987). Histiocytosis syndromes in children. *Lancet*, **1**, 208–209.

Cline, M.J. (1994). Histiocytes and histiocytosis. *Blood*, **84**, 2840–2853.

Corry, A., Russell, W., McPhillips, M., *et al.* (2004). Comment on: Imashuku *et al.* Pineal dysfunction (low melatonin production) as a cause of sudden death in a long-term survivor of Langerhans cell histiocytosis? *Med Pediatr Oncol* 2003; **41**: 151–153. *Pediatr Blood Cancer*, **43**, 93–94.

Cunningham, M.J., Curtin, H.D., Jaffe, R., *et al.* (1989). Otologic manifestations of Langerhans' cell histiocytosis. *Arch Otolaryngol Head Neck Surg*, **115**, 807–813.

Daras, C., Grayson, W., Mayet, I., *et al.* (1995). Langerhans' cell histiocytosis of the eyelid. *Br J Ophthalmol*, **79**, 91–92.

Dattani, M.T. (2001). Tests in paediatric endocrinology and normal values. In: Brook, C.G.D. and Handmarsh, C., eds, *Endocrinology*. Blackwell Science Cambridge, pp. 467–490.

Debray, D. (2003). Sclerosing cholangitis in children: an overview. *Proceedings of the XIX Meeting of the Histiocyte Society*, Philadelphia, 17.

Dehner, L.P. (2003). Juvenile xanthogranulomas in the first two decades of life: a clinicopatho-logic study of 174 cases with cutaneous and extracutaneous manifestations. *Am J Surg Pathol*, **27**, 579–593.

Dimentberg, R.A. and Brown, K.L. (1990). Diagnostic evaluation of patients with histiocytosis X. *J Pediatr Orthop*, **10**, 733–741.

Dogan, A.S., Conway, J.J., Miller, J.H., *et al.* (1996). Detection of bone lesions in Langerhans cell histiocytosis: complementary roles of scintigraphy and conventional radiography. *J Pediatr Hematol Oncol*, **18**, 51–58.

Donadieu, J., Rolon, M.A., Pion, I., *et al.* (2004a). Incidence of growth hormone deficiency in pediatric-onset Langerhans cell histiocytosis: efficacy and safety of growth hormone treatment. *J Clin Endocrinol Metab*, **89**, 604–609.

Donadieu, J., Rolon, M.A., Thomas, C., *et al.* (2004b). Endocrine involvement in pediatric-onset Langerhans' cell histiocytosis: a population-based study. *J Pediatr*, **144**, 350.

Donadieu, J., Piguet, F., Bernard, M., *et al.* (2004c). A new clinical score for disease activity in Langerhans cell histiocytosis. *Ped Blood Cancer*, **43**, 770–776.

Dunger, D.B., Broadbent, V., Yeoman, E., *et al.* (1989). The frequency and natural history of diabetes insipidus in children with Langerhans-cell histiocytosis. *New Engl J Med,* **321,** 1157–1162.

Duranay, M., Aribas, O.K., Erbilen, M., *et al.* (1996). Histiocytosis X and glomerulonephritis: a case report. *Nephron,* **73,** 329–330.

Edgar, J.D., Smyth, A.E., Pritchard, J., *et al.* (2001). Interferon-gamma receptor deficiency mimicking Langerhans' cell histiocytosis. *J Pediatr,* **139**(4), 600–603.

Egeler, R.M., Schipper, M.E. and Heymans, H.S.A. (1990). Gastrointestinal involvement in Langerhans' cell histiocytosis (histiocytosis X): a clinical report of three cases. *Eur J Pediatr,* **149,** 325–329.

Egeler, R.M., de Kraker, J. and Voûte, P.A. (1993). Cytosine–arabinoside, vincristine, and prednisolone in the treatment of children with disseminated Langerhans cell histiocytosis with organ dysfunction: experience at a single institution. *Med Pediatr Oncol,* **21,** 265–270.

Emile, J.F., Wechsler, J., Brousse, N., *et al.* (1995). Langerhans' cell histiocytosis. Definitive diagnosis with the use of monoclonal antibody O10 on routinely paraffin-embedded samples. *Am J Surg Pathol,* **19,** 636–641.

Favara, B.E., Jaffe, R. and Egeler, R.M. (2002). Macrophage activation and hemophagocytic syndrome in Langerhans' cell histiocytosis. A report of 30 cases. *Pediatr Dev Pathol,* **5,** 130–140.

Gabbay, E., Dark, J.H., Ashcroft, T., *et al.* (1998). Recurrence of Langerhans' cell granulomatosis following lung transplantation. *Thorax,* **53,** 326–327.

Gadner, H., Heitger, A., Grois, N., *et al.* (1994). Treatment strategy for disseminated Langerhans cell histiocytosis. *Med Pediatr Oncol,* **23,** 72–80.

Gadner, H., Grois, N., Aricò, M., *et al.* (2001). A randomized trial of treatment for multisystem Langerhans' cell histiocytosis. *J Pediatr,* **138,** 728–734.

Geissmann, F., Thomas, C., Emile, J.F., *et al.* (1996). Digestive tract involvement in Langerhans cell histiocytosis. The French Langerhans Cell Histiocytosis Study Group. *J Pediatr,* **129,** 836–845.

Greenberger, J.S., Cassady, J.R., Jaffe, N., *et al.* (1979). Radiation therapy in patients with histiocytosis: management of diabetes insipidus and bone lesions. *Int J Radiat Oncol Biol Phys,* **5,** 1749–1755.

Grois, N., Flucher-Wolfram, B., Heitger, A., *et al.* (1995). Diabetes insipidus in Langerhans cell histiocytosis: results from the DAL-HX 83 study. *Med Pediatr Oncol,* **24,** 248–256.

Grois, N.G., Favara, B.E., Mostbeck, G.H., *et al.* (1998). Central nervous system disease in Langerhans cell histiocytosis. *Hematol Oncol Clin North Am,* **12,** 287–305.

Grois, N., Prayer, D., Prosch, H., *et al.* (2004). Course of diabetes insipidus in Langerhans cell histiocytosis and clinical impact of associated magnetic resonance imaging findings in diabetes insipidus associated with Langerhans cell histiocytosis. *Ped Blood Cancer,* **43,** 59–65.

Ha, S.Y., Helms, P., Fletcher, M., *et al.* (1992). Lung involvement in Langerhans' cell histiocytosis: prevalence, clinical features, and outcome. *Pediatrics,* **89,** 466–469.

Hamada, K., Teramoto, S., Narita, N., *et al.* (2000). Pulmonary veno-occlusive disease in pulmonary Langerhans' cell granulomatosis. *Eur Respir J,* **15,** 421–423.

Hand, A. (1893). Polyuria and tuberculosis. *Arch Pediatr,* **10,** 673–675

Hoeger, P.H., Diaz, C., Malone, M., *et al.* (2001). Juvenile xanthogranuloma as a sequel to Langerhans cell histiocytosis: a report of three cases. *Clin Exp Dermatol,* **26,** 391–394.

Howarth, D.M., Mullan, B.P., Wiseman, G.A., *et al.* (1996). Bone scintigraphy evaluated in diagnosing and staging Langerhans' cell histiocytosis and related disorders. *J Nucl Med*, **37**, 1456–1460.

Howarth, D.M., Gilchrist, G.S., Mullan, B.P., *et al.* (1999). Langerhans cell histiocytosis. Diagnosis, natural history, management and outcome. *Cancer*, **85**, 2278–2290.

Kelly, K.M. and Pritchard, J. (1994). Monoclonal antibody therapy in Langerhans cell histiocytosis-feasible and reasonable? *Br J Cancer*, **23**(Suppl), S54–S55.

Kilpatrick, S.E., Wenger, D.E., Gilchrist, G.S., *et al.* (1995). Langerhans' cell histiocytosis (histiocytosis X) of bone. *Cancer*, **76**, 2471–2484.

Klein, A., Corazza, F., Demulder, A., *et al.* (1999). Recurrent viral associated hemophagocytic syndrome in a child with Langerhans cell histiocytosis. *J Pediatr Hematol Oncol*, **21**, 554–556.

Komp, D.M., El Mahdi, A., Starling, K.A., *et al.* (1980). Quality of survival in histiocytosis X: a Southwest Oncology Group study. *Med Pediatr Oncol*, **8**, 35–40.

Lahey, E. (1975). Histiocytosis X – an analysis of prognostic factors. *J Pediatr*, **87**, 184–189.

Laman, J.D., Leenen, P.J., Annels, N.E., *et al.* (2003). Langerhans-cell histiocytosis 'insight into DC biology'. *Trend Immunol*, **24**, 190–196.

Lichtenstein, L. (1953). Histiocytosis X: integration of eosinophilic granuloma of bone, Letterer–Siwe disease and Schuller–Christian disease as related manifestations of a single nosologic entity. *Am Medl Assoc Arch Pathol*, **56**, 84–102.

Lieberman, P.H., Jones, C.R., Steinman, R.M., *et al.* (1996). Langerhans cell (eosinophilic) granulomatosis. A clinicopathologic study encompassing 50 years. *Am J Surg Pathol*, **20**, 519–552.

Maghnie, M., Cosi, G., Genovese, E., *et al.* (2000). Central diabetes insipidus in children and young adults. *New Engl J Med*, **343**, 998–1007.

McLean, T.W. and Pritchard, J. (1996). Langerhans cell histiocytosis and hypercalcemia: clinical response to indomethacin. *J Pediatr Hematol Oncol*, **18**(3), 318–320.

McLelland, J., Broadbent, V., Yeomans, E., *et al.* (1990). Langerhans cell histiocytosis: the case for conservative therapy. *Arch Dis Child*, **65**, 301–303.

Minkov, M., Grois, N., Heitger, A., *et al.* (2000). Treatment of multisystem Langerhans cell histiocytosis. Results of the DAL-HX 83 and DAL-HX 90 studies. *Klin Padiatr*, **212**, 139–144.

Mogul, M., Hartman, G., Donaldson, S., *et al.* (1993). Langerhans cell histiocytosis presenting with the superior vena cava syndrome: a case report. *Med Pediatr Oncol*, **21**, 456–459.

Moore, A.T., Pritchard, J. and Taylor, D.S. (1985). Histiocytosis X: an ophthalmological review. *Br J Ophthalmol*, **69**, 7–14.

Muwakkit, S., Gharagozloo, A., Souid, A.K., *et al.* (1994). The sonographic appearance of lesions of the spleen and pancreas in an infant with Langerhans' cell histiocytosis. *Pediatr Radiol*, **24**, 222–223.

Nanduri, V.R., Pritchard, J., Chong, W.K., *et al.* (1998). Labyrinthine involvement in Langerhans' cell histiocytosis. *Int J Pediatr Otorhinolaryngol*, **46**, 109–115.

Nanduri, V.R., Kelly, K., Malone, M., *et al.* (1999). Colon involvement in Langerhans' cell histiocytosis. *J Pediatr Gastroenterol Nutr*, **29**, 462–466.

Nanduri, V.R., Barelle, P., Pritchard, J., *et al.* (2000). Growth and endocrine disorders in multisystem Langerhans cell histiocytosis. *Clin Endocrinol*, **53**, 509–515.

Nanduri, V.R., Lillywhite, L., Chapman, C., *et al.* (2003). Cognitive outcome of long-term survivors of multisystem langerhans cell histiocytosis: a single-institution, cross-sectional study. *J Clin Oncol*, **21**, 2961–2967.

Nezelof, C., Frileux-Herbert, F. and Cronier-Sachot, J. (1979). Disseminated histiocytosis X. Analysis of prognostic factors based on a retrospective study of 50 cases. *Cancer*, **44**, 1824–1838.

Nondahl, S.R., Finlay, J.L., Farrell, P.M., *et al.* (1986). A case report and literature review of 'primary' pulmonary histiocytosis X of childhood. *Med Pediatr Oncol*, **14**, 57–62.

Ottaviano, F. and Finlay, J.L. (2003). Diabetes insipidus and Langerhans cell histiocytosis: a case report of reversibility with 2-chlorodeoxyadenosine. *J Pediatr Hematol Oncol*, **25**, 575–577.

Papagelopoulos, P.J., Currier, B.L., Galanis, E., *et al.* (2002). Vertebra plana caused by primary Ewing sarcoma: case report and review of the literature. *J Spinal Disord Tech*, **15**(3), 252–257.

Pinckney, L. and Parker, B.R. (1977). Myelosclerosis and myelofibrosis in treated histiocytosis-X. *Am J Roentgenol*, **129**, 521–523.

Pritchard, J., Foley, P. and Wong, H. (2003). Langerhans and Langhans: what's misleading in a name? *Lancet*, **362**, 922.

Raney Jr, D.B. and D'Angio, G.J. (1989). Langerhans' cell histiocytosis (histiocytosis X): experience at the Children's Hospital of Philadelphia, 1970–1984. *Med Pediatr Oncol*, **17**, 20–28.

Réfabert, L., Rambaud, C., Mamou-Mani, T., *et al.* (1996). CD1a-positive cells in bronchoalveolar lavage samples from children with Langerhans cell histiocytosis. *J Pediatr*, **129**, 913–915.

Rivera-Luna, R., Alter-Molchadsky, N., Cardenas-Cardos, R., *et al.* (1988). Langerhans cell histiocytosis in children under 2 years of age. *Med Pediatr Oncol*, **26**, 334–343.

Sartoris, D.J. and Parker, B.R. (1984). Histiocytosis X: rate and pattern of resolution of osseous lesions. *Radiology*, **152**, 679–684.

Sartoris, D.J. and Resnick, D. (1985). Myelofibrosis arising in treated histiocytosis X. *Eur J Pediatr*, **144**, 200–202.

Sheils, C. and Dover, G.J. (1989). Frequency of congenital anomalies in patients with histiocytosis X. *Am J Hematol*, **31**, 91–95.

Slater, J.M. and Swarm, O.J. (1980). Eosinophilic granuloma of bone. *Med Pediatr Oncol*, **8**, 151–164.

Surico, G., Muggeo, P., Muggeo, V., *et al.* (2000). Ear involvement in childhood Langerhans' cell histiocytosis. *Head Neck*, **22**, 42–47.

The French LCH Study Group (1996). A multicentre retrospective survey of LCH: 348 cases observed between 1983 and 1993. *Arch Dis Child*, **75**, 17–24.

Titgemeyer, C., Grois, N., Minkov, M., *et al.* (2001). Pattern and course of single-system disease in Langerhans cell histiocytosis data from the DAL-HX 83 and 90 study. *Med Pediatr Oncol*, **37**, 108–114.

Trouillas, P., Takayanagi, T., Hallett, M., *et al.* (1997). International Cooperative Ataxia Rating Scale for pharmacological assessment of the cerebellar syndrome. The Ataxia Neuropharmacology Committee of the World Federation of Neurology. *J Neurol Sci*, **145**, 205–211.

Tsuchiya, H., Ishibashi, F., Migita, M., *et al.* (1995). Perirenal mass of Langerhans cell histiocytosis. *Eur J Pediatr*, **154**, 117–119.

Vassallo, R., Ryu, J.H., Schroeder, D.R., *et al.* (2002). Clinical outcomes of pulmonary Langerhans'-cell histiocytosis in adults. *New Engl J Med*, **346**, 484–490.

Wang, K.H., Cheng, C.J., Hu, C.H., *et al.* (2002). Coexistence of localized Langerhans cell histiocytosis and cutaneous Rosai–Dorfman disease. *Br J Dermatol*, **147**, 770–774.

Werner, K., Pritchard, J., Lappi, M., *et al.* (2003). Chronic papilloedema due to intra-orbital Langerhans cell histiocytosis. *Med Pediatr Oncol*, **41**, 580–583.

Willis, B., Ablin, A., Weinberg, V., *et al.* (1996). Disease course and late sequelae of Langerhans' cell histiocytosis: a 25 year experience at the University of Southern California, San Francisco. *J Clin Oncol*, **14**, 2073–2082.

Willman, C.L., Busque, L., Griffiths, B.B., *et al.* (1994). Langerhans cell histiocytosis – a clonal proliferation of Langerhans cells. *New Engl J Med*, **331**, 154–160.

Witters, G., Baert, L., D'Hoedt, M., *et al.* (1991). Eosinophilic granuloma of bladder. *Urology*, **37**, 72–74.

Yu, C.P., Tseng, H.H. and Tu, Y.C. (1990). Congenital Letterer–Siwe disease with intrauterine fetal death: a case report and review of the literature. *J Formos Med Assoc*, **89**, 806–810.

Yu, R.C., Attra, A., Quinn, C.M., *et al.* (1993). Multisystem Langerhans' cell histiocytosis with pancreatic involvement. *Gut*, **34**, 570–572.

7

Histiocytosis of the skin in children and adults

Bernice Krafchik, Elena Pope and Scott R.A. Walsh

The histiocytoses are a group of rare disorders that involve an abnormal accumulation of a specific cell type (the histiocyte) in various organs. Histiocytes are mainly derived from the bone marrow, developing from a common hematopoetic progenitor into two distinct types, the monocyte/macrophage system and the dendritic cells (DC), of which Langerhans cells (LCs) are one cell type. Despite advances in the study of the histiocytoses, their etiology remains elusive, their pathogenesis is poorly understood, their classification is constantly changing and their treatment is far from standardized. Of the histiocytoses, the DC group affects the skin more frequently than the hemophagocytic or malignant variants, particularly in children. The two most frequent dendritic histiocytoses are an accumulation of pathologic LCs, that manifests as LC histiocytosis (LCH), and a proliferation of dermal/interstitial dendrocytes, that presents in the skin and other organs as xanthogranulomas. Histiocytosis affects the skin more commonly than any other organ except bone. Due to the ease of skin biopsy, it is the most useful way of establishing the diagnosis of LCH. LCH of the skin has a wide range of presentations, but neither the type of lesion nor the histology is helpful in evaluating the prognosis.

This chapter will discuss the pathology, clinical appearance, appropriate investigations, treatment and prognosis of skin histiocytosis in children and adults.

LCH in infancy and childhood

Epidemiology

LCH is a rare disease affecting 2–7 children per million per year (Carstensen and Ornvold, 1993; Nicholson *et al.*, 1998) or 1 in 25,000 children per year (Favara *et al.*, 1997). Due to the known spontaneous resolution of lesions, particularly those affecting bone and skin, it is likely that this figure may be higher. The disease is most common in the 0–4-year-old age group, but any age may be affected.

Pathology (see also Chapter 2)

The cellular infiltrate is confined to the upper dermis presenting as a lichenoid band and/or having the appearance of pagetoid spread. The presence of numerous LCs in the lesions is typical (Van Heerde and Egeler, 1991). Morphologically pathologic LCs (unlike normal LCs) do not demonstrate dendrites. LCs are large cells with an abundant eosinophilic cytoplasm and numerous vacuoles. The nuclei are kidney shaped, and eccentrically placed with a grooved appearance and an irregular, granular chromatin pattern. There is often an admixture of eosinophils, mast cells, polymorphonuclear leukocytes and lymphocytes, all part of a reactive process. Mitotic figures are rare. Epidermotropism (infiltration into the epidermis) is typical and granulomas may be formed in older lesions. There may be micro-abscesses containing histiocytes in various layers of the epidermis. Partial effacement of the dermo-epidermal junction and multinucleated giant cells are common. The epidermis overlying the infiltrate may be attenuated and focally eroded (Eady, 1979; Wells, 1979; Crowe *et al.*, 1981; Kuttner *et al.*, 1987). Adult cases, in particular, may show a more prominent periadnexal infiltrate (Helm *et al.*, 1993). As lesions progress, there is often increasing fibrosis (Santillan *et al.*, 2003).

On electron microscopy (EM), LCs are recognized by the presence of racket-shaped organelles called Birbeck granules. Birbeck granules are found in 2–40% of LCs in an LCH lesion (Eady, 1979; Kuttner *et al.*, 1987), but these organelles are specific to LCs. Other organelles are also found in LCs, none as diagnostic as Birbeck granules. Birbeck granules are involved in the non-classical antigen-processing pathway mediated by Langerin, a calcium-dependent lectin, with mannose-binding specificity. Langerin facilitates antigen capture and routes it to the Birbeck granule (Valladeau *et al.*, 2000). The presence of Birbeck granules is the definitive diagnostic criterion for the diagnosis of LCH, but nowadays EM is seldom performed, and the diagnosis is readily made by clinical presentation, histology and immunomarkers.

Immunohistochemical typing helps distinguish LCs from other cells of the mononuclear/phagocytic system. The presence of a CD1a positive immunostain is characteristic of LCs, but rarely may be positive in diseases other than LCH. CD4 may be positive, but stains are negative for factor XIIIa, CD68 and CD163, the former being the hallmark of the xanthogranuloma family and the latter two of the monocyte/macrophage line. S100 staining is another feature typical of LCH but is also found on neural cells and melanocytes.

Classification

Despite enormous efforts to categorize histiocytic disease, the lack of understanding of the pathogenesis has undermined efforts at precise classification. Histiocytoses are broadly classified into dendritic and macrophage-related disorders but in the recent classification juvenile xanthogranuloma (JXG), thought to be derived from dermal/interstitial dendrocytes, are now classified in the dendritic group (Munn and Chu, 1998).

Clinical presentation

Skin lesions are common and occur in 20–40% of patients with LCH (the French Langerhans' Cell Histiocytosis Study Group, 1996). In disseminated disease the skin is involved in 75–100% of cases (Hamre *et al.*, 1997). Children usually present between the ages of 0 and 4 years, with at least 50% occurring under 1 year. In a questionnaire study involving three centers, LCH affected bone most commonly, being found in 74% of cases, skin in 38%, lymph nodes in 14% and other organs in less than 10% (Yu and Chu, 1995). Pulmonary lesions affect adults more frequently (Hamre *et al.*, 1997; Howarth *et al.*, 1999) and were only seen in 10–12% of children in two studies (the French Langerhans' Cell Histiocytosis Study Group, 1996; Hamre *et al.*, 1997).

The skin may be the only organ involved (skin-only LCH), there may be skin and a few other organs affected, or the disease may be generalized. Skin manifestations are the presenting feature in up to 50% of patients (Magana-Garcia, 1986; Munn and Chu, 1998). In a study conducted at Northwestern University in Chicago, in children who presented with LCH from birth to 4 weeks of age, the diagnosis was not made until an average of 3.5 months of age, because of the non-specific nature of the eruption (Stein *et al.*, 2001).

In another study of 314 patients, skin and/or mucous membranes were affected in 77 (25%) of patients. Of these, 66 (82%) had coexisting lesions in other areas, 64% had bone disease, 25% had pulmonary and 17% had lymph node involvement. Mucosal lesions were seen in 21% of patients with isolated skin involvement and 52% of multisystem (MS) disease (Howarth *et al.*, 1999).

Children often present with recurrent ear infections (related to temporal bone or external auditory canal lesions) or with skin lesions that fail to heal, or that heal only to re-erupt in other areas. The lesions occur anywhere on the body, but are most common on the scalp and diaper area. Pruritus is variable and a burning sensation may be experienced.

Skin lesions vary enormously, from erythematous and crusted macules, to papules and nodules, with or without ulceration (Figure 7.1). Petechiae are common and represent a valuable clue to the diagnosis. Papulovesicles that become crusted were the most common presentation in the Chicago series of infants from 0 to 4 weeks (Stein *et al.*, 2001). A seborrhea-like picture is another common presentation; the scalp lesions are erythematous, scaly and crusted with petechiae scattered in the lesions (Figures 7.2, 7.4 and 7.5). The area behind the ears often ulcerates. In the diaper area, there can be marked erythema in the intertriginous region, with

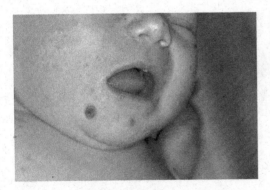

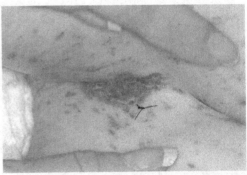

Figure 7.1   Necrotic papule in a 3-month-old baby with congenital self-healing reticulohistiocytosis. See also color plates

Figure 7.2   Ulceration, petechiae and papules in 6-month-old baby with disseminated LCH. See also color plates

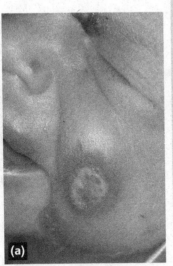

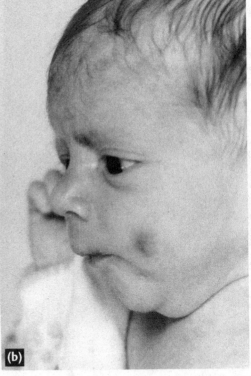

Figure 7.3   (a) Neonate born with deep ulceration on cheek and (b) at 1 month of age the lesion shows healing with scarring, at the same time as MS LCH developed. See also color plates

peripheral petechiae (Figures 7.6–7.9); deep ulceration in the erythema is typical. Small petechiae may also dot the whole diaper area intermingled with non-specific papules and nodules. Although petechiae and ulceration are suggestive of LCH, most of these clinical manifestations are non-specific and the diagnosis is easily missed.

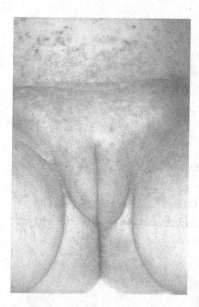

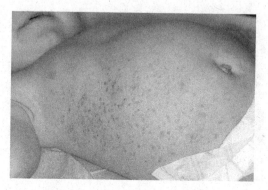

Figure 7.5   Petechial papules diagnostic of LCH.
See also color plates

Figure 7.4   Seborrheic pattern of
histiocytosis with petechiae at
peripheral edge. See also color plates

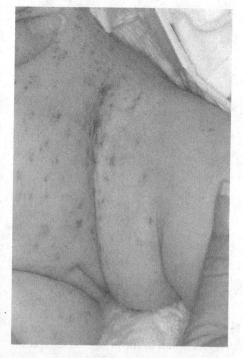

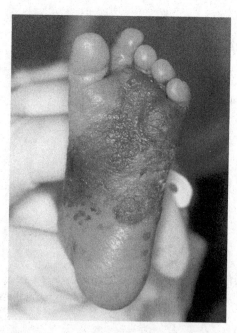

Figure 7.7   Deep hemorrhagic bulla in a
child with skin-only LCH who later progressed
to fatal MS disease. See also color plates

Figure 7.6   Scattered petechiae in LCH in
diaper area. See also color plates

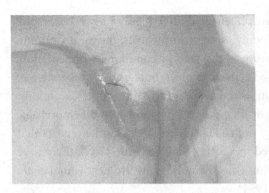

Figure 7.8   Typical deep seborrheic pattern of LCH in diaper area. See also color plates

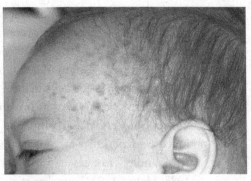

Figure 7.9   LCH crusting and petechiae on scalp. See also color plates

The mucous membranes can be involved, with nodules and ulcerations that may cause premature tooth eruption or loosening of the teeth. Nail changes have been the presenting sign in some patients with dystrophy, bleeding under the nail and paronychia (De Berker *et al.*, 1994). A chronic otitis externa from involvement of the mastoid bones has been described.

Specific forms of skin involvement

Skin-only LCH

LCH can affect the skin alone, without other organ involvement. In infants from birth to 4 weeks of age, this is known as the Hashimoto–Pritzker or congenital self-healing reticulohistiocytosis (CSRH) variant, but skin-only involvement can occur at any age. Patients have lesions that come and go, with or without itch. The lesions vary, having no specific clinical picture, except that they are usually polymorphous (varying in morphology) (see description above). The child usually appears healthy, but this does not preclude other organ involvement at presentation or later, and it is extremely important to investigate for this, and to continue frequent monitoring for at least 5 years, or longer.

Hashimoto–Pritzker variant: CSRH

In 1973, a new form of LCH was reported, which was characterized by an early age of onset (birth to a few weeks), a healthy child, minimal systemic involvement, papulonodules confined to the skin, a distinct histology and regression of the skin lesions within a few months (Hashimoto and Pritzker, 1973). In a retrospective review of infants from 0 to 4 weeks of age, at a single large institution, 14 of 19 patients had skin lesions noted at birth (Stein *et al.*, 2001). Lesions may occur anywhere on the skin, appearing commonly as vesiculo-pustules, the most common presentation. A seborrheic-like picture is the second commonest presentation. Petechiae (extravasation of red blood cells) and ulceration are very suggestive of LCH and their presence is helpful in distinguishing LCH from other conditions. Lesions may also present as brown or blue papules or nodules and hemorrhagic bullae (Stein *et al.*, 2001; Inuzuka *et al.*, 2003) (Figure 7.7). Despite reports that mucous membranes are not involved in CSRH (Bouillie *et al.*, 1988), there have been a number of case reports with mucous membrane involvement (Pujol *et al.*, 1988; Maher, 1993; Longaker *et al.*, 1994).

The diagnosis of CSRH is made on skin biopsy, where the characteristic pattern of LCH is seen. The histology of CSRH is not specific but organelles, such as laminated or non-laminated bodies, may be present on EM. They may represent senescent mitochondria, suggesting spontaneous regression. Birbeck granules are less prominent (affecting about 10% of cells), or may even be absent (Levinsohn *et al.*, 1993).

Since the original description there have been many case reports confirming the benign nature of this disease, and others suggesting that the diagnosis of CSRH can only be made in retrospect. Whilst it is true that lesions confined to the skin, with an early age of onset, may regress spontaneously and have an excellent prognosis, there have been many case reports of skin-only LCH that progress and evolves into MS disease, or regress initially only to recur up to years later, either on the skin or with other organ involvement, such as diabetes insipidus (DI) (Hoeger *et al.*, 1997; Stein *et al.*, 2001). Death has been reported in these infants. Even if the diagnosis of CSRH is made, it is important to monitor these patients for at least 5 years, to rule out progression/recurrence of disease (Figure 7.3a,b).

Skin LCH as part of limited MS disease (previously known as Hand–Schuller–Christian syndrome)

This entity is a chronic, multifocal form of LCH, and is typified by lytic bone lesions and the possible presence of exophthalmos, DI and skin lesions. Not all these features are necessary for the diagnosis. The age of onset is usually between 2 and 6 years, somewhat later than isolated skin disease. Exophthalmus, if present, is due to retro-orbital accumulation of LCs. Patients may present with DI with polyuria and polydipsia, or these symptoms may develop months or even years after the disease is diagnosed (Stein *et al.*, 2001).

The skin is involved with nodules and tumors that are yellow-brown in color or with the typical seborrhea-like picture. The gingiva and gums may also be affected, manifesting as gingival ulceration and hemorrhage. Premature tooth eruption may be the first manifestation of the disease (McDonald *et al.*, 1980).

Skin involvement as part of disseminated disease (previously known as Letterer–Siwe disease)

This variant of LCH is the most extensive and severe; it is usually seen under the age of 2 years, often in the neonatal period. It constitutes less than 15% of cases (Ladisch and Jaffe, 1997). In addition to the skin, affected in 75–100% of cases, multiple organs are involved including bones, liver, spleen, lungs, central nervous system (CNS) and bone marrow. This form of LCH carries the worst prognosis and is the least likely to resolve spontaneously. Skin lesions may be the presenting feature, the scalp and diaper area (seborrhea-like pattern) are usually affected, but any area of the body may be involved. Lesions are often polymorphous and resemble other clinical forms of LCH. Extensive ulceration may be seen. Petechiae and purpura are common and super-infection of the lesions may occur.

Diagnosis

The diagnosis of LCH is often missed for many months because of the non-specific clinical presentation. The clinical appearance, with the typical histology, positive S100 and CD1a immunostains and/or EM changes are all helpful in making the diagnosis. Histologic confirmation is the only certain way of establishing the diagnosis. A presumptive diagnosis is made on the characteristic histologic findings; a probable diagnosis is dependent on the finding of S100 cells with the typical hematoxylin and eosin (H&E) histology, and CD1a immunostaining or EM showing Birbeck granules is diagnostic of LCH (Chu and LeBoit, 1992). Others assert that in the typical clinical setting and characteristic histology, a positive S100 stain is sufficient to make the diagnosis (Munn and Chu, 1998); however, Rosai–Dorfman disease can involve skin and is typically S100 positive. Positive immunohistochemical staining with anti-Langerin antibodies confirm the presence of Birbeck granules, without the necessity for EM.

Differential diagnosis

Due to the diversity of clinical features, LCH of the skin can be mistaken for a number of other conditions. Nodules that resemble LCH and that occur at birth or early infancy can be mistaken for mastocytosis, neuroblastomas, vascular lesions and congenital leukemia.

In early infancy, LCH that presents with vesicles and bullae can be confused with a large number of vesiculo-bullous diseases of infancy including erythema toxicum, neonatal pustular melanosis, miliaria crystallina or rubra, incontinentia pigmenti, herpes simplex and varicella infection.

In late infancy and early childhood the lesions may resemble dermatitis. The most commonly mistaken condition is seborrheic dermatitis, it is not uncommon for LCH to be missed for months while treating for this condition. Both affect the scalp and diaper area, but while there is often marked scaling, there is not as much crusting in seborrheic dermatitis as in LCH, and there are no petechiae, a most helpful diagnostic feature of LCH. *The possibility of LCH should be considered in any patient with persistent scalp or diaper dermatitis*, as childhood lesions can be polymorphous.

It is important to rule out LCH while considering scabies. Although LCH can be pruritic, this is not usually as severe as in scabies. Petechiae are not present in scabies and finding the characteristic mite between the finger webs is diagnostic. In scabies it is usual to have other family members who are itchy.

Skin lesions may be seen in lymphomas, and lymphadenopathy with skin lesions can occur in LCH. Other histiocytic disorders, such as xanthogranulomas and benign cephalic histiocytosis (BCH), may also be confused with LCH.

Investigations

Skin biopsy is the easiest method of confirming the diagnosis of skin LCH. When this diagnosis is made it is important to thoroughly evaluate the patient, to rule out other organ involvement (see Chapter 6 for recommended investigations).

Prognosis

Neither the clinical presentation nor the histology is helpful as a prognostic indicator. The prognosis of LCH is generally benign but it is related to numerous factors that include age of onset, number of organs involved and the initial response to treatment (Stephan, 1995; French Langerhans' Cell Histiocytosis Study Group, 1996). Organ dysfunction is no longer independently prognostic (Gadner *et al.*, 2001).

In the study of infants with skin lesions at 0–4 weeks of age, the prognosis was excellent with a 90% survival at 4 years despite a median diagnosis at 3.5 months (Stein *et al.*, 2001). Bone-only involvement has the best prognosis, followed by skin-only involvement. Most studies report a survival rate of only 50% in disseminated disease under the age of 2 years (Greenberger *et al.*, 1981; Rivera-Luna *et al.*, 1996). Continuous monitoring of patients is important as progression to MS disease or to DI may occur years after diagnosis of skin-only LCH (Stein *et al.*, 2001).

Treatment

There is no good data on the definitive treatment for skin LCH. Whether it is better to monitor single-system disease or treat when the diagnosis is made is unknown. Treatment is geared toward the general well-being of the patient, the number of organs involved and the desire to minimize late effects. When LCH involves multiple organs, systemic therapy is indicated (Ladisch and Gadner, 1994) (see Chapters 11 and 12 for details of treatment programs).

Skin-only involvement may not require treatment other than observation, or therapy may be considered because of symptoms or even cosmetic concerns. The use of topical corticosteroids may be sufficient; it is often the first therapy given for skin LCH. Failure of complete response, fear of systemic effects when corticosteroids are used for long periods over a large surface area and recrudescence, often dictate a change of therapy. Topical nitrogen mustard has shown success in skin lesions (Wong *et al.*, 1986; Sheehan *et al.*, 1991), but despite a study that showed no premalignant or malignant changes in the mustine-treated skin of 20 children with a median follow-up of 8.3 years (Hoeger *et al.*, 2000), there continues to be concern in many centers regarding late malignancy.

Similarly, both ultraviolet-B (UV-B) and psoralen with UV (PUVA) therapy (Kaudewitz *et al.*, 1986; Selch and Parker, 1990) have been used effectively and have been considered by some to be the first-line therapy, but fear of late skin malignancy particularly in fair-skinned patients has limited their use.

Chemotherapy is usually effective in skin LCH but is usually limited to widespread symptomatic disease. Radiation therapy appears to be of limited value (Munn and Chu, 1998). Finally, topical administration of tacrolimus and related drugs, such as sirolimus, has produced rapid responses in patients with refractory skin lesions (Egeler, personal communication). Experience with this drug in LCH is anecdotal at present. The safety profile of tacrolimus in atopic dermatitis is excellent. It is recommended in children over 2 years of age (Patel *et al.*, 2003; Shainhouse and Eichenfield, 2003). Neither the US Food and Drug Administration nor the Canada Health Protection Branch support the use of tacrolimus in children under 2 years of age, despite studies showing safety in that age group, as little is known about long-term toxicity.

Histiocytic disorders of the skin, other than LCH (see also Chapter 15)

Juvenile Xanthogranuloma (JXG)

Juvenile xanthogranuloma is caused by an increase in cells related to dermal/interstitial dendrocytes. JXG presents at birth (in 20% of patients), or in infancy and early childhood. Most lesions are seen in children but adults may be affected. Parents notice the development of asymptomatic lesions, most commonly on the head, neck and face (Figure 7.10). They may increase in number for 1–2 years. JXG may be solitary or multiple red to yellow papules or nodules that can be difficult to differentiate from LCH (Figure 7.11). Lesions less than 10 mm in size are termed

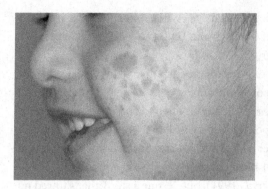

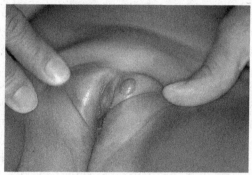

Figure 7.10 Micronodular lesions of JXG. See also color plates

Figure 7.11 JXG on labia

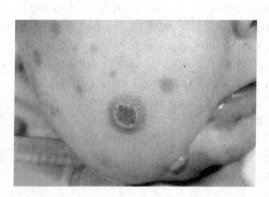

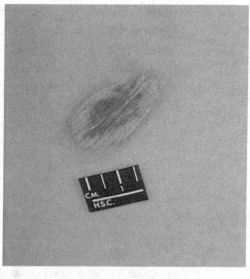

Figure 7.12 Ulceration of large lesion of JXG

Figure 7.13 Wrinkling after disappearance of large JXG. See also color plates

micronodular and those larger than 10 mm macronodular. Single nodules may be very large and may ulcerate (Figures 7.12–7.14).

The majority of lesions are confined to the skin, but other organs are occasionally affected, including the lung where a honeycomb appearance can be seen on X-ray, mucous membranes, testis, liver, CNS, bone and eye. In a study that involved ophthalmologists and dermatologists the incidence of eye involvement was 0.3%, occurring before the age of 2 years in children with multiple skin lesions (Chang *et al.*, 1996). Eye findings include erythema, irritation and photophobia related to iris involvement which can lead to acute hyphema, glaucoma and blindness (Shields *et al.*, 1990; Hernandez-Martin *et al.*, 1997). Cases of eye JXG can occur without

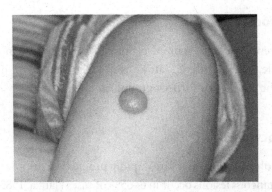

Figure 7.14 Xanthogranuloma: a typical red-yellow nodule. See also color plates

skin lesions. The figure of 0.3% reported by dermatologists is slightly higher when ophthalmologists are surveyed (Selch and Parker, 1990).

The histology of JXG is typical with a polymorphous granuloma mixed with lipid-laden histiocytes that are factor XIIIa positive but S100 and CD1a negative, and lack typical Birbeck granules. In mature lesions histiocytes have foamy cytoplasm and have the typical diagnostic feature of JXG, multinucleated Touton giant cells.

The prognosis is excellent, with resolution occurring in 2–6 years, usually without therapy. Ocular JXG and some forms of systemic JXG require therapy, however (see Chapter 15). Larger lesions may heal with atrophy or scarring (Figure 7.13). JXG associated with neurofibromatosis type 1 has a significantly increased incidence of juvenile chronic myelocytic leukemia (Jensen et al., 1971; Bestak et al., 1979; Mays et al., 1980).

Other forms of histiocytosis should be entertained in the differential diagnosis of JXG.

Benign cephalic histiocytosis

BCH is a rare non-LCH histiocytosis first described in 1971 (Gianotti et al., 1971). It is characterized by an asymptomatic eruption on the head, face and neck of infants and young children with no systemic or mucosal involvement. Forty-five percent of cases occur before 6 months of age. The lesions are small red-brown or yellow-tan macules and papules which resolve spontaneously (De Luna et al., 1989; Jih et al., 2002). The histology shows a well-circumscribed proliferation of histiocytes in the superficial and mid-dermis associated with a mixed inflammatory cell infiltrate. The cells are S100, CD1a and Birbeck granule negative. In at least two cases rebiopsy of the lesions later showed the typical histology of JXG (Zelger et al., 1995; Rodriguez-Jurado et al., 2000). BCH has an excellent prognosis with regression usually occurring within 2 years of onset, although some lesions may take up to 4 years to completely disappear (Gianotti et al., 1971).

Generalized eruptive histiocytomas

There have been rare reports of generalized eruptive histiocytomas in children (Alsowaidi and Sasseville, 2004). Differentiation from LCH is made on immunochemical staining and the absence of Birbeck granules.

Hemophagocytic lymphohistiocytosis

Hemophagocytic lymphohistiocytosis is a rare, rapidly progressive disorder of nondendritic histiocytes. Cutaneous lesions occur in 6–65% of cases (Janka, 1983; Henter *et al.*, 1991). Lesions present in the skin with petechiae, mostly on the upper body. The most commonly described skin manifestation is a non-specific maculo-papular eruption (Morrell *et al.*, 2002). Skin biopsy is not helpful. The diagnosis is made on clinical and laboratory criteria; hemophagocytosis is often absent at initial presentation (see Chapter 18). Survival rates vary, but treatment with chemotherapy and allogeneic bone marrow transplant have improved survival in the familial form of the disease.

LCH of the skin in adults

Between 10% and 30% of LCH cases have adult-onset (Baumgartner *et al.*, 1997; Singh *et al.*, 2003). As in children, LCH encompasses a spectrum of morphologies characterized by infiltration of various organs by aberrant LCs. Involvement can vary from the less common (in adults) single-system disease involving bone, lung or skin, primarily, to the more frequent MS disease where skin is one component. The International Registry of the Histiocyte Society (2003) reports that 7% of adults with single-system disease present with cutaneous involvement, while approximately 51% of those with MS disease report skin lesions (Aricò *et al.*, 2003). Overall, it is estimated that 37% of adults with LCH have cutaneous involvement. This is frequently the presenting feature of the disease (Helm *et al.*, 1993; Aricò *et al.*, 2003).

Among 31 cases reported in the literature, the average age of adults with skin-limited LCH was 60 years (range 29–88) (Kwong *et al.*, 1997; Singh *et al.*, 2003). Although variable in presentation, skin-limited disease is similar to that seen in children. Oral mucous membranes are not typically involved; however, genital mucous membrane involvement is not unusual (Santillan *et al.*, 2003). Localized cutaneous lesions have been reported to develop at sites of previously excised non-melanoma skin cancers (Simonart *et al.*, 2000). In general, the distribution and morphology of lesions can mimic other diseases including seborrheic dermatitis, dermatophytosis, Mucha–Haberman disease, Paget's disease, sexually transmitted diseases, mastocytosis, hidradenitis suppurativa, granuloma annulare or even rare genodermatoses presenting in adulthood, such as benign familial pemphigus

(Hailey–Hailey disease) and keratosis follicularis (Darier–White disease). Skin biopsy will distinguish amongst these disease entities.

Clinical appearance

All cases of LCH of the skin in adults should be evaluated for possible MS involvement. Cutaneous involvement in MS disease is identical to the lesions of single-system disease and lesions in adults are clinically similar to those in children (Figure 7.15). Additionally in adults, perivulvar or inguinal erythematous and purpuric plaques (Novice et al., 1989; Meunier et al., 1995; Santillan et al., 2003); orange-red and purpuric papules, and pustules beneath the breasts, axillary folds and in the groin may be seen (Novice et al., 1989; Thomas et al., 1993). Other presentations include pustules in the groin, scalp and axillae (Rodriguez-Valdes, 1982; Helm et al., 1993), purpuric vesicles on the upper and lower extremities (Mejia et al., 1997); xanthomatous-like yellowish-red papules widespread over the face and body (Chang et al., 2002); keratotic papules with follicular plugging (Helm et al., 1993); lichenoid papules (Vollum, 1979), sheeted and scaling erythema (Vollum, 1979; Lindelof, 1991), firm erythematous smooth papules on the scalp (Chang and Somach, 2001); poikilodermatous lesions (Zachary and MacDonald, 1983); prurigo-nodularis-like nodules on the arms, scalp and thighs (Kato et al., 1981; Holme and Mills, 2002); and large, polypoid and pedunculated tumors in the axillae and inguinal folds (Santhosh-Kumar et al., 1990). Cutaneous lesions can also involve the nails and mucous membranes (Misery et al., 1999).

As in children, oral mucosal lesions are often a sign of underlying bone involvement. Severe alveolar bone resorption can present as gingival swelling, hypertrophy and necrosis, ulcerations over the hard palate or buccal mucosa, and loosening of the teeth (Hashimoto et al., 1985; Eckardt and Schultze, 2003). The mandible is involved more commonly than the maxilla, and this can result in the appearance of 'floating teeth' on panoramic radiographs. Approximately 30% of adults with bony involvement can present with mucosal lesions (Baumgartner et al., 1997). Similarly, ulceronecrotic lesions of the scalp have been reported adjacent to underlying skull bone disease (Zachary and MacDonald, 1983).

Cutaneous lesions may be pruritic, have a burning quality or be asymptomatic (Wright et al., 1985; Santhosh-Kumar et al., 1990; Tsambaos et al., 1995; Chang et al., 2002; Holme and Mills, 2002).

Prognosis

In adult LCH, the prognosis is related to the extent of systemic disease and not to the extent of cutaneous involvement (Vollum, 1979). The prognosis for adult patients with isolated cutaneous disease is excellent with 100% probability of 5-year survival (Aricò et al., 2003). Survival in MS disease with cutaneous involvement is somewhat

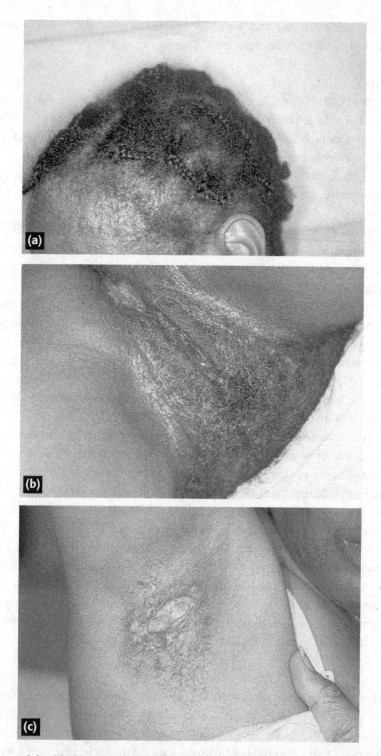

Figure 7.15   Adult with skin LCH. (a) Involving scalp, (b) vulva and (c) axillary lesion
(Figures courtesy of Algin B. Garrett, MD., Richmond, VA.). See also color plates

less, with 5-year survival ranging from 87.5% to 93.6% depending on co-morbid pulmonary involvement (Aricò et al., 2003). Due to the often few systems involved, MS LCH appears to be more benign in adults than in infants (Kolde et al., 2002).

Treatment

Surgical excision should be undertaken for small isolated lesions, but mutilating surgery should be avoided.

Skin-limited disease in adults has been treated with corticosteroids (topical, intralesional and oral), with variable results. Nitrogen mustard and both UV-B and PUVA have also had some success in skin-limited disease (see earlier discussion). Interferon (INF) alpha (six megaunits daily for up to 9 months with tapering thereafter) has been successful in a few cases (Kwong et al., 1997; Chang et al., 2002). Oral thalidomide (200 mg po q.d to q.i.d.) or isotretinoin (40 mg po q.d.) has achieved complete resolution of refractory cutaneous lesions (Thomas et al., 1993; Meunier et al., 1995; Tsambaos et al., 1995; Misery et al., 1999; Kolde et al., 2002; Santillan et al., 2003; Singh et al., 2003). Relapse after thalidomide treatment does occur, but may respond to retreatment (Moraes and Russo, 2001; Claudon et al., 2002). Long-term use of thalidomide may be limited due to the potential for development of irreversible peripheral neuropathy.

Dramatic responses of cutáneous and ano-genital lesions to combination of thalidomide plus INF have been reported (Montero et al., 2003). As in pediatric skin LCH, chemotherapy has been efficacious in adults, including successful use of prolonged oral etoposide, without adverse effects (Helmbold et al., 1998). The use of chemotherapy is usually limited to skin disease associated with MS LCH or to severe unresponsive disease.

As discussed earlier, topical tacrolimus and its derivatives may prove to be a useful addition to the armamentarium for skin LCH, although its use to date is limited to anecdotal reports (Egeler, personal communication).

Indeterminate cell histiocytosis in adults

Cutaneous indeterminate cell histiocytosis (CICH) is a rare neoplastic disorder presenting primarily in adults. The diagnosis is confirmed by immunophenotyping whereby the profile of the neoplastic cells includes a mixture of both LC (CD1a positive, S100 positive) and non-LC (CD68, HAM56, factor XIIIa) markers, and the cells lack Birbeck granules on EM (Manente et al., 1997; Rosenberg and Morgan, 2001).

Clinically, this entity presents with sudden onset of asymptomatic, firm, flesh-colored to reddish-brown papulonodules distributed diffusely over face and body or confined to the flexural areas and trunk (Kolde and Brocker, 1986; Contreras et al., 1990; Manente et al., 1997).

Dermatopathology reveals a superficial and deep dermal infiltrate of vacuolated and xanthomatized histiocytes with less marked epidermotropism than observed in LCH. There may be an interposed Grenz zone and lymphocytes admixed with the infiltrate (Kolde and Brocker, 1986). Although some have reported an associated hematologic malignancy (Kolde and Brocker, 1986), this is rare and lesions commonly self-resolve over a period of years without treatment (Contreras *et al.*, 1990). Lesions can be confused with generalized eruptive histiocytosis which it resembles clinically and pathologically, only differing with respect to immuno-markers (see below).

Non-LCH in adults

This group contains sufficiently rare entities that in most cases, isolated case reports or photographic reproductions must substitute for clinical experience as the basis for diagnosis. Members in this group are all S100 and CD1a negative and lack Birbeck granules. They have various dermal dendritic or monocyte/macrophage markers, but many entities have such overlapping pathologic features that distinction among this group is often by clinical context (Caputo *et al.*, 2003).

Many terms have been used in attempts to split entities within this group. Accepted distinctions that appear to predominate in the adult population include the benign cutaneous entity of generalized eruptive histiocytosis, the possibly paraneoplastic entities of xanthoma disseminatum and necrobiotic xanthogranuloma, and the systemic disease of multicentric reticulohistiocytosis (MRH).

Generalized eruptive histiocytosis

Generalized eruptive histiocytosis is considered to be primarily a benign, self-healing disease characterized by sudden onset of successive crops of asymptomatic, firm, dark red to bluish papulonodules located symmetrically over the face, trunk and proximal limbs (Sohi *et al.*, 1979; Caputo *et al.*, 1981; Seward *et al.*, 2004). Histopathology is variable and may show a pattern similar to indeterminate cell histiocytosis with vacuolated histiocytes in the superficial and mid-dermis Caputo *et al.*, 1981; Zelger and Burgdorf, 2001). Immuno-markers are usually positive for CD68 and factor XIIIa, and negative for CD1a and S100 (Seward *et al.*, 2004). No treatment is required for this self-healing condition.

Xanthoma disseminatum

Xanthoma disseminatum (Montgomery syndrome) is a clinically characteristic disease that often presents in young adult males (Weiss and Keller, 1993). Typically multiple brownish-red to yellowish-red papules appear on the eyelids, flexural areas and mucous membranes. Lesions coalesce to form verrucous plaques. There may be associated dyspnea, dysphagia with oro-pharyngeal involvement, blindness with conjunctival/corneal involvement and transient DI. Underlying multiple myeloma and/or monoclonal gammopathies have been reported in a few cases (Caputo *et al.*, 1995). Dermatopathology reveals foamy cells, Touton giant cells, siderosis and a mixed inflammatory infiltrate. Immuno-markers are positive for CD68 and factor XIIIa. The prognosis varies from spontaneous self-healing, through persistent disease to a progressive form with CNS involvement. Treatment of life-threatening mucosal or disfiguring cutaneous lesions has included Grenz rays, cyclophosphamide and cyto-destructive methods (Caputo *et al.*, 1995).

Necrobiotic xanthogranuloma

Necrobiotic xanthogranuloma is an extremely rare inflammatory histiocytoxan-thomatosis of the dermis and subcutaneous tissue, frequently associated with a paraproteinemia or cryoglobulinemia (Burdick *et al.*, 2003; Chang *et al.*, 2003). It usually presents in the middle age to elderly as reddish-orange papulonodules in the periorbital region which progress to become large ulcerated, atrophic plaques with telangiectasias (Burdick *et al.*, 2003). Dermatopathology reveals a granuloma-tous infiltrate including foamy cells, lymphocytes and Touton giant cells mixed with areas of necrobiosis containing cholesterol crystals. Histiocytic cells are CD68 positive, but factor XIIIa negative (Goodman and Barrett, 2003). Therapy is usu-ally aimed towards the underlying hematologic abnormality (Venencie *et al.*, 1995; Machado *et al.*, 2001).

Multicentric reticulohistiocytosis

MRH is a systemic granulomatous disease characterized by cutaneous nodules with an acral predominance and a destructive arthritis affecting distal interpha-langeal joints most frequently (Hiramanek *et al.*, 2002). In addition, some patients may show periungual 'coral beading' of lesions. These are not pathognomonic and may occur in sarcoid or cutaneous Crohn's disease. However, beading on the pinna and violaceous lesions on the nostrils may be pathognomonic (Gorman *et al.*, 2000). MRH predominates in middle-aged women and is usually self-limited, burning itself out in 5–10 years. The arthritis can be severely mutilating, destroying both cartilage and bone (Santilli *et al.*, 2002). Dermatopathology shows bizarre-shaped histiocytes and multinucleated giant cells with a characteristic ground-glass cyto-plasmic appearance that is positive with periodic acid–Schiff staining. They are CD68 positive but usually factor XIIIa negative (Goodman and Barrett, 2003). Several cases have had associated hematologic or solid tumor malignancies, or concomitant connective tissue disease (Cox *et al.*, 2001; Hsiung *et al.*, 2003). Treatment is aimed at identifying and correcting any co-morbid systemic disease. In the absence of an underlying cause, systemic immunosuppression is used to control disease progression (Hiramanek *et al.*, 2002) (see also Chapter 15).

REFERENCES

Alsowaidi, M. and Sasseville, D. (2004). Histiocytic disorders. Part 2: Non-Langerhans cell histiocytosis. *Dermatology Rounds*, Division of Dermatology, McGill University, **3**(3). http://www.dermatologyrounds.ca

Aricò, M., Girschikofsky, M., Genereau, T., *et al.* (2003). Langerhans cell histiocytosis in adults. Report from the International Registry of the Histiocyte Society. *Eur J Cancer*, **39**, 2341–2348.

Baumgartner, I., Von Hochstetter, A., Baumert, B., *et al.* (1997). Langerhans'-cell histiocytosis in adults. *Med Ped Oncol*, **28**, 9–14.

Bestak, M., Miller, D. and Mouradian, J. (1979). Juvenile chronic myelogenous leukemia and dermal histiocytosis in Von Recklinghausen's disease. *Am J Dis Child*, **133**, 831–833.

Bouillie, M.C., Thomine, E., Fessard, C., *et al.* (1988). Self-limited neonatal histiocytosis. Report of two cases and a review of the literature. *Ann Pediatr (Paris)*, **35**, 339–344.

Burdick, A.E., Sanchez, J. and Elgart, G.W. (2003). Necrobiotic xanthogranuloma associated with a benign monoclonal gammopathy. *Cutis*, **72**, 47–50.

Caputo, R., Alessi, E. and Allegra, F. (1981). Generalized eruptive histiocytoma: a clinical, histological, ultrastructural study. *Arch Dermatol*, **117**, 216–221.

Caputo, R., Veraldi, S. Grimalt, R., *et al.* (1995). The various clinical patterns of xanthoma disseminatum. Consideration on seven cases and review of the literature. *Dermatol*, **190**, 19–24.

Caputo, R., Passoni, E. and Cavicchini, S. (2003). Papular xanthoma associated with angiokeratoma of fordyce: consideration on the nosography of this rare non-Langerhans cell histiocytoxanthomatosis. *Dermatol*, **206**, 165–168.

Carstensen, H. and Ornvold, K. (1993). The epidemiology of LCH in children in Denmark, 1975–89. *Med Pediatr Oncol*, **21**, 387–388.

Chang, C. and Somach, S.C. (2001). Firm erythematous papules of scalp in a woman with a history of breast cancer. *Arch Pathol Lab Med*, **125**, 1379–1380.

Chang, M.W., Frieden, I.J. and Good, W. (1996). The risk of intraocular juvenile xanthogranuloma: survey of current practices and assessment of risk. *J Am Acad Dermatol*, **34**(3), 445–449.

Chang, S.E., Koh, G.J., Choi, J.H., *et al.* (2002). Widespread skin-limited adult Langerhans cell histiocytosis: long-term follow-up with good response to interferon alpha. *Clin Exp Dermatol*, **27**, 135–137.

Chang, S.E., Lee, W.S., Lee, M.W., *et al.* (2003). A case of necrobiotic xanthogranuloma without paraproteinemia presenting as a solitary tumor on the thigh. *Int J Dermatol*, **42**, 470–472.

Chu, P. and LeBoit, P.E. (1992). Histologic features of cutaneous sinus histiocytosis (Rosai–Dorfman disease): cases with and without systemic involvement. *J Cutan Pathol*, **19**, 201–206.

Claudon, A., Dietemann, J.L., Hamman De Compte, A., *et al.* (2002). Interest in thalidomide in cutaneo-mucous and hypothalamo–hypophyseal involvement of Langerhans cell histiocytosis. *Revue de Medecine Interne*, **23**, 651–656.

Contreras, F., Fonseca, E., Gamallo, C. *et al.* (1990). Multiple self-healing indeterminate cell lesions of the skin in an adult. *Am J Dermatopath*, **12**, 396–401.

Cox, N.H., West, N.C. and Popple, A.W. (2001). Multicentric reticulohistiocytosis associated with idiopathic myelofibrosis. *Br J Dermatol*, **145**, 1022–1036.

Crowe, M.J., O'Loughlin, S., Noel, J., et al. (1981). Histiocytosis X with pulmonary and cutaneous manifestations. *Irish J Med Sci*, **150**, 278–281.

De Berker, D., Lever, L.R. and Windebank, K. (1994). Nail features in Langerhans' cell histiocytosis. *Br J Dermatol*, **130**, 523–527.

De Luna, M.L., Glikin, I., Golberg, J., et al. (1989). Benign cephalic histiocytosis: report of four cases. *Pediatr Dermatol*, **6**(3), 198–201.

Eady, R.A.J. (1979). Letterer–Siwe disease in an elderly patient: histological and ultrastructural findings. *Clin Exp Dermatol*, **4**, 413–420.

Eckardt, A. and Schultze, A. (2003). Maxillofacial manifestation of Langerhans cell histiocytosis: a clinical and therapeutic analysis of 10 patients. *Oral Oncol*, **39**, 687–694.

Egeler, R.M. (1993). Genetic predisposition in Langerhans cell histiocytosis? An hypothesis (PhD thesis). In: Haveka, B.V., ed. *Langerhans Cell Histiocytosis and Other Histiocytic Disorders*, University of Amsterdam, Amsterdam, pp. 181–197.

Favara, B.E. (1991). Langerhans cell histiocytosis: pathobiology and pathogenesis. *Sem Oncol*, **18**, 3.

Favara, B.E., Feller, A.C., Pauli, M., et al. (1997). Contemporary classification of histiocytic disorders. The WHO Committee on Histiocytic/Reticulum Cell Proliferations. Reclassification Working Group of the Histiocyte Society. *Med Pediatr Oncol*, **29**(3), 157–166.

The French Langerhans' Cell Histiocytosis Study Group. (1996). A multicentre retrospective survey of Langerhans' cell histiocytosis: 348 cases observed between 1983 and 1993. *Arch Child Dis*, **75**, 17–24.

Gadner, H., Grois, N., Aricò, M., et al. (2001). A randomized trial of treatment for multisystem Langerhans cell histiocytosis. *J Pediatr*, **138**, 728–734. *Erratum J Pediatr*, **139**, 170.

Gianotti, R., Caputo, R. and Ermacora, E. (1971). Singuliere histiocytose infantile a cellules avec particules vermiformes intracytoplasmiques. *Bull Soc Fr Dermatol Syphil*, **78**, 232–233.

Goodman, W.T. and Barrett, T.L. (2003). Histiocytoses. In: Bolognia, J.L., Jorizzo, J.L. and Rapini, R.P., et al., eds. *Dermatology*, Mosby, Toronto. pp. 1429–1445.

Gorman, J.D., Danning, C., Schumacher, H.R., et al. (2000). Multicentric reticulohistiocytosis. *Arthritis Rheum*, **43**, 930–938.

Greenberger, J., Crocker, A., Vawter, G., et al. (1981). Results of treatment of 127 patients with systemic histiocytosis (Letterer–Siwe syndrome, Schuller–Christian syndrome and multifocal eosinophilic granuloma). *Medicine*, **60**, 311–338.

Hamre, M., Hedberg, J., Buckley, J., et al. (1997). Langerhans cell histiocytosis: an exploratory epidemiologic study of 177 cases. *Med Pediatr Oncol*, **28**, 92–97.

Hashimoto, K. and Pritzker, M.S. (1973). Electron microscopic study of reticulohistio-cytoma: an unusual case of congenital self-healing reticulohistiocytosis. *Arch Dermatol*, **107**, 263–270.

Hashimoto, K., Takahashi, S., Fligiel, A., et al. (1985). Eosinophilic granuloma. *Arch Dermatol*, **121**, 770–774.

Helm, K.F., Lookingbill, D.P. and Marks Jr, J.G. (1993). A clinical and pathologic study of histiocytosis X in adults. *J Am Acad Dermatol*, **29**, 166–170.

Helmbold, P., Hegemann, B., Holzhausen, H.-J., et al. (1998). Low dose oral etoposide monotherapy in adult Langerhans cell histiocytosis. *Arch Dermatol*, **134**, 1275–1278.

Henter, J.I., Elinder, G., Soder, O. et al. (1991). Incidence in Sweden and clinical features of familial hemophagocytic lymphohistiocytosis. *Acta Paediatr Scand*, **80**, 428–435.

Hernandez-Martin, A., Baselga, E., Drolet, B.A., *et al.* (1997). Juvenile xanthogranuloma. *J Am Acad Dermatol*, **36**, 355–367.

Hiramanek, N., Kossard, S. and Barnetson, R.S. (2002). Multicentric reticulohistiocytosis presenting with a rash and arthralgia. *Australas J Dermatol*, **43**, 136–139.

Hoeger, P.H., Janka-Schaub, G. and Mensing, H. (1997). Late manifestation of diabetes insipidus in 'pure' cutaneous Langerhans cell histiocytosis. *Eur J Pediatr*, **156**, 524–527.

Hoeger, P.H., Nanduri, V.R., Harper, J.L., *et al.* (2000). Long term follow up of topical mustine treatment for cutaneous Langerhans cell histiocytosis. *Arch Dis Child*, **82**, 483–487.

Holme, S.A. and Mills, C.M. (2002). Adult primary cutaneous Langerhans' cell histiocytosis mimicking nodular prurigo. *Clin Exp Dermatol*, **27**, 247–251.

Howarth, D.M., Gilchrist, G.S., Mullan, B.P., *et al.* (1999). Langerhans cell histiocytosis: diagnosis, natural history, management, and outcome. *Cancer*, **85**(10), 2278–2290.

Hsiung, S.H., Chan, E.F., Elenitsas, R., *et al.* (2003). Multicentric reticulohistiocytosis presenting with clinical features of dermatomyositis. *J Am Acad Dermatol*, **48**, S11–S14.

Inuzuka, M., Tomita, K., Tokura, Y., *et al.* (2003). Congenital self-healing reticulohistiocytosis presenting with hemorrhagic bullae. *J Am Acad Dermatol*, **48**(5 Suppl), S75–S77.

Janka, G.E. (1983). Familial hemophagocytic lymphohistiocytosis. *Eur J Pediatr*, **140**, 221–230.

Jensen, N.E., Sabharwal, S. and Walker, A. (1971). Naevoxanthoendothelioma and neurofibromatosis. *Br J Dermatol*, **85**, 326–330.

Jih, D.M., Salcedo, S.L. and Jaworsky, C. (2002). Benign cephalic histiocytosis: a case report and review. *J Am Acad Dermatol*, **47**(6), 908–913.

Kato, T., Matsuda, M., Ando, H., *et al.* (1981). A case of multifocal proliferations of histiocytic cells containing Langerhans' cell granules. *Am J Clin Pathol*, **76**, 480–485.

Kaudewitz, P., Przybilla, B., Chmoeckel, C., *et al.* (1986). Cutaneous lesions in histiocytosis X: successful treatment with PUVA. *J Invest Dermatol*, **86**, 324–325.

Kolde, G. and Brocker, E.-B. (1986). Multiple skin tumors of indeterminate cells in an adult. *J Am Acad Dermatol*, **15**, 591–597.

Kolde, G., Schulze, P. and Sterry, W. (2002). Mixed response to thalidomide therapy in adults: two cases of multisystem Langerhans' cell histiocytosis. *Acta Dermatol Venereol*, **82**, 384–386.

Kuttner, B.J., Friedman, K.J., Burton, C.S., *et al.* (1987). Letterer-Siwe disease in an adult. *Cutis*, **39**, 142–146.

Kwong, Y.L., Chan, A.C. and Chan, T.K. (1997). Widespread skin-limited Langerhans cell histiocytosis: complete remission with interferon alfa. *J Am Acad Dermatol*, **36**, 628–629.

Ladisch, S. and Gadner, H. (1994). Treatment of Langerhans' cell histiocytosis: evolution and current approaches. *Br J Cancer*, **70**, S41–S46.

Ladisch, S. and Jaffe, E.S. (1997). The histiocytoses. In: Pizzo, P.A. and Poplack, D.G., eds. *Principles and Practice of Pediatric Oncology*, 3rd edn. Lippincott, Philadelphia, pp. 613–631.

Levinsohn, D., Siedel, D., Phelps, A., *et al.* (1993). Solitary congenital indeterminate cell histiocytoma. *Arch Dermatol*, **129**, 81–85.

Lindelof, B., Forslind, B., Hilliges, M., *et al.* (1991). Langerhans' cell histiocytosis in an adult. *Acta Dermatol Venereol*, **71**, 178–180.

Longaker, M.A., Frieden, I.J., Leboit, P.E., *et al.* (1994). Congenital 'self-healing' Langerhans cell histiocytosis: the need for long-term follow-up. *J Am Acad Dermatol*, **31**, 910–916.

Machado, S., Alves, R., Lima, M., *et al.* (2001). Cutaneous necrobiotic xanthogranuloma (NXG) – successfully treated with low dose chlorambucil. *Eur J Dermatol*, 11, 458–462.

Magana-Garcia, M. (1986). Pure cutaneous histiocytosis X. *Int J Dermatol*, 25, 106–108.

Maher, D. (1993). Congenital Langerhans cell histiocytosis (histiocytosis X). *Br J Hosp Med*, 49, 500.

Manente, L., Cotellessa, C., Schmitt, I., *et al.* (1997). Indeterminate cell histiocytosis: a rare histiocytic disorder. *Am J Dermatopath*, 19, 276–283.

Mays, J.A., Neerhout, R.C., Bagby, C., *et al.* (1980). Juvenile chronic granulocytic leukemia: emphasis on cutaneous manifestations and underlying neurofibromatosis. *Am J Dis Child*, 134, 654–658.

McDonald, J.S., Miller, R.L., Bernstein, M.L., *et al.* (1980). Histiocytosis X: a clinical presentation. *J Oral Pathol*, 9, 342–349.

Mejia, R., Dano, J.A., Roberts, R., *et al.* (1997). Langerhans' cell histiocytosis in adults. *J Am Acad Dermatol*, 37, 314–317.

Meunier, L., Marck, Y., Ribeyre, C., *et al.* (1995). Adult cutaneous Langerhans cell histiocytosis: remission with thalidomide treatment. *Br J Dermatol*, 132, 168.

Misery, L., Rougier, N., Crestani, B., *et al.* (1999). Presence of circulating abnormal CD34+ progenitors in adult Langerhans cell histiocytosis. *Clin Exp Immunol*, 117, 177–182.

Montero, A.J., Diaz-Montero, C.M., Malpica, A., *et al.* (2003). Langerhans cell histiocytosis of the female genital tract: a literature review. *Int J Gynecol Cancer*, 13, 381–388.

Moraes, M. and Russo, G. (2001). Thalidomide and its dermatologic uses. *Am J Med Sci*, 321, 321–326.

Morrell, D.S., Pepping, M.A., Scott, J.P., *et al.* (2002). Cutaneous manifestations of hemophagocytic lymphohistiocytosis. *Arch Dermatol*, 138(9), 1208–1212.

Munn, S. and Chu, A.C. (1998). Langerhans cell histiocytosis of the skin. *Hematol Oncol Clin North Am*, 12(2), 269–286.

Nicholson, H.S., Egeler, R.M. and Nesbit, M.E. (1998). The epidemiology of Langerhans cell histiocytosis. *Hematol Oncol Clin North Am*, 12, 379–384.

Novice, F.M., Collison, D.W., Kleinsmith, D.M., *et al.* (1989). Letterer–Siwe disease in adults. *Cancer*, 63, 166–174.

Patel, R.R., Vander Straten, M.R. and Korman, N.J. (2003). The safety and efficacy of tacrolimus therapy in patients younger than 2 years with atopic dermatitis. *Arch Dermatol*, 139, 1184–1186.

Pujol, R.M., Moreno, A., Lopez, D., *et al.* (1988). Childhood self-healing histiocytosis X. *Pediatr Dermatol*, 5, 97–102.

Rivera-Luna, R., Alter-Molchadsky, N., Cardenas-Cardos, R., *et al.* (1996). Langerhans cell histiocytosis in children under 2 years of age. *Med Pediatr Oncol*, 26, 334–343.

Rodriguez-Jurado, R., Duran-McKinster, C. and Ruiz-Maldonado, R. (2000). Benign cephalic histiocytosis progressing into juvenile xanthogranuloma: a non-Langerhans cell histiocytosis transforming under the influence of a virus? *Am J Dermatopathol*, 22, 70–74.

Rodriguez-Valdes. J., Cordoba, M. and Perez-Espinosa, J. (1982). Hand–Schuller–Christian disease. *Cutis*, 29, 256–258; 268.

Rosenberg, A.A. and Morgan, M.B. (2001). Cutaneous indeterminate cell histiocytosis: a new spindle cell variant resembling dendritic cell sarcoma. *J Cut Pathol*, 28, 531–537.

Santillan, A., Montero, A.J., Kavanagh, J.J., *et al.* (2003). Vulvar Langerhans cell histiocytosis: a case report and review of the literature. *Gynec Oncol*, **9**, 241–246.

Santilli, D., Lo Monaco, A., Cavazzini, P.L., *et al.* (2002). Multicentric reticulohistiocytosis: a rare cause of erosive arthropathy of the distal interphalangeal finger joints. *Ann Rheum Dis*, **61**, 485–487.

Santhosh-Kumar, C.R., Al Momen, A., Ajarim, D.S., *et al.* (1990). Unusual skin tumors in Langerhans' cell histiocytosis. *Arch Dermatol*, **126**, 1617–1620.

Selch, M.T. and Parker, R.G. (1990). Radiation therapy in the management of Langerhans' cell histiocytosis. *Med Pediatr Oncol*, **18**, 97–102.

Seward, J.L., Malone, J.C. and Callen, J.P. (2004). Generalized eruptive histiocytosis. *J Am Acad Dermatol*, **50**, 116–120.

Shainhouse, T. and Eichenfield, L.F. (2003). Long-term safety of tacrolimus ointment in children treated for atopic dermatitis. *Expert Opin Drug Safety*, **2**, 457–465.

Sheehan, M.P., Atherton, D.J., Broadbent, V., *et al.* (1991). Topical nitrogen mustard: an effective treatment for cutaneous Langerhans' cell histiocytosis. *J Pediatr*, **119**, 317–321.

Shields, C.L., Shields, J.A. and Buchanon, H.W. (1990). Solitary orbital involvement with juvenile xanthogranuloma. *Arch Ophthalmol*, **108**, 1587–1589.

Simonart, T., Urbain, F., Verdebout, J.-M., *et al.* (2000). Langerhans' cell histiocytosis arising at the site of basal cell carcinoma excision. *J Cutan Pathol*, **27**, 476–478.

Singh, A., Prieto, V.G., Czelusta, A., *et al.* (2003). Adult Langerhans cell histiocytosis limited to the skin. *Dermatol*, **207**, 157–161.

Sohi, A.S., Tiwari, V.D., Subramaman, C.S., *et al.* (1979). Generalized eruptive histiocytoma. *Dermatologica*, **159**, 471–475.

Stein, S.L., Paller, A.S., Haut, P.R., *et al.* (2001). Langerhans cell histiocytosis presenting in the neonatal period: a retrospective case series. *Arch Pediatr Adolesc Med*, **155**, 778–783.

Stephan, J.L. (1995). Histiocytoses. *Eur J Pediatr*, **154**, 600–609.

Thomas, L., Ducros, B., Secchi, T., *et al.* (1993). Successful treatment of adult's Langerhans cell histiocytosis with thalidomide. *Arch Dermatol*. **129**, 1261–1264.

Tsambaos, D., Georgiou, S., Kapranos, N., *et al.* (1995). Langerhans' cell histiocytosis: complete remission after oral isotretinoin therapy. *Acta Dermatol Venereol*, **7**, 62–64.

Valladeau, J., Ravel, O., Dezutter-Dambuyant, C., *et al.* (2000). Langerin, a novel C-type lectin specific to Langerhans cells, is an endocytic receptor that induces the formation of Birbeck granules. *Immunity*, **12**, 71–81.

Van Heerde, P. and Egeler, R.M. (1991). Cytology of Langerhans' cell histiocytosis (histiocytosis X). *Cytopathology*, **2**, 149–158.

Venencie, P.Y., Le Bras, P., Toan, N.D., *et al.* (1995). Recombinant interferon alfa-2b treatment of necrobiotic xanthogranuloma with paraproteinemia. *J Am Acad Dermatol*, **32**, 666–667.

Vollum, D.I. (1979). Letterer–Siwe in the adult. *Clin Exp Dermatol*, **4**, 395–406.

Weiss, N. and Keller, C. (1993). Xanthoma disseminatum: a rare normolipemic xanthomatosis. *Clin Invest*, **71**, 233–238.

Wells, G.C. (1979). The pathology of adult type Letterer–Siwe disease. *Clin Exp Dermatol*, **4**, 407–412.

Wong, E., Holden, C.A., Broadbent, V., *et al.* (1986). Histiocytosis X presenting as intertrigo and responding to topical nitrogen mustard. *Clin Exp Dermatol*, **11**, 183–187.

Wright, A.L., Tucker, W.F.G., Slater, D.N., *et al.* (1985). Letterer–Siwe disease in the ninth decade. *J Am Acad Dermatol*, **12**, 369–371.

Yu, R.C. and Chu, A.C. (1995). Lack of T-cell receptor gene rearrangements in cells involved in Langerhans cell histiocytosis. *Cancer*, **75**, 1162–1166.

Zachary, C.B. and MacDonald, D.M. (1983). Hand–Schuller–Christian disease with secondary cutaneous involvement. *Clin Exp Dermatol*, **8**, 177–183.

Zelger, B. and Burgdorf, W.H. (2001). The cutaneous histiocytoses. *Adv Dermatol*, **17**, 77–114.

Zelger, B.G., Selger, B., Steiner, H., *et al.* (1995). Solitary giant xanthogranuloma and benign cephalic histiocytosis – variants of juvenile xanthogranuloma. *Br J Dermatol*, **133**, 598–604.

8

Langerhans cell histiocytosis of bone

Sheila Weitzman and R. Maarten Egeler

Bone is the commonest single organ involved in Langerhans cell histiocytosis (LCH) in children. Of 154 consecutive children admitted to a single large institution, 126 (81%) had bone involvement, of whom 80% had single system (SS) disease and 20% bone disease as part of multisystem (MS) LCH. A single bone was involved in 76% – unifocal bone (UFB) and two or more bones – multifocal bone (MFB) in 24% (Stuurman *et al.*, 2003), correlating almost exactly with the 78% UFB and 22% MFB found by the DAL-HX group (Titgemeyer *et al.*, 2001).

The commonest presentation of LCH in children is thus with UFB. The picture is different in adults in whom SS skin and lung disease predominate, and in whom bone is more often part of MS disease (Malpas, 1998; Aricò *et al.*, 1999, 2003).

Clinical aspects

The bones most commonly involved are skull, spine, lower extremity, pelvis, ribs and upper extremity (Table 8.1). Proximal long bones are commoner than distal (Figure 8.1) (Egeler *et al.*, 1999), and hands and feet are rarely involved. In adults the flat bones are involved more frequently, with jaw involved in 30% (Baumgartner *et al.*, 1997). The ribs accounted for only 6% of lesions in Baumgartner's series but was the second commonest bone affected in two other adult series (Kilpatrick *et al.*, 1995; Islinger *et al.*, 2000) (Figure 8.2). In the long bones diaphysis and metaphysis are equally involved, epiphysis is commonly spared, but epiphyseal location does not exclude LCH (Ghanem *et al.*, 2003).

Spontaneous healing of bone lesions is well known and healing at one site at the same time as, or followed by, progression in another is not uncommon.

Clinical presentation

The majority of patients present with pain and/or swelling. Symptoms are present during activity and at rest. Depending on the area involved, there may be additional

Table 8.1 Sites of bone involvement in adult and pediatric LCH patients

Series	Baumgartner[a] (adult) (%)	DAL-HX[b] (pediatric) (%)	Slater[c] (all ages) (%)
Skull	21	40	36
Extremity lower	17	17	14
Extremity upper		8	6
Ribs	6	7	12
Pelvis	13	10	10
Spine	13	18	8
Mandible	30	included with skull	7
Other			7

[a]Baumgartner *et al.* (1997), [b]Titgemeyer *et al.* (2001), [c]Slater and Swarm (1980).

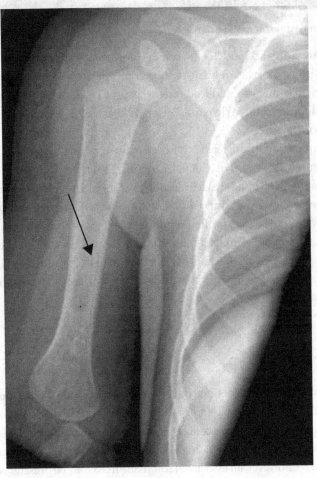

Figure 8.1   LCH – 'typical' lytic lesion in diaphysis of a long bone

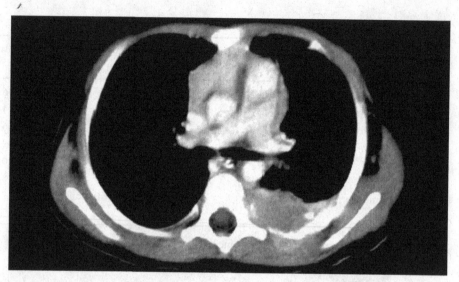

Figure 8.2   LCH involving rib, with soft tissue extension

symptoms. Jaw pain and loose teeth is a common complaint particularly in adult patients. Persistent otorrhea refractory to therapy, particularly with dermatitis of the outer auricular canal should lead one to suspect LCH, as should hypertrophic gingivitis and loose teeth (Aricò and Egeler, 1998). Lower extremity lesions may cause a limp or fracture.

A rare complication of calvarial LCH is an acute epidural hematoma, unrelated to biopsy or curettage (Lee *et al.*, 2000; Cho *et al.*, 2001).

Most patients with SS bone are afebrile, but fever should not exclude the diagnosis. Blood counts may show mild eosinophilia, but are otherwise normal and the erythrocyte sedimentation rate (ESR) is often mildly elevated (Slater and Swarm, 1980).

Bone lesions may be completely asymptomatic, and because of the different prognosis and therapy of UFB and MFB, every patient should have a complete work-up at first diagnosis, irrespective of presentation (see Chapter 6 for recommended investigations).

Special sites

Spine

Spine LCH comprises 7–15% of bone disease (Guzey *et al.*, 2003), and includes vertebral body (VB), pedicle, lamina and/or transverse process (Ghanem *et al.*, 2003). Presentation is with pain, kyphoscoliosis and/or neurologic symptoms. LCH is the commonest cause of vertebra plana in children (Villas *et al.*, 1993; Kamimura *et al.*, 2000) (Figure 8.3), however, an associated soft tissue mass may be present. Neurologic complications arise from extension of tumor into the extradural space, rather than

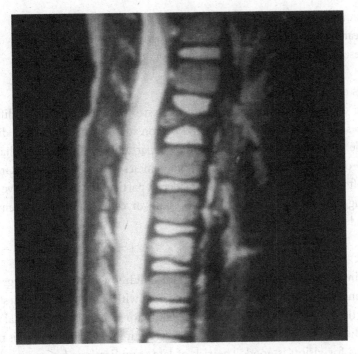

Figure 8.3   LCH spine – vertebra plana

compression from bone (Haggstrom *et al.*, 1998), although a patient became para-plegic from involvement of two adjacent VBs (Turgut and Gurcay, 1992).

Characteristically LCH does not disturb endochondral ossification thereby allowing some recovery of vertebral height (Raab *et al.*, 1998). Recovery does not only occur in the youngest patients as previously published (Ippolito *et al.*, 1984).

Differential diagnosis of spine LCH

Other causes of the 'characteristic' finding of vertebra plana are osteomyelitis, infantile myofibromatosis (Dautenheimer *et al.*, 1995), juvenile xanthogranuloma (Dehner, 2003) aneurysmal bone cyst, osteogenesis inperfecta, leukemia, lymph-oma and malignant sarcomas, such as Ewings and osteogenic sarcoma (Yeom *et al.*, 1999). Several cases are reported where misdiagnosis as LCH led to significant delay in therapy of Ewings sarcoma (Emir *et al.*, 1999; Kager *et al.*, 1999). In adults myeloma must be considered.

Temporal bone

Temporal bone involvement may be unilateral or bilateral, and may include involve-ment only of the petrous bone. Extensive bony destruction and an associated soft tis-sue mass are frequent. The commonest presentation is with mucopurulent otorrhea, a post-auricular swelling (Koch, 2000), aural polyps and peri-auricular skin disease. Hearing loss, vertigo and facial nerve paralysis are rare. Petrous involvement may present with proptosis and diplopia.

Differential diagnosis of temporal bone lesions

Chronic otitis media, mastoiditis and cholesteatoma are the major differential diagnoses. Temporal bone LCH should be considered whenever these diagnoses are made in children less than 3 years of age, particularly if radiologic changes are out of proportion to clinical findings. Malignancies such as rhabdomyosarcoma or other soft tissue sarcomas should be considered, particularly if cranial nerve involvement suggests extension to the base of skull or central nervous system (CNS) (Fernández-Latorre et al., 2000).

Orbit

Orbital involvement was seen in 14% of 275 children with LCH at a large institution (Nanduri et al., 2003). It is often associated with significant bony destruction and soft tissue swelling. Presentation is usually with proptosis, peri-orbital swelling and erythema, diplopia and ophthalmoplegia (Figure 8.4). Loss of vision is rare, and prognosis for vision is good. The risk of late complications however, is high. In Nanduri's series, diabetes insipidus (DI) developed in 40%, anterior pituitary deficiency in 26% and CNS abnormalities in 23%.

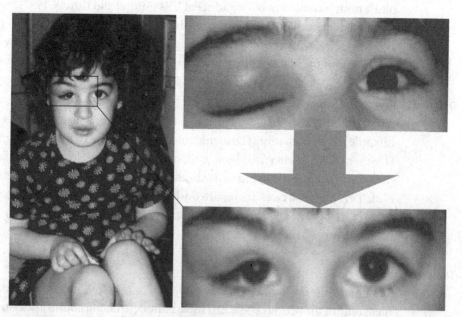

Figure 8.4   LCH bone presenting as peri-orbital cellulitis

Differental diagnosis of orbital LCH

Differential diagnosis of unilateral orbital LCH is acute infection, dermoid cyst, inflammatory pseudotumor, lymphangioma, hemangioma, rhabdomyosarcoma, lymphoma, and anterior optic glioma, while bilateral involvement would suggest infection, metastatic neuroblastoma, nasopharyngeal rhabdomyosarcoma or rarely

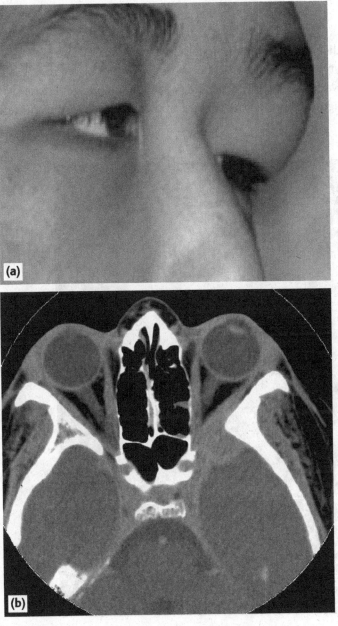

Figure 8.5   LCH involving orbital margin (a) clinical presentation, (b) CT scan

acute leukemia with orbital infiltration (Figure 8.5(a) and (b)). Erdheim–Chester disease is another histiocytic disorder that classically involves orbit as may other forms of xanthogranuloma and sinus histiocytosis with massive lymphadenopathy.

Radiologic investigation of bone LCH

Plain radiographs

Plain radiographs remain the first investigation in LCH patients.

The typical appearance is a 'punched-out' lytic lesion, but the radiologic characteristics vary considerably depending on site, and phase of disease (Potepan *et al.*, 1996) (Figure 8.6 (a) and (b)). In the commonest site, the calvarium, lesions usually

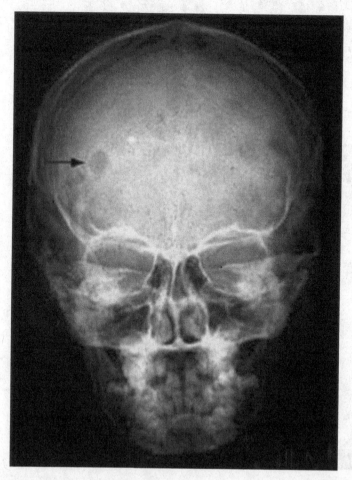

Figure 8.6a   LCH – 'Punched-out' lytic lesion in skull

appear osteolytic with sharply demarcated margins and little or no peri-osteal reaction. Beveling, or asymmetric involvement of the inner and outer skull tables, is characteristic. There is commonly an associated mass, which may extend extra-cranially or intracranially and may cause compression of brain (Figure 8.7).

By contrast, lesions which involve orbit, mastoid or other areas of skull base are often extensive and irregular, with a soft tissue component that may strongly resemble a malignant tumor (Potepan *et al.*, 1996) (Figure 8.8). In one series, 14 of 15 children with lesions involving skull base or facial bones had destructive lesions with soft tissue masses (Meyer *et al.*, 1995). In the mandible, the bone may be completely destroyed and the teeth left with no visible support, so-called 'floating teeth'.

Similarly in long bones, LCH may present as classic lytic lesions or may present with aggressive radiologic features with poorly-defined borders, a significant peri-osteal reaction and a large soft tissue mass that must be differentiated from a malignancy (Ruppert *et al.*, 1989; Potepan *et al.*, 1996) (Figure 8.9). With healing there is disappearance of the mass with recalcification and development of a well-defined sclerotic rim.

Bone scintigraphy

Technetium-99 nuclear medicine scans appear to be less sensitive than radiography for detection of LCH lesions (Ruppert *et al.*, 1989; Meyer *et al.*, 1995). In the series from the DAL-HX group, 97% of lesions were visible on radiographs, 82%

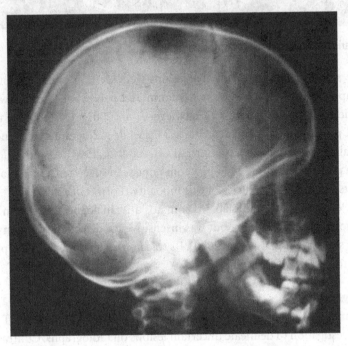

Figure 8.6b Typical lytic lesion in calvarium

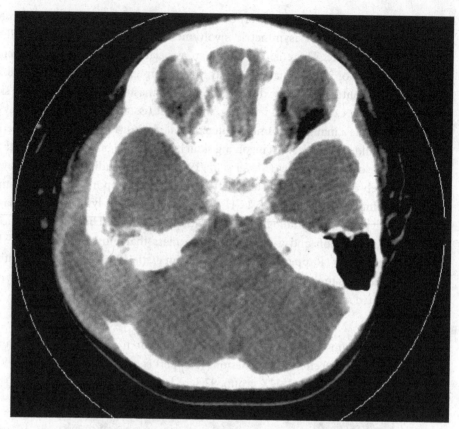

Figure 8.7   LCH calvarium, soft tissue mass compressing brain

on bone scan ($P \leqslant 0.001$). Only five lesions were seen on bone scan but not on radiograph, and in particular spinal column and pelvic bone lesions were more readily detected by radiographs (Titgemeyer *et al.*, 2001). It is possible that bone scans are positive in early and evolving lesions while radiographs continue to show abnormalities until healing has occurred (Meyer *et al.*, 1995). As well as lower sensitivity, a patient with spine LCH in whom bone scan suggested a malignant lesion, highlights the lack of specificity of this modality (Porn *et al.*, 2003).

[111]In-Pentetreotide, a radiolabeled somatostatin analogue, was shown to detect LCH lesions in lung and bone but was insensitive for detection of lesions in CNS, liver and skin (Weinmann *et al.*, 2000). Its role in investigation and therapy of LCH remains to be determined.

Computerized tomography

Lesions are usually well seen on computerized tomography (CT) and CT skull is a useful investigation to delineate uncertain lesions on radiographs. Contrast images delineate the soft tissue involvement and peri-osteal reaction.

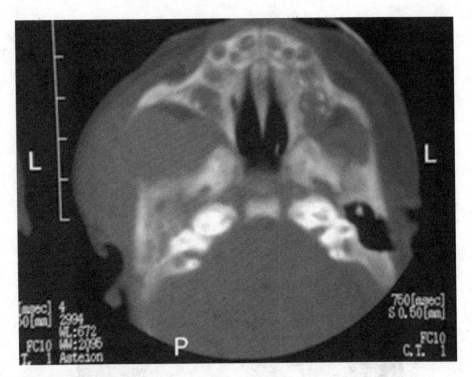

Figure 8.8   Radiologically aggressive bone LCH

Magnetic resonance imaging

Magnetic resonance imaging (MRI) findings include a hypo- or isointense mass on T1 weighted images, becoming hyperintense on T2, with moderate to intense gadolinium uptake (Koch, 2000). MRI abnormalities are prominent in bone marrow and surrounding soft tissues where a poorly-defined signal hyperintensity with irregular margins may be present (Potepan *et al.*, 1996). With healing the sclerotic rim seen on radiographs, is seen as an area of lucency surrounding the lesion. MRI is most useful for evaluating the extraosseous extent of disease and planning of biopsies or surgery, however neither CT nor MRI is useful in distinguishing benign from malignant disease in radiologically aggressive lesions (Hayes *et al.*, 1992). Bone lesions that are indistinguishable clinically and radiologically from malignant tumors, have the same favorable outcome as more typical LCH lesions (Lau *et al.*, 2003). Clinicians must be aware of the less common radiologic appearances to avoid over-treatment (Figure 8.9).

In addition, occasional patients with radiologically 'typical' LCH have proven on biopsy to have osteomyelitis, myofibromatosis (Dautenheimer *et al.*, 1995), Juvenile xanthogranuloma (Dehner, 2003) and lymphoma. There is no radiologic appearance that is absolutely specific for LCH (Fisher *et al.*, 1995). The diagnosis should be proven pathologically whenever possible.

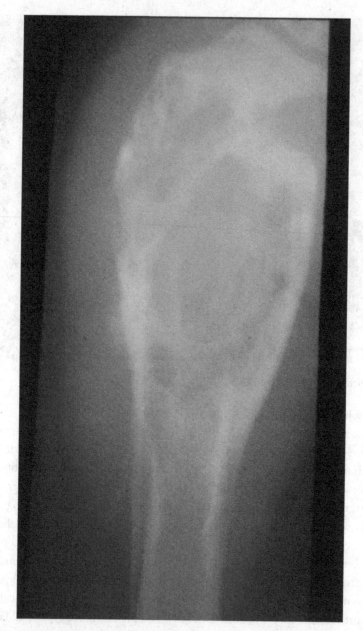

Figure 8.9   LCH involving proximal humerus with peri-osteal reaction

Coincidence FDG PET scan

Positron emission tomography (PET) is a sensitive technique for identifying active lesions. In a study of three patients with LCH, PET scans identified all active osseous lesions, differentiated active from healed lesions and demonstrated normalization of uptake in a treated lesion earlier than bone scan and radiography

(Binkovitz *et al.*, 2003). Further study is needed. PET may be a useful modality to evaluate therapy but cost and availability limit its usefulness.

Therapy

Effective therapies for bone LCH include observation, biopsy, curettage, intralesional steroids, non-steroidal anti-inflammatory drugs (NSAIDS), bisphosphonates, chemotherapy, low-dose radiation therapy and various forms of immunotherapy.

Observation is limited to lesions in 'non-risk' bones, in patients in whom a pathologic diagnosis has been previously made. Patients who have intense pain, restriction of motion, unacceptable deformity, involvement of a growth plate or involvement of a bone likely to fracture, usually require some form of therapy (Egeler *et al.*, 1992).

In patients presenting with vertebra plana, a decision may be made to observe the patient without therapy and without a firm diagnosis. Those patients should be carefully followed (see later).

Intralesional steroid

Intralesional steroid may be used for solitary bone lesions, or as adjunctive therapy for MFB, and is best inserted under radiographic control. Generally there is rapid relief of pain, followed by predictable healing. Yasko *et al.* utilized fine needle aspirate or percutaneous biopsy for solitary lesions, and inserted intralesional methylprednisolone (100–150 mg) at the same procedure in the majority. Only 10% required open biopsy for diagnosis. Between 10% (Yasko *et al.*, 1998) and 27% (Egeler *et al.*, 1992) require a repeat injection. Other steroids such as triamcinolone have been utilized (Fernández-Latorre *et al.*, 2000). The method is cost-effective when compared to surgery or radiation therapy. Possible complications include infection, necrosis, bleeding, impaired healing and thinning of the skin, however few serious complications have been reported (Egeler *et al.*, 1992; Yasko *et al.*, 1998).

Non-steroidal anti-inflammatory drugs

Indomethacin, a potent prostaglandin-2 inhibitor, resulted in CR in 8 of 10 patients treated in one series, six with UFB, four with MFB (Munn *et al.*, 1999). Dose ranged from 1–2.5 mg/kg/day for 1–16 weeks (mean 6). Many more anecdotal cases have been treated with good responses, and with other NSAIDS including naproxen and ibuprofen (Arceci *et al.*, 1998). Uncertainty remains regarding its role in promoting healing versus a pure analgesic effect (Munn *et al.*, 1999), as well as its role in preventing disease reactivation.

Radiation therapy

The use of radiation therapy has decreased in recent years, because of concerns regarding late effects, including second tumors. However, low-dose radiation (6–10 Gy) remains an effective modality when the disease threatens the function of a critical organ such a spinal cord or optic nerve (Ladisch and Gadner, 1994). It is unlikely that interference with skeletal growth or second tumors will occur at the recommended dose, but no completely safe dose for thyroid problems or second tumors is known.

Bisphosphonate therapy

Bisphosphonates are osteoclast inhibitors and have been shown to decrease cytokine/prostaglandin production. Their activity in LCH is likely through reduction in LCH cell proliferation and reduced formation, and function of osteoclasts (Brown, 2001; Farran et al., 2001). The analgesic effect is likely through increase in bone structure, and decrease in inflammatory mediators (Farran et al., 2001). Despite a theoretical advantage for second- and third-generation amine-bisphosphonates such as pamidronate and alendronate (Brown, 2001), the non-amine bisphosphonate etidronate 200 mg/m^2/day $\times$ 14 days every 3 months (Kamizono et al., 2002), as well as intravenous (iv) pamidronate 2 mg/kg daily for 3 days/month (Farran et al., 2001) have been shown to be effective in bone LCH in children and adults.

It has been suggested that pamidronate will act synergistically with interferon-α to treat LCH osteolytic lesions, because of activity against different pathways which induce osteoclastogenesis (Brown, 2003). Toxicity has been tolerable in most patients. One patient developed nephrotic syndrome and renal failure after pamidronate therapy for LCH (Lockridge et al., 2002). In rare instances these drugs can cause serious ocular adverse effects, visual or ocular symptoms should be referred immediately for consultation (Fraunfelder and Fraunfelder, 2003).

The long-term effects of bisphosphonates on growing bones are not known, and it is unclear whether bisphosphonates ± Interferon-α would prevent progression to CNS/endocrine complications.

Chemotherapy

Patients with MFB or bone LCH in MS disease, are usually treated with chemotherapy.

Many combinations have been used, the commonest is the combination of vinblastine and prednisone ± a third drug, although many drugs have demonstrated efficacy.

It has been suggested that the vinca alkaloid/steroid combination is not as effective in adults as in children, and that alternative drugs such as azathioprine and prolonged oral etoposide, have produced responses when other drugs have failed (Munn et al., 2001). Cladribine (2CdA) is a nucleoside analogue shown to have activity in multiple pretreated patients, with a favorable short-term toxicity profile (Saven and Burian, 1999). This drug appears to be effective against active CNS LCH (Watts and Files, 2001) and was shown to reverse DI in a recent patient (Ottaviano and Finlay, 2003). Due to good CNS penetration, 2-CdA may have the potential for reducing late CNS toxicity. This remains to be proven in prospective randomized trials which also evaluate long-term effects of the drug (see Chapter 13).

Effective chemotherapy usually results in immediate relief of pain, followed by healing of bone lesions, although healing is not accelerated (see below).

In MS disease, chemotherapy is warranted for treatment of lesions other than bone. In MFB disease, the natural history, plus the availability of therapy which appears to be effective in treating pain and accelerating healing such as NSAIDS and bisphosphonates, means that the use of chemotherapy requires more justification than pain, or regression of bone lesions.

Overview of therapeutic decision-making

Decisions with regard to therapy are confounded by the fact that bone lesions may resolve without therapy or with minimal local therapy such as biopsy, curettage or intralesional steroids. It might be expected that getting rid of active LCH with adjuvant therapy would accelerate healing, however chemotherapy alone, chemotherapy with radiation or radiation alone does not appear to alter the rate of healing (Sartoris and Parker, 1984; Womer et al., 1985; Bollini et al., 1991).

In this era however, resolution of bone lesions is only one of the criteria to be considered when making a treatment decision. Late sequelae were seen in 64% of patients with more than 3 years follow-up. These included skeletal defects 42%, dental problems 30%, DI 25%, growth failure 20%, sex hormone deficiency 16%, hypothyroidism 14%, hearing loss 16% and other CNS dysfunction 14% (Willis et al., 1996), as well as hyperprolactinemia and morbid obesity (Municchi et al., 2002). It appears that late effects are commoner with facial bone or skull-base disease, especially if associated with an intracranial soft tissue mass.

The permanent and sometimes devastating nature of the late effects described, must figure into therapeutic decision-making.

Therapy of 'non-risk' bones

In solitary calvarial lesions (the commonest presentation of childhood LCH), solitary extremity, pelvic or rib lesions, initial therapy is usually by curettage, which performs the dual function of supplying diagnostic tissue and initiating healing. Surgeons should be discouraged from attempting complete excisions, thereby leaving large defects which often require secondary repair, and is unnecessary for cure. For most patients with UFB lesions, no adjuvant therapy is required.

Therapy of 'risk' bones

Spine

The optimal treatment for spinal LCH is still debated and includes observation, prolonged immobilization, radiation therapy, chemotherapy and curettage with a reconstructive bone graft (Guzey et al., 2003). When vertebra plana occurs with intact intravertebral disks above and below, without an associated mass or signs of infection, the relative risk of biopsy means that observation without biopsy and with careful follow-up is appropriate (Yeom et al., 1999; Guzey et al., 2003). Due to the potential for disaster if an infection or malignancy is missed, the presence of a soft tissue mass, neurologic deficit or systemic symptoms should be an indication for biopsy, despite the good result reported by Kamimura et al. (2000), who treated two patients with spinal cord compression conservatively, one without biopsy confirmation, with good results.

Generally curettage is not recommended because it leads to decreased potential for vertebral reconstitution (Guzey et al., 2003), an opinion confirmed by Yeom et al. (1999) who found that the worst results occurred in patients who underwent surgery. These authors felt that prolonged bracing and casting was unnecessary once pain had subsided and the VB had begun to regain height.

For patients with neurologic deficit there is controversy regarding the best therapy, Yeom et al. (1999) feel that low-dose radiation therapy gives a rapid response and the least long-term effects. Other investigators prefer a surgical approach for patients with neurologic symptoms or spinal instability (Raab et al., 1998; Kamimura et al., 2000; Guzey et al., 2003). It is unlikely that low-dose radiation (below 1000 cGy) will produce long-term problems, and in the absence of recent onset of complete paralysis, radiation may be a reasonable option.

For those with two adjacent vertebrae involved or who are not likely to comply with activity restriction or follow-up, short-segmental fusion and internal fixation may be indicated (Guzey et al., 2003).

Treatment of temporal bone LCH

Treatment of temporal bone lesions with surgical excision resulted in a high morbidity that included transient facial nerve palsy, sensorineural or conductive hearing loss, post-auricular fistulas (Irving et al., 1994; Koch, 2000). Use of more conservative approaches such as biopsy and intralesional steroids is effective with a much lower morbidity. Temporal bone surgery should be avoided except for occasional débridement (Koch, 2000).

The worrying finding of chronic mastoid disease on MRI scans of patients with CNS abnormalities, suggests the possibility that these lesions should be treated early with systemic therapy (Grois N, Personal Communication). However in a series of 14 patients, only four with MS disease developed DI after reactivation (Fernández-Latorre et al., 2000).

Therapy of orbital and facial bone LCH

Aggressive surgery is contraindicated in LCH of orbit or face. Fine needle aspirate or percutaneous biopsy is indicated in all cases, as most have an aggressive appearance radiologically. If isolated and accessible, intralesional steroid has been used successfully, as has low-dose radiation therapy, particularly if the optic nerve is involved. Chemotherapy is recommended for facial/orbital involvement with intra-cranial extension, or if part of MS or MFB disease, in view of the high risk of late complications.

For other unifocal face/orbital LCH chemotherapy could likely be delayed until reactivation.

Reactivation of disease

Reactivation of disease, defined as recurrence after achieving a complete remission, is one of the most difficult problems in LCH. Recent review of 563 patients from the Histiocyte Society LCH data-base, showed that 134 reactivated, all within 2 years of diagnosis, giving a 5-year cumulative risk of 29%. The risk of second reactivation was much lower, being 8%, while the 5-year cumulative risk of a third or subsequent reactivation was 3% or less (Minkov et al., 2003). The risk is significantly higher in MS (70%) than in SS disease, and in MFB (26%) than UFB (12%) (Stuurman et al., 2003). It is clear from many studies that the rate of late neuro/ endocrine complications increases with the reactivation rate, with the highest incidence in patients with MS disease.

Possibly if reactivations could be prevented, these major late sequelae might be prevented as well. Except for the minority of patients who present initially with DI, most patients with DI have had previous chemotherapy and many investigators feel that therapy does not alter the natural history of LCH. This may be a reflection of the chemotherapy used or the duration, however. In the DAL-HX studies utilizing five drugs and 12 months of chemotherapy for MS patients, the reactivation rate was reduced to 27%, compared to a reactivation rate of 53% and 61%, respectively with 6 months of therapy given on the LCH-1 and -2 protocols (Gadner et al., 2001). Similar results were found when 'risk' and 'low-risk' patients were evaluated separately, raising the possibility that longer duration therapy would also decrease reactivations in SS patients.

Furthermore although recommendations for therapy of MFB patients were not included in the LCH-2 protocol, 104 patients were registered with the study center. Of the 104, 68 were treated with systemic therapy and 36 with local therapy, the risk of reactivation was 52% for local therapy, 45% for monotherapy, 20% for two drug therapy and 10% for DAL-HX 83 combination therapy (Gadner et al., 2001). In the DAL studies, DI occurred in only one patient with localized disease and 10% of patients with disseminated disease when DAL therapy was promptly instituted (Grois et al., 1995).

While these suffer from the problems of retrospective studies, there is suggestive evidence that combination therapy given for a longer duration may decrease the reactivation and late complication rates.

An anecdotal report of daily oral 6-Mercaptopurine and weekly oral methotrexate given for a 24-month period preventing reactivations in a small number of Swedish patients (Henter, Personal Communication) raises the possibility of trying 24 months of low toxicity oral maintenance therapy, for those patients who have a second reactivation. A preliminary report of 11 cases from Denmark confirms the potential utility and low toxicity of this combination in children with recurrent LCH (Ibsen Bank *et al.*, 2002).

Conclusions

UFB LCH is the commonest presentation of LCH in childhood. Most cases, but possibly excluding the 'risk' bones described above, need no therapy other than local therapy.

Very few fatalities are seen in patients with SS bone LCH, whether they have UFB or MFB disease. Progression to widespread MS disease, as seen in young infants with SS skin disease, does not appear to occur, even in younger patients with SS bone.

Patients with MFB or bone involvement as part of MS disease, have a much higher risk of reactivation and of progression to major late sequelae.

It is unclear whether chemotherapy alters the course of the disease, but the high incidence and severity of the consequences makes finding a solution mandatory.

The findings of the DAL studies suggest that limiting the period of disease activity by early and effective therapy reduces the permanent consequences. Utilization of chemotherapy later in the course of the disease when hypothalamic pituitary adrenal (HPA) abnormalities are established likely does not. For these reasons, members of the Histiocyte Society decided to recommend systemic therapy for patients with 'risk' bone involvement at diagnosis, even if unifocal, if associated with a large soft tissue mass. In addition, the decision was made to change the recommendation for patients presenting with DI, so that those patients also receive systemic therapy as early as possible after diagnosis, in order to try to reverse the DI (likely in a minority of patients only), but also to try to prevent the progression to anterior pituitary disease, and neurologic and neuropsychologic dysfunction.

The best drugs to use and the duration of therapy required are the focus of ongoing studies.

REFERENCES

Arceci, R.J., Brenner, M.K. and Pritchard, J. (1998). Controversies and new approaches to treatment of LCH. *Hematol Oncol Clin North Am*, **12**, 339–357.

Aricò, M. and Egeler, R.M. (1998). Clinical aspects of Langerhans' cell histiocytosis. *Hematol Oncol Clin North Am*, **12**, 247–258.

Aricò, M., Nichols, K., Whitlock, J.A., *et al.* (1999). Familial clustering of Langerhans' cell histiocytosis. *Br J Haematol*, **107**, 883–888.

Aricò, M., Girschikofsky, M., Généreau, T., *et al.* (2003). Langerhans' cell histiocytosis in adults report from the International Registry of the Histiocyte Society. *Eur J Cancer*, **39**, 2341–2348.

Baumgartner, I., von Hochstetter, A., Baumert, B., *et al.* (1997). Langerhans' cell histiocytosis in adults. *Med Pediatr Oncol*, **28**, 9–14.

Binkovitz, L.A., Olshefski, R.S. and Adler, B.H. (2003). Coincidence FDG-PET in the evaluation of Langerhans' cell histiocytosis: preliminary findings. *Pediatr Radiol*, **33**, 598–602.

Bollini, G., Jouve, J.L., Gentet, J.C., *et al.* (1991). Bone lesions in Histiocytosis X. *J Pediatr Orthop*, **11**, 469–477.

Brown, R.E. (2001). More on pamidronate in Langerhans' cell histiocytosis. *New Engl J Med*, **345**, 1503.

Brown, R.E. (2003). Interferon-alpha therapy, protein kinase C-alpha and Langerhans' cell histiocytosis. *Med Pediatr Oncol*, **41**, 63–64.

Cho, D.-Y., Liau, W.-R. and Chiang, I.-P. (2001). Eosinophilic granuloma with acute epidural hematoma. *Pediatr Neurosurg*, **35**, 266–269.

Dautenheimer, L., Blaser, S.I., Weitzman, S., *et al.* (1995). Infantile myofibromatosis as a cause of vertebra plana. *Am J Neuroradiol*, **16**(Suppl. 4), 828–830.

Dehner, L.P. (2003). Juvenile xanthogranulomas in the first two decades of life: a clinicopathologic study of 174 cases with cutaneous and extracutaneous manifestations. *Am J Surg Pathol*, **27**, 579–593.

Egeler, R.M., Thompson, R.C., Voûte, P.A., *et al.* (1992). Intralesional infiltration of corticosteroids in localized Langerhans' cell histiocytosis. *J Pediatr Orthop*, **12**, 811–814.

Egeler, R.M., Favara, B.E., van Meurs, M., *et al.* (1999). Differential *in situ* cytokine profiles of Langerhans'-like cells and T cells in Langerhans' cell histiocytosis: abundant expression of cytokines relevant to disease and treatment. *Blood*, **94**, 4195–4201.

Emir, S., Akyüz, C., Yazici, M., *et al.* (1999). Vertebra plana as a manifestation of Ewing Sarcoma in a child-letter to the editor. *Med Pediatr Oncol*, **33**, 594–595.

Farran, R.P., Zaretski, E. and Egeler, R.M. (2001). Treatment of Langerhans' cell histiocytosis with Pamidronate. *J Pediatr Hematol Oncol*, **23**, 54–56.

Fernández-Latorre, F., Menor-Serrano, F., Alonso-Charterina, S., *et al.* (2000). Langerhans' cell histiocytosis of the temporal bone in pediatric patients. *Am J Roentg*, **174**, 217–221.

Fisher, A.J., Reinus, W.R., Friedland, J.A., *et al.* (1995). Quantitative analysis of the plain radiographic appearance of eosinophilic granuloma. *Invest Radiol*, **8**, 466–473.

Fraunfelder, P.W. and Fraunfelder, F.T. (2003). Bisphosphonates and ocular inflammation. *New Engl J Med*, **348**, 1187–1188.

Gadner, H., Grois, N., Aricò, M., *et al.* (2001). A randomized trial of treatment for multisystem Langerhans' cell histiocytosis. *J Pediatr*, **138**, 728–734.

Ghanem, I., Tolo, V.T., D'Ambra, P., *et al.* (2003). Langerhans' cell histiocytosis of bone in children and adolescents. *J Pediatr Orthop*, **23**, 124–130.

Grois, N., Flucher-Wolfram, B., Heitger, A., *et al.* (1995). Diabetes Insipidus in Langerhans' cell histiocytosis: results from the DAL-HX 83 study. *Med Pediatr Oncol*, **24**, 248–256.

Guzey, F.K., Bas, N.S., Emel, E., *et al.* (2003). Polyostotic monosystemic calvarial and spinal Langerhans' cell histiocytosis treated by surgery and chemotherapy. *Pediatr Neurosurg*, **38**, 206–211.

Haggstrom, J.A., Brown, J.C. and Marsh, P.W. (1998). Eosiniphilic Granuloma of the spine: MR demonstration. *J Comput Assist Tomogr*, **12**, 344–345.

Hayes, C.W., Conway, W.F., and Sundaram, M. (1992). Misleading aggressive MR imaging appearance of some benign musculoskeletal lesions. *Radiographics*, **12**, 1119–1134.

Ibsen Bank, M., Rengtved, P., Carstensen, H., *et al.* (2002). High expression of markers of apoptosis and proliferation in Langerhans' cell histiocytosis. *J Pediatr Hematol Oncol*, **24**, 733–738.

Ippolito, E., Farsetti, P., and Tudisco, C. (1984). Vertebra plana, long term follow up in five patients. *J Bone Joint Surg (Am)*, 1364–1368.

Irving, R.M., Broadbent, V., and Jones, N.S. (1994). Langerhans' cell histiocytosis in childhood: management of head and neck manifestations. *Laryngoscope*, **104**, 64–70.

Islinger, R.B., Kuklo, T.R., Owens, B.D., *et al.* (2000). Langerhans' cell histiocytosis in patients older than 21 years. *Clin Orthop*, **379**, 231–235.

Kager, L., Zoubek, A., Kotz, R., *et al.* (1999). Misleading leads. Vertebra plana due to a Ewing tumor. *Med Pediatr Oncol*, **32**, 57–59.

Kamimura, M., Kinoshita, T., Itoh, H., *et al.* (2000). Eosinophilic granuloma of the spine: early spontaneous disappearance of tumor detected on magnetic resonance imaging. *J Neurosurg*, **93**(Suppl. 2), 312–316.

Kamizono, J., Okada Y., Shirahata, A., *et al.* (2002). Bisphosphonate induces remission of refractory osteolysis in Langerhans' cell histiocytosis. *J Bone Joint Surg*, **17**, 1926–1928.

Kilpatrick, S.E., Wenger, D.E., Gilchrist, G.S., *et al.* (1995). Langerhans' cell histiocytosis (histiocytosis X) of bone. *Cancer*, **76**, 2471–2484.

Koch, B. (2000). Langerhans' cell histiocytosis of temporal bone: role of magnetic resonance imaging. *Top Magn Reson Imaging*, **11**, 66–74.

Ladisch, S. and Gadner, H. (1994). Treatment of Langerhans' cell histiocytosis-evolution and current approaches. *Br J Cancer*, **70**(Suppl. XXIII), S41–S46.

Lau, L., Stuurman, K.E., Doda, W., *et al.* (2003). Radiologically aggressive Langerhans' cell histiocytosis (LCH) bone lesions in children. *Proc XIX meeting Histiocyte Society,* Philadelphia.

Lee, K.-W., McCleary, M.S., Zuppan, C.W., *et al.* (2000). Langerhans' cell histiocytosis presenting with an intracranial epidural hematoma. *Pediatr Radiol*, **30**, 326–328.

Lockridge, L., Papac, R.J. and Perazella, M.A. (2002). Pamidronate-associated nephrotoxicity in a patient with Langerhans's histiocytosis. *Am J Kidney Dis*, **40**, E2.

Malpas, J.S. (1998). Langerhans' cell histiocytosis in adults. *Hematol Oncol Clin North Am*, **12**, 259–268.

Meyer, J.S., Harty, M.P., Mabboubi, S., *et al.* (1995). Langerhans' cell histiocytosis: presentation and evolution of radiologic findings with clinical correlation. *Radiographics*, **15**, 1135–1146.

Minkov, M., Grois, N., Braier, J., *et al.* (2003). Immunosuppressive therapy for chemotherapy-resistant multisystem Langerhans' cell histiocytosis. *Med Pediatr Oncol*, **40**, 253–256.

Municchi, G., Marconcini, S., D'Ambrosio, A., *et al.* (2002). Central precocious puberty in multisystem Langerhans' cell histiocytosis: a case report. *Pediatr Hematol Oncol*, **19**, 273–278.

Munn, S., Murray, S. and Chu, A.C. (2001). Adult Langerhans' cell histiocytosis – a review of 46 cases. *Med Pediatr Oncol*, **38**, 222.

Munn, S.E., Olliver, L., Broadbent, V., *et al.* (1999). Use of Indomethacin in Langerhans' cell histiocytosis. *Med Pediatr Oncol*, **32**, 247–249.

Nanduri, V., Titgemeyer, C. and Brock, P. (2003). Long term outcome of orbital involvement in Langerhans' cell histiocytosis. *Med Pediatr Oncol*, **40**, 176.

Ottaviano, F. and Finlay, J.L. (2003). Diabetes Insipidus and Langerhans' cell histiocytosis: a case report of reversibility with 2-Chlorodeoxyadenosine. *J Pediatr Hematol Oncol*, **25**, 575–577.

Porn, U., Howman-Giles, R., Onkel, E., *et al.* (2003). Langerhans' cell histiocytosis of the lumbar spine. *Clin Nuclear Med*, **28**, 52–53.

Potepan, P., Tesoro-Tess, J.D., Laffranchi, A., *et al.* (1996). Langerhans' cell histiocytosis mimicking malignancy: a radiologic appraisal. *Tumori*, **82**, 603–609.

Raab, P., Hohmann, F., Kühl, J., *et al.* (1998). Vertebral remodeling in eosinophilic granuloma of the spine. *Spine*, **23**, 1351–1354.

Ruppert, D., Oria, R.A., Kumar, R., *et al.* (1989). Radiologic features of eosinophilic granuloma of bone. *Am J Roentgenol*, **153**, 1021–1026.

Sartoris, D.J. and Parker, B.R. (1984). Histiocytosis X: rate and pattern of resolution of osseous lesions. *Radiology*, **152**, 679–684.

Saven, A. and Burian, C. (1999). Cladribine activity in adult Langerhans' cell histiocytosis. *Blood*, **93**, 4125–4130.

Slater, J.M. and Swarm, O.J. (1980). Eosinophilic granuloma of bone. *Med Pediatr Oncol*, **8**, 151–164.

Stuurman, K.E., Lau, L., Doda, W., *et al.* (2003). Evaluation of the natural history and long term complications of patients with Langerhans' cell histiocytosis of bone. *Proc XIX meeting Histiocyte Society*, Philadelphia.

Titgemeyer, C., Grois, N., Minkov, M., *et al.* (2001). Pattern and course of single-system disease in Langerhans' cell histiocytosis data from the DAL-HX 83 and 90 study. *Med Pediatr Oncol*, **37**, 108–114.

Turgut, M. and Gurcay, O. (1992). Multifocal histiocytosis X of bone in two adjacent vertebrae causing paraplegia. *Aust NZ J Surg*, **62**, 241–244.

Villas, C., Martinez-Peric, R., Barrios, R.H., *et al.* (1993). Eosinophilic granuloma of the spine with and without vertebra plana. *J Spinal Disord*, **36**, 260–268.

Watts, J. and Files, B. (2001). Langerhans' cell histiocytosis: central nervous system involvement treated successfully with 2-Chlorodeoxyadenosine. *Pediatr Hematol Oncol*, **18**, 199–204.

Weinmann, P., Crestani, B., Tazi, A., *et al.* (2000). ^{111}In-Pentetreotide scintigraphy in patients with Langerhans' cell histiocytosis. *J Nucl Med*, **41**, 1808–1812.

Willis, B., Ablin, A., Weinberg, V., *et al.* (1996). Disease course and late sequelae of Langerhans' cell histiocytosis: a 25 year experience at the University of Southern California, San Francisco. *J Clin Oncol*, **14**, 2073–2082.

Womer, R.B., Raney, R.B. and D'Angio, G.J. (1985). Healing rates of treated and untreated bone lesions in Histiocytosis X. *Pediatrics*, **76**, 286–288.

Yasko, A.W., Fannng, C.V., Ayala, A.G., *et al.* (1998). Percutaneous techniques for the diagnosis and treatment of localized Langerhans' cell histiocytosis (Eosinophilic granuloma of bone). *J Bone Joint Surg*, **80**, 219–228.

Yeom, J.S., Lee, C.K., Shin, H.Y., *et al.* (1999). Langerhans' cell histiocytosis of the spine. Analysis of 23 cases. *Spine*, **24**, 1740–1749.

9

Special aspects of Langerhans cell histiocytosis in the adult

Maurizio Aricò, Emanuela De Juli, Thierry Généreau and Alan Saven

Introduction

Langerhans cell histiocytosis (LCH) may affect patients of any age, from the newborn to the elderly (Nezelof *et al.*, 1979; Aricò and Egeler, 1998; Aricò *et al.*, 2003). For several reasons this disease has been more familiar to pediatricians than to specialists of adult patients, and in adults the features of this disease are still poorly defined. Thus, most of the available information concerning clinical features, pathogenesis, and treatment outcome derives from the pediatric experience. Several features of the disease are common to pediatric and adult patients who may both have either localized or disseminated disease. The proportion of cases with lung involvement is much higher in adults, however. This can be partly explained by cigarette smoking, but other differences between pediatric and adult LCH still require elucidation.

Background and clinical features

Only a limited number of literature reports are available which describe series of patients with LCH diagnosed during adulthood, and only a few describe relatively large series of patients. Furthermore, most of these reports derive from single-specialty experiences, which may carry an inherent selection bias. In addition, continued uncertainty with regard to the pathogenesis of adult LCH has limited our current ability to devise optimal therapy, and no randomized clinical trials have been conducted in adults so far. Thus, most information derives from the descriptions of single or a few cases, often reported retrospectively. Forty years ago, Lewis reported 12 patients with 'eosinophilic granuloma and its variants with special reference to lung involvement' (Lewis, 1964). In 1991, Axiotis *et al.* reported a review of 42 females with LCH involving the genital tract, either as 'pure' genital LCH, genital LCH with subsequent multi-organ involvement, oral or cutaneous LCH with subsequent genital and multi-organ involvement, or diabetes insipidus (DI) with subsequent genital and multi-organ disease. The outcome of the disease was variable, with complete regression, partial improvement, persistent lesions, and recurrences occurring in all four groups of patients. Although treatment was highly individualized, including surgery, irradiation, topical corticosteroids, topical nitrogen mustard, systemic chemotherapy, as well as combinations of these treatments, no modality was shown to yield a superior outcome. The authors suggested, surprisingly enough, complete surgical excision as initial therapy (Axiotis et al., 1991).

In 1995, the Mayo Clinic group reported clinical and pathologic features of 263 patients with LCH and bone involvement, including 91 adults, reviewed over an 80-year period. The most common presenting complaint was pain, often worse at night. The skull was the most frequent osseous site in children and adults. Follow-up times varied from 3 months to 50 years, but three adults died either directly or indirectly from LCH and one developed systemic amyloidosis. Recrudescence of LCH in children, but not in adults, strongly correlated with the development of DI (Kilpatrick et al., 1995).

In 1996, 47 patients with LCH with onset as late as the ninth decade were described. Females were slightly preponderant, the skin was the commonest site of presentation, but pulmonary and bone involvement were also frequent. Patients with single-site disease fared best, and the worst prognosis was seen in the elderly or those with organ 'dysfunction'. There was a high incidence of various associated cancers observed either before, simultaneously or after the diagnosis of LCH (Malpas and Norton, 1996). In 1997, Baumgartner et al. reported 19 patients whose biopsies met the histopathologic criteria for presumptive LCH and who were followed for 1.5–20 years (average 7.7). Skeletal lesions were most frequent, followed by pulmonary disease and DI. Lesions of the skull and axial skeleton were associated with adjacent soft tissue infiltration in 10/16 patients (61%). Liver, lymph node, and bone marrow involvement were also noted. Localized disease had a good prognosis while multifocal and multisystem (MS) LCH had a more aggressive course. Bone lesions with adjacent soft tissue showed a >80% relapse rate, independent of the treatment. Pulmonary involvement caused greater morbidity than other 'single-system' (SS) disease, and systemic treatment yielded no convincing effect. In three patients with liver or bone marrow involvement, LCH resulted in persistent, serious deficits. One patient died after acute myelo-monocytic leukemia developing 18 months after diagnosis, without preceding chemotherapy. The authors concluded that in adults, LCH was usually limited to a few organ systems. Multifocal LCH represents the more aggressive form, with an unfavorable prognosis especially in patients with osseous lesions spreading into adjacent soft tissue, and liver or bone marrow involvement (Baumgartner et al., 1997). A large series of 314 patients from the Mayo Clinic, all with histologically proven LCH was reported in 1999. They were followed for a median of 4 years and included patients up to 83-year old. An MS

LCH was identified in 96 patients, of whom 25 (26%) had continuing 'active' disease after treatment. Single-bone LCH lesions were observed in 114, of whom 111 (97%) were alive and disease-free after treatment. The commonest sites of osseous LCH were the skull and proximal femur. Of the 87 patients with 'SS' pulmonary involvement, only three were non-smokers. After treatment with corticosteroids (with or without cyclophosphamide or busulphan), 74 patients survived apparently disease-free, but 10 patients died. DI developed in 44 patients (14%), of whom 30 were alive, disease-free after treatment, though all required long-term replacement therapy with desmopressin. Lymph node involvement was found in 21 (16%) patients, and muco-cutaneous involvement in 77 (24%) patients. Those with SS-bone lesions had the best prognosis compared to patients with LCH involving other systems. By contrast, 20% of patients with MS involvement had progressive disease, despite treatment (Howarth *et al.*, 1999).

In 2000, Kaltsas *et al.* described 12 adults with LCH and DI, followed for a median of 11.5 years. The median age at diagnosis of DI was 34 years; four patients presented with DI, whereas the other 18 developed DI at 1–20 years (median 2 years) after the diagnosis of LCH. All patients developed other sites of disease, outside the hypothalamus, during the course of the study and no fluctuation of disease activity was noted in the hypothalamo–pituitary region. Anterior pituitary hormone deficiencies developed in 8 of 12 patients with hypothalamo–pituitary LCH over the course of 20 years (see further discussion later in the chapter). Radiotherapy was useful in achieving local control of tumor extent, but established anterior or posterior pituitary and hypothalamic dysfunction did not improve (Kaltsas *et al.*, 2000).

LCH in children and adults: really the same disease?

Although most of the clinical features of LCH are very similar in children and adults, it appears from published reports, that the incidence of some manifestations is different (Tables 9.1 and 9.2). This may be related to the differences connected with the growth process in children. Yet, the lack of prospective comparisons means that we are not able at present to assess with confidence whether the incidence of tissue and organ involvement in adults completely overlap those in children. A direct comparison can perhaps be done on the basis of the findings of the International Histiocyte Society Registry, in which 274 adults from 12 countries, with biopsy-proven LCH were registered. These results may represent the current standard since the data was collected through the cooperation of specialists from a number of different medical fields, which may have reduced most selection biases, thus contributing to a more realistic picture of the disease. For example, the proportion of patients with LCH restricted to the lungs was limited to 16%, while 69% had MS disease (Aricò *et al.*, 2003). In this series, bone involvement, the most frequent

Table 9.1 Organ involvement in adult LCH

References	Bone	Lung (SS)	Skin (SS/MS muco-cutaneous)	MS	DI
Howarth *et al.* (1999), Mayo Clinic, *n* = 314 (adult)	36% (SS)	21%	24%	31%	14%
Aricò *et al.* (2003), Histiocyte Society Adult Registry, *n* = 274	57% (SS/MS)	16%	40%	69%	29.6%

Table 9.2 Major clinical features of LCH in children and adults

Manifestation	Adult	Children
Bone disease	Frequent	Very frequent
Skin disease	Frequent	Frequent
Dental involvement	Infrequent	Frequent
Pulmonary disease	Very frequent	Infrequent
Isolated pulmonary disease	Very frequent	Exceptional
Genital involvement	Frequent	Exceptional
DI	Frequent	Frequent

manifestation of LCH reported in at least 80% of children, was observed in 57% of adults; skin involvement was observed in 37%, exactly the same percentage observed in a large number of children from the French series (The French Langerchans' cell histiocytosis Study Group, 1996). When patients with MS disease alone are evaluated, skin involvement is present in 50% of adults versus 75% of children. It is important to note that 40% of all adult patients show 'muco-cutaneous' involvement of any type. The ear involvement, resulting from adjacent osteolytic lesions and from external ear dermatitis in about 65% of children with MS disease, is far less frequently reported in adults (5%). Lymphadenopathy is also less frequent in adults (6%). Hepatosplenomegaly was recorded in only 16% of the patients, which raised to 23% the number of patients with MS disease; this incidence appears somewhat lower than the 35–45% incidence of liver and spleen enlargement in children with MS disease enrolled in the Histiocyte Society trials (Gadner *et al.*, 2001; Minkov *et al.*, 2003). DI was diagnosed in 29.6% of adult patients, a proportion which is not significantly different from 22.7% and 24.2% at 5 and 10 years, respectively, reported in a large pediatric series (Donadieu *et al.*, 2004). Remarkably, hypothyroidism was recorded in 6.6% of the adult patients but is extremely rare in children. Overall, the pattern of disease involvement in this adult cohort was the following: SS lung disease in 16.1%; SS, unifocal in any other tissue in 10.6%; SS, multifocal in 4.7%; MS in 68.6%. Although this is a very large series, we cannot exclude that these proportions are somewhat biased by selection criteria.

Correlation with the pattern of disease distribution observed in children may be attempted by using the data reported by the German-Austrian group. In the DAL-HX 83/90 studies a total of 324 patients were enrolled, 63 (19.4%) fulfilled the criteria for MS LCH (i.e. involvement of two or more organ/systems) (Minkov *et al.*, 2000). In another report, the pattern of disease in 170 patients with SS LCH from the same studies showed single-bone lesions in 68%; multiple bone lesions in 19%; isolated skin disease in 11%; isolated lymph node involvement in only four patients (Titgemeyer *et al.*, 2001).

The apparently higher frequency of MS disease in the adult population enrolled in the registry is likely influenced, even in such a large series, by the inherent bias due to the characteristic of the disease, with localized LCH being more frequently under-diagnosed, and also to the registration bias which might have induced participating investigators to report more frequently the more severe cases.

A few points seem to be clear, however. The major difference between children and adults is the much higher incidence of isolated pulmonary disease, particularly occurring in adults who smoke. Other differences include the more frequent involvement of genital and oral mucosa (see also Chapter 7), and possibly some differences in the distribution of bone lesions in adults compared to children (Table 8.1). Whether these reflect differences in pathogenesis or only age-driven differences in adaptation in the host remains to be assessed.

Interestingly, one small study suggests that not only the distribution of bone involvement at diagnosis may be different, but that the natural history may also be different in mature versus immature bones. The authors followed single-bone lesions prospectively for a mean of 5 years, and found no recurrences in children with immature bones, whereas 4 of 13 skeletally mature patients had a recurrence (Plasschaert *et al.*, 2002). This small study needs to be repeated in a larger group of patients before the significance can be appreciated.

What is the standard treatment of LCH in adults?

The uncertainties concerning the pathogenesis of LCH have certainly limited our ability to design rational treatment options. Furthermore, compared to children, only limited information is available for adult patients. There are no trials, for example of testing the standard chemotherapy drugs vinblastine and corticosteroids in adult patients. The lack of trials in adult patients may have resulted in different attitudes compared to the pediatric experience. In pediatric LCH for instance, the role of etoposide has been greatly reduced by the combination of the risk of secondary leukemia and the lack of improved efficacy when compared to vinblastine in the Histiocyte Society LCH-I trial, or when added to vinblastine and corticosteroid in the LCH-II trial (Ladisch *et al.*, 1994; Gadner *et al.*, 2001) (see Chapter 12). This drug nevertheless, remains quite popular among some adult specialists. In 1992, Tsele *et al.* reported their evaluation of three adult patients with severe or resistant LCH (one SS skin disease, two with MS disease), treated with intravenous (IV) etoposide, $100 \, mg/m^2/day$, for 3 days, repeated every 3 or 4 weeks for three to four cycles. All patients achieved clinical remission for 12–14 months of follow-up. No serious immediate side effects were noted (Tsele *et al.*, 1992).

More recently, Helmbold *et al.* (1998) reported the successful use of prolonged oral administration of etoposide, and Munn *et al.* (2001), reviewing 46 adult cases found the best responses with azathioprine in localized disease and with etoposide in refractory or MS disease. In 1997, Giona *et al.* reported a retrospective single-center study of 11 adults with LCH. Of six patients with recurrent unifocal ($n = 3$) or multifocal ($n = 3$) bone disease, five received chemotherapy with vinblastine and high-dose methylprednisolone (HDMP), and one received α-interferon (IFN); of four patients with MS disease, two with bone and visceral disease were treated with etoposide and HDMP, and two with lung and lymph node involvement received multiagent chemotherapy, with good results (Giona *et al.*, 1997). Despite the results, the lack of uniformity in the therapy does not allow for recommendations regarding the best therapy.

Another drug which appears to be fairly commonly used in front-line therapy in adult patients, and which thus requires consideration when designing a treatment program for adult LCH, is the nucleoside analog 2-chlorodeoxyadenosine (2-CdA/cladribine).

Following the observation that patients treated with cladribine for hairy cell leukemia developed monocytopenia, it was suggested that the drug would be of value in the treatment of LCH (Saven *et al.*, 1994), Hampshire and Saven recently updated the results of a phase II trial of cladribine in adults with LCH conducted at the Scripps Clinic. Cladribine was administered at $0.14 \, mg/kg/day$ IV over 2 h for five consecutive days every 4 weeks, for a maximum of six cycles. Sixteen patients (nine females and seven males) with a median age of 44 years (range 19–72 years) were treated. The median time from diagnosis to start of cladribine was 82 months (range 1–288). Fourteen of the 16 patients (88%) had been pre-treated with a median number of three treatments (range 1–6). At the time of enrollment in the study, 11 patients (69%) had stage I, four patients (25%) had stage II, and one patient (6%) had stage III disease, as defined in the study. Organ involvement included skin in 10 patients, bone in six, lung in six, adenopathy in five, DI in four, colon in two, and thyroid in one. A median of three cycles of cladribine (range 1–6) was administered. Sixteen patients were evaluable for toxicity, 15 for response; one was removed from the study after an allergic reaction during the first infusion.

Complete response (CR) was achieved in seven patients (44%) and partial response in three patients (19%), giving as overall response rate of 63%. Median response duration was 36.2 months (range 0.9–112.5); five of the patients who achieved CR remain in remission at 97.1+ months (range 40.8+ to 114.8+). Leukopenia was the principal toxicity with eight patients (50%) experiencing grade 3/4 neutropenia – apparently in contrast to the lower toxicity in the pediatric cases when similar doses were given to LCH patients without hematopoietic involvement (Stine *et al.*, 1997; Rodriguez-Galindo *et al.*, 2002). Febrile neutropenia developed in two patients and one patient developed dermatomal zoster. Three patients developed a malignancy: recurrent thyroid cancer, non-melanoma skin cancer, chronic myelo-monocytic leukemia (CMMoL) (>3 years from cladribine); one additional patient developed refractory anemia at 9 years from treatment. With a median follow-up of 105.6 months (range 8.5–149.3), three patients died (two from progressive LCH and one from CMMoL), and 13 remain alive (seven disease-free, two on salvage therapy, and four who were alive with disease at last contact) (Saven and Burian, 1999; Hampshire and Saven, 2004).

Single-agent cladribine clearly has major activity in the treatment of adults with previously treated LCH. Its position in the hierarchical management schema of adults with LCH remains to be determined, given its potential for severe, and sometimes long lasting, myelotoxicity and immunosuppression. Since the number of adults with LCH treated with cladribine is relatively small, caution should be exercised before making predictions about which patterns and sites of disease involvement will be more susceptible to, and therefore more appropriate for, cladribine treatment. Nevertheless, there have been individual patients with osseous, cutaneous, visceral and pulmonary involvement by LCH who have responded.

Treatment of LCH in adults: where do we go from here?

An MS LCH is associated, in adults as in children, with a 10% risk of fatal disease progression at 5 years (Aricò *et al.*, 2003). Systemic chemotherapy may reduce this number. Since the 1960s, a number of small single- and multicentre studies for children with MS LCH showed a clear benefit from therapy with cytotoxic drugs and/or steroids, alone or in combination. On the basis of these preliminary findings, an international cooperative effort by the Histiocyte Society, including the two randomized trials mentioned above (Gadner *et al.*, 2001; Minkov *et al.*, 2003), have produced considerable information regarding LCH and the response to therapy in childhood. Much of this information may potentially be transferable to adult patients, although this cannot be taken for granted. Due to the lack of significant long-term toxicity, the therapeutic efficacy of the standard regimen for

MS LCH in children (i.e. the combination of vinblastine and prednisone) should be explored first in adult MS patients. We have to keep in mind, however, that despite the fact that vinblastine has been associated with little toxicity in most pediatric patients, this is not necessarily true for adults. Adults have unfortunately demonstrated increased neurotoxicity and more profound bone marrow suppression, as compared to children. Unlike the pediatric experience, the administered vinblastine dose is therefore likely to often require adjustment in individual adult patients, and the inability to administer weekly doses to some patients, may also adversely affect the efficacy of the therapy. Clearly, in order to find the best therapy for adult patients, clinical trials are needed.

The Histiocyte Society Registry was the first step toward a cooperative effort in adult LCH (Aricò *et al.*, 2003). Of over 250 patients registered, SS disease was found in 86 (31%). This included isolated pulmonary involvement in 44 cases while 188 patients (69%) had MS disease. The data collected support the great uncertainty and the lack of a therapeutic standard at least for front-line treatment, and further supports the need for a common approach in a prospective, cooperative trial. To address this issue, several requirements still have to be achieved. Uniform initial evaluation and stratification of patients are necessary for evaluation of disease course and of treatment results, for a disease in which, on the one hand, spontaneous resolution and improvement, and on the other, reactivation are common. Furthermore, the aims of the study should be appropriate for the different patient groups. For example, most patients with localized disease are not at risk for disease-related death and the therapeutic plan should reflect this. For isolated skin diseases, specific therapeutic approaches have been developed by dermatologists. Surgical excision may be appropriate for localized skin lesions but mutilating surgery is not considered appropriate, as a number of active therapies are available (see Chapter 7). For patients with isolated pulmonary disease, the treatment should be directed at reduction in the frequency and severity of reactivations, with the intent of reducing the degree of eventual disability and improving the quality of life (see Chapter 10).

In SS lung patients with disease progression on corticosteroids, it seems logical to evaluate the efficacy of standard chemotherapy (vinblastine and prednisone), as used for patients with MS disease. Although the results obtained in MS children are promising, an incomplete knowledge of the pathogenesis of LCH would suggest caution in directly extrapolating to pulmonary LCH in adults. Furthermore, in adult patients additional features have to be considered, among them the possibility that the patient may have associated, pre-existing conditions which may influence disease manifestations and drug metabolism. In adults with diabetes mellitus, for example, glucose intolerance may require modification of steroid dosage; auto-immune disorders may require immune modulation; pregnancy may affect the immune system and thus the disease course and its treatment. There is also an increased risk of other malignancies in adults with LCH.

For patients with multiple reactivations in bone, it will be necessary to compare the results obtained with standard chemotherapy, with the good results and moderate toxicity seen with the use of cladribine as described above. This comparison will of necessity take many years, as the comparative late effects of the two therapies need to be documented in this patient group.

Finally, preliminary reports have been published of the efficacy of cladribine in active central nervous system (CNS) disease (Watts and Files, 2001; Giona *et al.*, 2002) although in the absence of any comparison with standard chemotherapy. This too warrants further investigation. It must be clear that there is no evidence of activity of this, or any other drug, against neurodegenerative disease.

On the basis of these considerations, the Histiocyte Society has launched the first international cooperative trial for diagnosis and treatment of LCH in adults. This trial, known as 'LCH-A1', is aimed at: defining and implementing uniform initial evaluation and stratification of patients; defining a common therapeutic strategy for patients with MS and pulmonary LCH; exploring the therapeutic efficacy in adult patients of the standard pediatric regimen (vinblastine and pred-nisone); defining the natural history of 'isolated' pulmonary disease and in particular the role of smoking cessation on the disease course; and exploring the efficacy of steroid monotherapy in adults with isolated pulmonary disease and disease progression. Research studies, ancillary to this trial, offer unique opportunities to address some of the unanswered questions in LCH, including the genetic component of the disease as supported by evidence of familial clustering and chromosomal instability, the issue of clonality (which might be different in isolated lung LCH from other forms of LCH), the relationship of pulmonary disease to cigarette smoking, and the immune system polymorphisms that might increase individual susceptibility to LCH (Nezelof and Basset, 2004).

The results of this study will hopefully contribute to a better understanding of the characteristics of LCH in adults, and will help establish the first 'therapeutic standard' for this intriguing disease. Participation in this trial by national cooperative groups and large institutions should be encouraged.

Permanent consequences in adults with LCH

Pediatric specialists have learned much about the late effects of LCH, as well as of its treatment, on the growing body and growing brain (see also Chapter 14). In adult patients who develop LCH, the pattern of sequelae may be different, in particular the bone, endocrine and CNS consequences may depend more on the natural course of the disease, rather than on treatment-induced toxicity.

In a small series of 19 adult patients, bone lesions with associated soft tissue infiltration in the orodental and otomastoid region ($n = 14$) were manifest with loss of teeth in six patients, and hearing loss in three. Dyspnea on exertion and a non-productive cough was seen in three patients and cor pulmonale in two with chronic progressive lung disease. One patient treated with radiation therapy alone, died from myelo-monocytic leukemia 18 months after diagnosis of LCH. In this series, the late consequences appeared to be significantly associated with MS disease (Baumgartner *et al.*, 1997).

Patients with an extended duration of the disease may develop the full pattern of pituitary dysfunction; that is, DI followed by thyroid and gonadal insufficiency. Of 12 adult patients with LCH and DI followed for a median of 11.5 years (range 3–28), eight patients developed one or more anterior pituitary deficiencies at a median of 4.5 years (range 2–22 years), growth hormone deficiency in eight, follicle-stimulating hormone–luteinizing hormone (FSH–LH) deficiency in seven, and adrenocorticotrophic hormone (ACTH) and thyroid-stimulating hormone (TSH) in five. In addition, seven patients with anterior pituitary deficiency developed other symptoms of hypothalamo–pituitary dysfunction: morbid obesity in five, short-term memory deficits in five, sleeping disorders in four, disorders of thermoregulation in two, and adipsia in one (Kaltsas *et al.*, 2000). The lack of obvious growth and pubertal problems in adult LCH patients does not negate the importance of regular careful endocrine assessment and appropriate hormonal replacement, particularly in those with DI.

The natural history of the disease makes lung dysfunction, which is very unlikely in children with a much greater ability for alveolar regeneration, common in adults with pulmonary LCH. The clinical course of the disease (see also Chapter 10) may be variable and unpredictable although a large proportion of patients, particularly those with onset during early adulthood, may be candidates to develop end-stage disease. This is characterized by prominent fibrotic scarring, which may make lung transplantation essential for survival. Even those patients who do not have end-stage respiratory failure may be severely limited by their reduced pulmonary function (Delobbe *et al.*, 1996; Vassallo *et al.*, 2002).

Finally, the characteristics of LCH, its variable natural history and our limited ability to control the disease and its sequelae, make living with it difficult for patients and families. Psychological support may well be a necessity for patients who are affected with an 'obscure' disease, which is very likely not cancer but is likely to be chronic, with frequent reactivations and occasional severe limitation to normal living, and which may thus severely affect the self-esteem of the patient. As with the pediatric population, patients with LCH diagnosed in adulthood require careful, complete and long-term follow-up assessments, provided by an experienced, multidisciplinary team.

Conclusion

LCH in adults has been termed an 'orphan disease' based on the fact that pediatric LCH has long found a home in the world of pediatric oncology, while adult LCH is often treated by different, although expert, subspecialists. Thus, except in centers dedicated to this problem, the adult patient often suffers from the lack of a physician willing to coordinate the management. In addition, as with pediatric LCH, there remains incomplete information on the etiology and pathogenesis of both isolated and MS LCH in adults. The Histiocyte Society is working to transfer to the adult patients the bulk of the experience which has been accumulated in children and adolescents. The new LCH-A1 trial for adult patients with LCH, with its novel, collaborative effort between scientists, pediatricians and adult specialists, will hopefully provide a unique opportunity for researchers to gain access to uniformly collected and evaluated biologic material, as well as patient information. In this way it is hoped to address the many still unanswered questions in pivotal fields like epidemiology, pathogenesis, genetics and management of this puzzling disorder.

A concerted joint effort between pediatric and adult specialists could in this way be the key to the development of insights into LCH, in all age groups affected by this distressing and often debilitating condition.

REFERENCES

Aricò, M. and Egeler, R.M. (1998). Clinical aspects of Langerhans cell histiocytosis. *Hematol Oncol Clin North Am*, **12**, 247–258.

Aricò, M., Girschikofsky, M., Généreau, T., *et al.* (2003). Langerhans cell histiocytosis in adults. Report from the International Registry of the Histiocyte Society. *Eur J Cancer*, **39**, 2341–2348.

Axiotis, C.A., Merino, M.J. and Duray, P.H. (1991). Langerhans cell histiocytosis of the female genital tract. *Cancer*, **67**, 1650–1660.

Baumgartner, I., von Hochstetter, A., Baumert, B., *et al.* (1997). Langerhans'-cell histiocytosis in adults. *Med Pediatr Oncol*, **28**, 9–14.

Delobbe, A., Durieu, J., Duhamel, A. and Wallaert, B. (1996). Determinants of survival in pulmonary Langerhans' cell granulomatosis (histiocytosis X). Groupe d'Etude en Pathologie Interstitielle de la Societe de Pathologie Thoraci que du Nord. *Eur Respir J*, **9**, 2002–2006.

Donadieu, J., Rolon, M.A., Thomas, C., *et al.* (2004). French LCH Study Group. Endocrine involvement in pediatric-onset Langerhans' cell histiocytosis: a population-based study. *J Pediatr*, **144**, 344–350.

Gadner, H., Grois, N., Aricò, M., *et al.* (2001). A randomized trial of treatment for multisystem Langerhans' cell histiocytosis. *J Pediatr*, **138**, 728–734.

Giona, F., Caruso, R., Testi, A.M., *et al.* (1997). Langerhans' cell histiocytosis in adults: a clinical and therapeutic analysis of 11 patients from a single institution. *Cancer*, **80**, 1786–1791.

Giona, F., Annino, L., Bongarzoni, V., et al. (2002). Unifocal Langerhans cell histiocytosis involving the central nervous system successfully treated with 2-chlorodeoxyadenosine. Med Pediatr Oncol, 38, 223.

Hampshire, A.P. and Saven, A. (2004). Update of cladribine in the treatment of adults with Langerhans-cell histiocytosis (LCH). Proc Am Society Clin Oncol, 23, 6602.

Helmbold, P., Hegemann, B., Holzhausen, H.-J., et al. (1998). Low dose oral etoposide monotherapy in adult Langerhans cell histiocytosis. Arch Dermatol, 134, 1275–1278.

Howarth, D.M., Gilchrist, G.S., Mullan, B.P., et al. (1999). Langerhans cell histiocytosis: diagnosis, natural history, management, and outcome. Cancer, 85, 2278–2290.

Kaltsas, G.A., Powles, T.B., Evanson, J., et al. (2000). Hypothalamo–pituitary abnormalities in adult patients with Langerhans cell histiocytosis: clinical, endocrinological, and radiological features and response to treatment. J Clin Endocrinol Metab, 85, 1370–1376.

Kilpatrick, S.E., Wenger, D.E., Gilchrist, G.S., et al. (1995). Langerhans' cell histiocytosis (histiocytosis X) of bone. A clinicopathologic analysis of 263 pediatric and adult cases. Cancer, 76, 2471–2484.

Ladisch, S., Gadner, H., Aricò, M., et al. (1994). A randomized trial of etoposide vs. vinblastine in disseminated Langerhans cell histiocytosis. Med Pediatr Oncol, 23, 107–110.

Lewis, J.G. (1964). Eosinophilic granuloma and its variants with special reference to lung involvement. QJM New series, 131, 337–359.

Malpas, J.S. and Norton, A.J. (1996). Langerhans cell histiocytosis in the adult. Med Pediatr Oncol, 27, 540–546.

Minkov, M., Grois, N., Heitger, A., et al. (2000). Treatment of multisystem Langerhans cell histiocytosis. Results of the DAL-HX 83 and DAL-HX 90 studies. DAL-HX Study Group. Klin Padiatr, 212, 139–144.

Minkov, M., Grois, N., Aricò, M., et al. (2003). Preliminary results of the LCH-II clinical trial of the Histiocyte Society. Proceedings of the XXXV meeting of the International Society for Pediatric Oncology. Med Pediatr Oncol, 41, 263.

Munn, S.E., Murray, S. and Chu, A.T. (2001). Adult Langerhans cell histiocytosis – a review of 46 cases. Med Pediatr Oncol, 38, 222.

Nezelof, C. and Basset, F. (2004). An hypothesis Langerhans cell histiocytosis: the failure of the immune system to switch from an innate to an adaptive mode. Pediatr Blood Cancer, 42, 398–400.

Nezelof, C., Frileux-Herbet, F., Cronier-Sachot, J., et al. (1979). Disseminated histiocytosis X: analysis of prognostic factors based on a retrospective study of 50 cases. Cancer, 44, 1824–1838.

Plasschaert, F., Craig, C., Bell, R., et al. (2002). Eosinophilic granuloma. A different behaviour in children and adults. J Bone Joint Surg Br, 84, 870–872.

Rodriguez-Galindo, C., Kelly, P., Jeng, M., et al. (2002). Treatment of children with Langerhans cell histiocytosis with 2-chlorodeoxyadenosine. Am J Hematol, 69, 179–184.

Saven, A. and Burian, C. (1999). Cladribine activity in adult Langerhans-cell histiocytosis. Blood, 93, 4125–4130.

Saven, A., Foon, K. and Piro, L. (1994). 2-Chlorodeoxyadenosine induced complete remissions in Langerhans cell histiocytosis. Ann Intern Med, 21, 430–432.

Stine, K.C., Saylors, R.L., Williams, L.L., *et al.* (1997). 2-Chlorodeoxyadenosine (2-CDA) for the treatment of refractory or recurrent Langerhans cell histiocytosis (LCH) in pediatric patients. *Med Pediatr Oncol*, **29**, 288–292.

The French LCH Study Group (1996). A multicentre retrospective survey of LCH: 348 cases observed between 1983 and 1993. *Arch Dis Child*, **75**, 17–24.

Titgemeyer, C., Grois, N., Minkov, M., *et al.* (2001). Pattern and course of single-system disease in Langerhans cell histiocytosis data from the DAL-HX 83- and 90-study. *Med Pediatr Oncol*, **37**, 108–114.

Tsele, E., Thomas, D.M. and Chu, A.C. (1992). Treatment of adult Langerhans cell histiocytosis with etoposide. *J Am Acad Dermatol*, **27**, 61–64.

Vassallo, R., Ryu, J.H., Schroeder D.R., Decker P.A. and Limper, A.H. (2002). Clinical outcomes of pulmonary Langerhans'-cell histiocytosis in adults. *New Engl J Med*, **346**(7), 484–490.

Watts, J. and Files, B. (2001). Langerhans cell histiocytosis: central nervous system involvement successfully treated with 2-chlorodeoxyadenosine. *Pediatr Hematol Oncol*, **18**, 199–204.

10

Adult lung histiocytosis

Abdellatif Tazi, T. Jeroen N. Hiltermann and Roberto Vassallo

Introduction

Langerhans cell histiocytosis (LCH) encompasses a group of disorders of unknown origin with diverse clinical presentations and outcomes, characterized by infiltration of involved tissues by pathologic Langerhans cells (LCs). Acute disseminated LCH is a severe multisystem disease that predominantly affects young children. Multifocal LCH is seen mainly in older children and adolescents and runs a variable but usually more favorable course. Single-system disease (eosinophilic granuloma) is characterized by involvement of a single organ (bone, lungs, or skin) and often follows a benign course (Howarth *et al.*, 1999). Pulmonary involvement in patients with multisystem disease is rarely at the forefront of the clinical picture. Isolated or predominant pulmonary involvement is the pattern encountered by pulmonologists in adults and has a number of specific epidemiological and clinical features that warrant its individualization as a separate entity (Tazi *et al.*, 2000; Vassallo *et al.*, 2000; Sundar *et al.*, 2003).

Epidemiology

Adult lung LCH is an uncommon disorder that occurs almost exclusively in smokers. In an early series of more than 500 patients with diffuse infiltrating lung disease, surgical lung biopsy showed LCH in less than 5% of cases (Gaensler and Carrington, 1980). Several studies have documented comparable data thereafter as reviewed in Tazi *et al.* (2000) and Vassallo *et al.* (2000). The prevalence of pulmonary LCH (pLCH) is, however, probably underestimated because some patients are asymptomatic or experience spontaneous remission, and histological findings are nonspecific in advanced forms. The wide use of chest high-resolution computed tomography (HRCT) in the evaluation of patients may increase the number of patients in whom pLCH is diagnosed.

A few familial cases of LCH have been reported (Arico *et al.*, 2001), but pulmonary disease occurs sporadically. Although pLCH has been rarely described in black patients, no accurate epidemiological data are available on racial differences. Recently, the clinical and epidemiological features of pLCH in Asians have been described (Watanabe *et al.*, 2001).

Pulmonary LCH predominantly affects young adults, typically between 20 and 40 years of age (Tazi *et al.*, 2000; Vassallo *et al.*, 2000). Female patients may be slightly older. A marked male predominance was initially reported but recent studies suggest a similar proportion or even a slight predominance of women (Howarth *et al.*, 1999; Vassallo *et al.*, 2002). These differences probably reflect smoking habit changes over time. Indeed, the most striking epidemiological characteristic of adult pLCH is that 90–100% of patients are smokers (often smoking more than 20 cigarettes per day) (Tazi *et al.*, 2000; Vassallo *et al.*, 2000). No other epidemiological factors associated with pLCH have been identified. Cases of pLCH have been reported after radiation therapy and/or chemotherapy for lymphoma, most notably Hodgkin's disease (Egeler *et al.*, 1993; Unger *et al.*, 1994).

Lung pathology

Accumulation of activated LCs organized in loose granulomas that develop in, and destroy, the distal bronchiole walls is the pathological hallmark of pLCH (Tazi *et al.*, 2000; Vassallo *et al.*, 2000). Lymphocytes and inflammatory cells including eosinophils and macrophages are also found.

Under the light microscope, LCs are moderately sized cells (15 μm in diameter), with convoluted irregular nuclei and pale, weakly eosinophilic cytoplasm that contain few, if any, phagocytic particles. Cell type should always be confirmed by immuno-histochemical staining with monoclonal antibodies to the membrane antigen CD1a or by visualization under the electron microscope (EM) of Birbeck granules, which are more numerous than in normal LCs. The nature of LC present in the lesions can be also confirmed with an antibody to langerin (CD207), a type II mannose lectin specifically expressed by LCs including those in LCH lesions (Valladeau *et al.*, 1999; Geissmann *et al.*, 2001). Positive staining for the intracellular S100 protein is not specific and can also be observed in other cell types such as neuroendocrine cells and some macrophages.

The appearance of LCH lesions varies with the stage of the disease and with the tissue involved. In the lung, the lesions are focal, poorly demarcated, separated by apparently normal lung parenchyma, and centered on the terminal and respiratory bronchioles, destroying the airway walls (Tazi *et al.*, 2000; Vassallo *et al.*, 2000). In view of this feature, pLCH resembles bronchiolitis rather than a diffuse infiltrating lung disease. The granulomas are poorly demarcated, extend into adjacent alveolar structures, which often contain an abundance of pigmented macrophages, producing respiratory bronchiolitis/interstitial lung disease (RB/ILD)-like or a desquamative interstitial pneumonia (DIP)-like pattern (Vassallo *et al.*, 2003). In uninvolved areas, the lung architecture seems normal, despite the common presence of nonspecific smoking-related abnormalities (respiratory bronchiolitis, intra-alveolar accumulation of pigmented macrophages, and lymphoid clusters infiltrating the alveolar walls). Pathological features change over time, and lesions of various ages are often found in a same specimen. Early lesions are responsible for eccentric infiltration of the walls of terminal and respiratory bronchioles, which undergo gradual destruction (Figure 10.1). Due to their close anatomic association with bronchioles, spread to adjacent arterioles is common. LCs are abundant at this stage and form a compact central granuloma with a large number of lymphocytes. Inflammatory cells, mainly eosinophils and macrophages, are also present in variable numbers. Destruction of the bronchiolar epithelium occurs early in the disease process, so that the bronchiole-centered development of the lesions may be difficult to confirm on a single section. Three-dimensional reconstruction of the lesions from serial sections shows a granulomatous cuff spreading along the walls of the distal airways (Kambouchner *et al.*, 2002). Although early lesions often seem cavitated, the cavity is the residual lumen of the destroyed bronchiole and not tissue necrosis. Later in the process, the LCs are less abundant and form clusters surrounded by lymphocytes and other inflammatory cells. In advanced disease, there are few or no LCs. The lesions are replaced by stellar fibrotic scars or by confluent and adjacent cystic cavities, that can

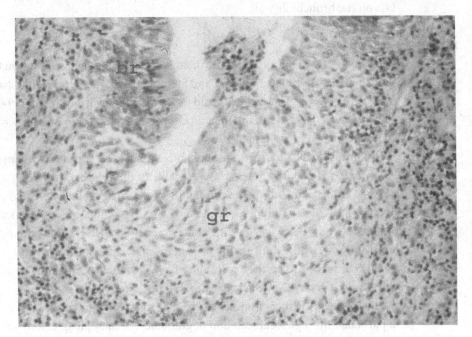

Figure 10.1 A characteristic florid pulmonary LC granuloma, a portion of the remnant bronchiole is still visible, hematoxylin and eosin (H&E) ×200

give a 'honeycomb' aspect. Traction emphysema contributes to the cystic appearance of advanced lesions.

Pathogenesis

As the etiology of LCH is unknown, the pathogenesis remains poorly understood (Egeler *et al.*, 2004; Nezelof and Basset, 2004). No animal model is available for this disease, and although the various clinical patterns share similar histopathological features, it is unclear whether similar mechanisms apply to all forms of LCH. The tremendous progress in the knowledge of dendritic cell (DC) biology provides important insight in the understanding of the mechanisms potentially involved in LCH (Banchereau *et al.*, 2000; Mellman and Steinman, 2001; Steinman *et al.*, 2003).

In pLCH, pathogenic hypotheses must try to explain at least three aspects:

1 The selective involvement of bronchioles by LCH lesions.
2 The ability of LC granulomas to destroy the bronchioles that they infiltrate.
3 The very strong epidemiological link with smoking, as well as the low incidence of pLCH as compared to the prevalence of smoking in the general population.

It should be stressed that a similar mechanism can be involved at these different steps, leading for example both to focal LC accumulation and to the destructive effects of LCs on the bronchiole wall.

Langerhans cells

LCs belong to the DC lineage whose main function is antigen presentation to T cells (Banchereau *et al.*, 2000; Mellman and Steinman, 2001). *In vitro* studies have identified various DC subsets which could be derived from various hematopoietic precursors when cultured with different growth factors and cytokines (Banchereau *et al.*, 2000; Mellman and Steinman, 2001).

In contrast to DCs that are present in most tissues (i.e. lymphoid organs, dermis, pulmonary parenchyma) LCs are specifically localized in the epidermis and other mucosal epithelia including the epithelium of the airways (Banchereau *et al.*, 2000; Knight *et al.*, 2002; Stumbles *et al.*, 2003). These cells differ morphologically from other DCs by the presence of cytoplasmic organelles called Birbeck granules, which are visible only by EM, and are involved in internalizing exogenous substances. LCs can also be identified by the expression of langerin that is constitutively associated with Birbeck granules (Valladeau *et al.*, 1999).

The epithelial microenvironment is essential to LC recruitment and differentiation, in particular through local secretion of granulocyte-macrophage colony stimulating factor (GM-CSF), transforming growth factor (TGF)-β, and the chemokine CCL20 (MIP-3α) (Burnham *et al.*, 2000; Godefroy *et al.*, 2001; Caux *et al.*, 2002). Transgenic mice with TGF-β gene deficiency have no intraepidermal LCs but have normal dermal DC counts. More recently, the chemokine CCL20 (MIP-3α), produced predominantly by epithelial cells, strongly attracted LCs *in vitro* by interacting with the CCR6 receptor expressed on their surface and this chemokine is also involved in recruiting LCs *in vivo* (Dieu-Nosjean *et al.*, 2000; Homey *et al.*, 2000; Vanbervliet *et al.*, 2002). Other factors such as the expression of E-cadherin by epithelial cells and LCs are important for the tissue homing of these cells (Riedl *et al.*, 2000).

In the normal lung, LCs are virtually confined to the tracheobronchial epithelium, where they form a well-developed network (Tazi *et al.*, 2000; Stumbles *et al.*, 2003). Whereas LCs are extremely sparse in normal alveolar epithelium, these cells are present in the alveoli of smokers and patients with pulmonary inflammation, in areas of alveolar epithelial hyperplasia (Tazi *et al.*, 2000). In addition, abundant LC infiltrates may be found in lung cancer. The presence of these pathologic LCs correlated with local GM-CSF production by hyperplastic alveolar cells, or bronchial tumor cells, suggesting that GM-CSF plays a key role in the recruitment and/or differentiation of LCs in the human lung (Tazi *et al.*, 1993).

LCs, like other DCs found in peripheral tissues, are immature DCs and serve essentially as sentinels that uptake antigens but do not induce an immune response *in situ* (Banchereau *et al.*, 2000; Knight *et al.*, 2002). In response to various stimuli (particularly pro-inflammatory signals such as lipopolysaccharide (LPS), tumor necrosis factor (TNF)-α, interleukin(IL)-1β), these cells migrate via afferent lymph ducts to the regional lymphoid organs, where they stimulate the development of antigen-specific T cells (Geissmann *et al.*, 2002; Stoitzner *et al.*, 2003). This migration toward secondary lymphoid organs is crucial for induction of a specific immune response and is strongly influenced by the chemokine gradient between the afferent lymph ducts and the antigen introduction site (Sallusto and Lanzavecchia, 2000; Caux *et al.*, 2002). During their migration, LCs lose their Birbeck granules, and switch their surface expression of CCR6 to CCR7, the receptor of the CCL19 (MIP-3β) chemokine produced in secondary lymphoid tissues. These cells lose their ability to capture antigens, and in response to additional signals, particularly CD40–CD40L interaction, become fully mature DCs that are able to secrete large amounts of IL-12 and efficiently activate T lymphocytes (Trinchieri, 2003). Importantly, the microenvironment exerts a strong influence on DC function at all the steps of the immune response and influence the elicitation of an efficient immune response or tolerance. Thus, cytokines and membrane signals delivered to DCs influence the functional maturation of these cells, directing the immune response to an effective TH1 response or, on the contrary, to immune tolerance via activation of TH2 lymphocytes or regulatory T lymphocytes (Steinman *et al.*, 2003; Trinchieri, 2003).

Consistent with their functional abilities, LCs, including LCs in normal lung, express a surface phenotype of immature DCs. In particular, they show little or no expression of the costimulation molecules CD40, CD80 (B7-1) and CD86 (B7-2) (Tazi *et al.*, 1999; Stumbles *et al.*, 2003). Interestingly, although LC counts are substantially increased at sites of alveolar epithelial hyperplasia and in some lung cancers, these cells remain negative for CD80, CD86, and CD40 (Tazi *et al.*, 1999).

Accumulation of LCs in the lung of patients with LCH

In pLCH, numerous LCs accumulate in the bronchioles involved by the pathologic process. The lesions are focal, involving some distal bronchioles but sparing others. This distribution suggests that changes in the bronchiolar epithelial microenvironment, presumably induced by cigarette smoking, are essential for bronchiolar LC accumulation. This bronchiolar infiltration by numerous LCs may be related to LC recruitment of LCs precursors, local LC proliferation, and/or decreased LC sensitivity to apoptosis-inducing mechanisms.

As pointed out above, bronchiolar epithelial cells can produce a number of mediators, most notably GM-CSF, known to regulate the proliferation and differentiation of hematopoietic LC precursors and to enhance their survival *in vitro* (Tazi *et al.*, 1993). In early pLCH lesions, the epithelium of involved bronchioles produces larger amounts of GM-CSF (Tazi *et al.*, 2000). There are multiple lines of investigation that support a critical role for GM-CSF in the accumulation of LCs in normal tissue as well as within LCH lesions, particularly in the lungs (Burnham *et al.*, 2000; Tazi *et al.*, 2000; Wang *et al.*, 2000).

Other mediators produced by airway cells probably contribute to this process. Pulmonary neuroendocrine cell hyperplasia and the production of peptides analogous to bombesin has been reported in pLCH, but their role remains unclear (Dunzendorfer and Wiedermann, 2001; Lambrecht, 2001). Similarly, granulomatous lesions of pLCH produce abundant TGF-β, which is crucial to intraepithelial LC differentiation (Asakura *et al.*, 1996). Finally, in two recent studies, CCL20 (MIP-3α) was shown to be produced within bone and skin LCH lesions (Annels *et al.*, 2003; Fleming *et al.*, 2003). Interestingly, the LCs of these granulomas expressed both CCR6 but surprisingly also CCR7 in one study (Fleming *et al.*, 2003).

It is likely that nonepithelial factors play a role in maintaining LCs within the LCH granuloma. LCs themselves produce mediators, that may contribute to perpetuate the lesions via an autocrine and/or paracrine mechanism (Egeler *et al.*, 1999). In addition, immunohistochemistry studies of pulmonary LC granulomas have identified several cytokines, of which some (including TNF-α and IL-4) influence LC growth, survival, and differentiation *in vitro*, but their exact role in the pathogenesis of pLCH remains to be determined (Egeler *et al.*, 1999).

The ability of LCs to proliferate within LCH lesions is a matter of controversy. The division rate of LCs within pLCH granulomas is similar to that of normal bronchial epithelial cells and far lower than that of lung cancer cells, suggesting a limited role for cell division in LC accumulation within pLCH lesions (Brabencova *et al.*, 1998). Conversely, at other sites, particularly in the skin and bone, LCs within LCH lesions express the proliferation marker Ki67, as well as other peptides involved in the cell cycle (Schouten *et al.*, 2002).

A central point concerning LCH is whether the disease represents a neoplastic process or is reactive to yet unidentified stimuli. Whereas, LCs within lesions from patients with a variety of clinical presentations were clonal in origin, supporting a neoplastic origin (Willman and McClain, 1998), another study suggests polyclonal expansion of LCs in the lungs of patients with pLCH (Yousem *et al.*, 2001). Thus, pLCH seems to be rather a reactive process in response to one or more unknown stimuli.

Destruction of bronchioles by LCH lesions

In pathologic situations characterized by LC accumulation within the lungs (e.g. alveolar epithelial hyperplasia and some lung cancers), the LCs do not induce tissue destruction or inflammatory cell recruitment (Tazi *et al.*, 2000). A possible explanation for the bronchiolar destruction seen in pLCH is that the LCs are in a special functional state that allows them to induce a local T-cell immune response with cytotoxic effects on the bronchiolar epithelial wall and adjacent lung tissue. The abundance of T cells in early pLCH lesions is consistent with this hypothesis. As with cell-mediated immune responses secondary to antigen stimulation, these T cells are primarily CD4+ and express αβ antigen receptors, as well as early activation markers (Tazi *et al.*, 2000). Under EM, the LCs in pLCH lesions contain many more Birbeck granules than normal LCs (Tazi *et al.*, 2000). These lesional LCs have intimate contact with lymphocytes, sometimes a large number of lymphocytes surround a single LC forming a rosette (Tazi *et al.*, 2000). Finally, the structure of the granuloma, with central LCs surrounded by lymphocytes, closely resembles that of immune granulomas. More recently, LCs in pLCH lesions were shown to express activation markers. Unlike normal or other lesion-associated LCs, the pathologic LCs in pLCH lesions express CD80, CD86, and CD40 (Tazi *et al.*, 1999). In addition, T cells expressing the CD40 ligand are present in these lesions, supporting the existence of local interactions with LCs (Tazi *et al.*, 1999). These data, however, are not a definitive proof that these LCs are fully mature DCs that can induce T-cell proliferation.

The microenvironment surrounding LCs in pLCH lesions is conducive to local LC activation. The cytokine profile (with presence of GM-CSF, TNF-α, and IL-1β but absence of IL-10) is similar to the profile that promotes DC maturation *in vitro*, whereas in the other pathologic situations in which LCs exhibit an immature phenotype, the opposite cytokine profile is found (presence of IL-10 and absence of IL-1β) (Tazi *et al.*, 1999; Akbari *et al.*, 2001; Stumbles *et al.*, 2003; Steinman *et al.*, 2003). Studies of LCH lesions in the bone and skin suggest, however, that the activation status of LCs may be heterogeneous. Although at both sites the LCs express CD40, LCs phenotype in skin lesions are similar to that of lung granulomas and express CD80 and CD86, whereas those in bone lesions do not (Geissmann *et al.*, 2001). Increased IL-10 production has been electively found within bone LCH granulomas (Geissmann *et al.*, 2001). Consistently, functional studies of LCs isolated from bone lesions have shown that these cells are weak lymphostimulatory cells, but this defect was not an intrinsic deficiency since after stimulation via CD40, these cells effectively activated T cells *in vitro* (Geissmann *et al.*, 2001). In summary, LCs in LCH lesions exhibit an unusual surface phenotype, which suggests at least a partial maturation of these cells.

Many other cytokines are produced in LC granulomas and contribute to the accumulation and activation of the inflammatory cells that make up these lesions (Egeler *et al.*, 1999). Similarly, mediators such as TGF-β and some types of metalloproteinases are produced locally and are probably involved in the tissue remodeling and fibrous reaction seen as the lesions change over time (Hayashi *et al.*, 1997).

The hypothesis that pLCH lesions results from an uncontrolled immune response implies that one or more antigens induce this response. To date, no candidate antigens have been identified. A viral cause was hypothesized initially when intramitochondrial inclusions were found in some granuloma LCs, and a role for the HHV6 virus was suggested but not confirmed (Willman and McClain, 1998; Glotzbecker *et al.*, 2004). Testing for genomes of a broad array of viruses within LCH lesions has essentially been negative (Willman and McClain, 1998; Slacmeulder *et al.*, 2002).

Smoking and pLCH

The close association between smoking and pLCH strongly suggests a role for tobacco smoke in the pathogenesis. The role for smoking in triggering pLCH was highlighted recently by the finding that most children with systemic LCH who developed pLCH in adolescence or adulthood started to smoke before this event (Bernstrand *et al.*, 2001). In addition, in an animal model, one group reported accumulation of LC clusters in mouse lungs exposed to tobacco smoke, but this study has not been reproduced (Zeid and Muller, 1995).

How tobacco smoke triggers the formation of pLCH lesions remains unknown. An immune response to a component of tobacco was suggested, but surprisingly, proliferation of blood lymphocytes from patients with pLCH to tobacco-glycoprotein was found to be decreased compared to controls (Youkeles *et al.*, 1995). More recently, the effects of nicotine on DC function was evaluated and both increasing and inhibitory effects were reported (Nouri-Shirazi and Guinet, 2003; Aicher *et al.*, 2003). A direct effect of tobacco smoke, however, fails to explain the occurrence of pLCH in young children and, occasionally, in adult nonsmokers. Another possibility is that the bronchiolar epithelial cells are the target of the immune response in pLCH. Thus, the development of hyperplastic or dysplastic bronchiolar lesions may be involved in both the accumulation and the activation of LCs in bronchioles and, in addition, epithelial cells may express neoantigens, making them the target of an immune response. This hypothesis, which remains to be proved, would explain the bronchiole-centered distribution of the lesions, as well as the early destruction of the bronchiolar epithelium.

The low incidence of pLCH compared to the high prevalence of smoking in the population at large, strongly supports the existence of host-related factors that predispose to development of the disease. Reports of recurrent disease in lungs transplanted to patients with pLCH are further evidence in favor of patient-related factors, whose nature remains to be determined (Sulica *et al.*, 2001).

Clinical presentation

Pulmonary LCH is pleomorphic in its presentation (Tazi *et al.*, 2000; Vassallo *et al.*, 2000; Sundar *et al.*, 2003). Despite diffuse lung involvement, symptoms can be relatively minor or absent, and patients often attribute initial symptoms to smoking. The interval between the onset of symptoms and diagnosis varies but is approximately 6 months on average. The diagnosis is usually made in one of three circumstances:

1 In about 25% of cases, asymptomatic disease is detected on a routine chest radiograph.
2 Respiratory symptoms (dry cough and dyspnea on exertion) are present in two-thirds of cases and can be associated with constitutional manifestations.
3 Spontaneous pneumothorax leads to the diagnosis in about 10–20% of cases.

The occurrence of pneumothorax seems more common in young males, may occur at any time during the course of the disease and may be bilateral and/or recurrent (Mendez *et al.*, 2004).

Other infrequent presentations include chest pain resulting from an associated rib lesion or wheezing. Hemoptysis is uncommon and should not be attributed to pLCH until other causes (particularly lung cancer) have been ruled out (Tazi *et al.*, 2000; Vassallo *et al.*, 2000).

Pulmonary LCH in adults is a single-system disease in the large majority of patients. Bone lesions (<20% of patients), diabetes insipidus with polyuria and polydipsia, and skin lesions are the commonest extrapulmonary manifestations (Tazi *et al.*, 2000; Vassallo *et al.*, 2000).

Physical examination of the chest is usually normal, except in patients with pneumothorax, ribs lesions, or advanced disease with signs of cor pulmonale. Rales are rarely present and clubbing is exceedingly rare. In patients without extrapulmonary involvement, the remainder of the physical examination is typically unremarkable.

Radiology

Chest radiographs

The abnormalities on chest radiography vary with the stage of the disease. Reticulo-micronodular infiltration is the most common pattern (Tazi et al., 2000; Vassallo et al., 2000; Sundar et al., 2003). Cysts may be visible within the infiltrates, which symmetrically involve both lungs, predominating in the middle and upper lung fields and sparing the costophrenic angles. In contrast to most other diffuse pulmonary infiltrating diseases – except lymphoangioleiomyomatosis – lung volumes are normal or increased. Pneumothorax or, more rarely, a lytic lesion in a rib may be visible. Pleural effusion is not a feature, and mediastinal adenopathy is unusual, although hilar enlargement may occur in patients with pulmonary hypertension. In advanced disease, nodular lesions are sparse or absent, and cysts constitute the main radiographic abnormality, sometimes producing an emphysema-like appearance. In rare cases the chest radiograph may be normal (fewer than 10% of patients in an early series) (Epler et al., 1978).

High-resolution computed tomography

HRCT is very useful in the diagnosis of pLCH and is now mandatory when this condition is suspected (Tazi et al., 2000; Vassallo et al., 2000; Sundar et al., 2003). HRCT provides additional details on the parenchymal lesions such as cavitation of nodules. HRCT also permits the demonstration of parenchymal abnormalities in patients with normal chest radiographs. The typical HRCT pattern combines small poorly demarcated nodules, cavitated nodules, thick-walled cysts, and thin-walled cysts (Figure 10.2). These changes affect both the peripheral and the central parts of the lung fields. The lesions are focal, being separated by normal appearing parenchyma, usually predominate in the upper and middle lung fields and tend to spare the basal portions of the lungs. The distribution of the nodules is centrilobular, reflecting the bronchiole-centered development of pLCH lesions. As the disease evolves, cystic lesions become a predominant finding (Figure 10.3). They vary in size, although most are smaller than 1 cm, and may be isolated or confluent, sometimes mimicking centrilobular emphysema. Longitudinal studies involving serial computed tomography (CT) scans have shown that radiological lesions progress from nodules to cavitated nodules, then thick-walled cysts, and finally thin-walled cysts (Brauner et al., 1997). These studies have also shown that nodules and cavitated nodules can resolve, whereas cysts usually persist or enlarge over time (Brauner et al., 1997). Other findings in pLCH include ground-glass attenuation and linear densities

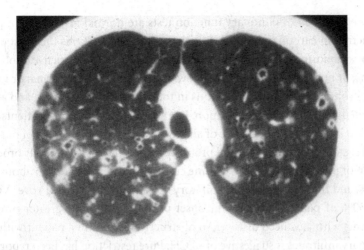

Figure 10.2   HRCT of the lung in a patient with pLCH, showing the typical association of nodules, cavitated nodules, thick-walled cysts, and thin-walled cysts

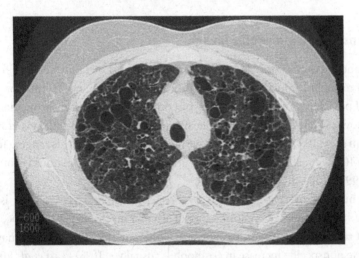

Figure 10.3   HRCT of the lung in a patient with advanced pLCH showing numerous variably sized pulmonary cysts

or emphysematous bulla secondary to cigarette smoke exposure. Pleural effusion is exceedingly rare and mediastinal adenopathy is unusual. Pulmonary artery enlargement has been reported. Finally, HRCT is crucial for selecting surgical biopsy sites in those patients who require this investigation.

Pulmonary function

Pulmonary function abnormalities are variable and depend both on the predominant anatomic lesions and on disease duration (Tazi *et al.*, 2000; Vassallo *et al.*, 2000;

Sundar *et al.*, 2003). Pulmonary function tests are normal in 10–15% of patients. A reduction in carbon monoxide diffusing capacity (D_LCO) is the most common functional abnormality, being found in 70–90% of patients. Restrictive or obstructive patterns, or both, has been reported. Low vital capacity (VC), normal or increased residual volume (RV), mild alterations in total lung capacity (TLC), and a normal or elevated RV/TLC ratio are common. In a sizeable proportion of patients, airflow limitation is observed. The degree of airway obstruction appears out of proportion to total cigarette consumption, and probably reflects the predominantly bronchiolar location of pLCH lesions. Flow/volume curve alterations are seen in about 50% of patients, and the ratio of forced expiratory volume in 1 min (FEV1) over VC is low in 20–30% of patients with recent-onset pLCH and in a far greater proportion of patients with advanced disease. An obstructive pattern in a patient with diffuse pulmonary infiltrates is suggestive of pLCH. Pure restriction has been reported too. Exercise testing often demonstrates alveolar-arterial oxygen gradient elevation and hypoxemia which has been ascribed to vascular impairment.

Bronchoscopy and bronchoalveolar lavage

The bronchial tree is normal to gross examination or shows only nonspecific inflammation related to smoking. Bronchial mucosa biopsies are not helpful for the diagnosis of pLCH but are useful in ruling out other diagnoses. Transbronchial biopsies may show pLCH, provided multiple specimens are obtained (Travis *et al.*, 1993; Houssini *et al.*, 1994). Some studies have reported diagnostic yields ranging from only 10% to 40%, reflecting the focal distribution of the parenchymatous lesions (Travis *et al.*, 1993; Houssini *et al.*, 1994).

The number of cells recovered by bronchoalveolar lavage (BAL) is usually increased, with a marked predominance of alveolar macrophages, a nonspecific finding that reflects cigarette smoke exposure. Differential BAL cell counts may show a moderate nonspecific increase in eosinophils (usually <10%) (Tazi *et al.*, 2000). The proportion of alveolar lymphocytes is normal or diminished, and the CD4/CD8 ratio is decreased, as is observed in smokers.

The identification of LC among BAL cells using anti-CD1a monoclonal antibodies (OKT6 or equivalent) is frequently suggested as a diagnostic test, but this test lacks sensitivity. Up to 3% LC can be recovered by lavage from smokers without diffuse lung disease, and increased numbers of LC (up to 4% in our series) can be seen in patients with diffuse interstitial lung disease associated with alveolar hyperplasia (particularly diffuse pulmonary fibrosis) (Tazi *et al.*, 2000). If one uses the threshold of 5% LC for the diagnosis of LCH in adults, the specificity is good, but sensitivity is low (<25% in our experience). In most adults with pLCH, the proportion of CD1a-positive LCs is similar to that in smokers without lung disease.

In practice, BAL rarely establishes the definite diagnosis of pLCH in adults. It is of greatest use in differential diagnosis of patients without typical radiologic findings. The test can be used to orient the diagnosis away from interstitial lung diseases with more characteristic lavage findings, and rule out certain pulmonary infections such as cavitated forms of *Pneumocystis* infection that may cause confusion in certain cases.

Routine laboratory tests

Standard laboratory tests are uninformative. In patients with constitutional symptoms, serological tests should be obtained to rule out human immunodeficiency virus (HIV) infection.

Unusual presentations

Atypical forms of pLCH are uncommon but raise major diagnostic challenges. A variety of atypical radiographic findings have been reported, including presentation as an isolated nodule, markedly asymmetric radiological abnormalities, presence of air-fluid levels in cystic lesions, focal 'alveolar' consolidation, pleural effusion and mediastinal adenopathy (Tazi *et al.*, 2000). Rare cases with extensive ground-glass opacities at lung HRCT have been reported (Vassallo *et al.*, 2003). This ground-glass pattern seems to reflect the extent of histologic respiratory bronchiolitis/interstitial lung (RB/ILD)-like changes related to smoking that are observed in the lung of these patients.

Pulmonary LCH can be associated with severe pulmonary arterial hypertension, and symptoms and hemodynamic features similar to those seen in primary pulmonary hypertension can dominate the clinical presentation (Fartoukh *et al.*, 2000). The pulmonary vascular lesions tend to predominate in the venules and may produce a picture reminiscent of pulmonary veno-occlusive disease (Fartoukh *et al.*, 2000; Hamada *et al.*, 2000). .

Diagnosis

The definite diagnosis of LCH rests on identification of an LC granuloma in involved tissue. Although transbronchial biopsy may show LC granulomas in pLCH, histological documentation is more often obtained by surgical biopsy (usually video-assisted thoracoscopy), and should be taken from sites where HRCT shows an abundance of nodules. As the lesions are focal, the specimens should be sufficiently large to ensure the availability of adequate material, an extensive search for specific lesions should be performed, and whenever possible a tissue fragment should be frozen for immunohistochemical studies. When no frozen tissue is available, the specimens can be tested with anti-CD1a O10 antibody, which reacts with LCs in formalin-fixed and paraffin-embedded tissue. Features of DIP-like or RB/ILD-like patterns may mask LCH lesions, and the presence of these findings should not discourage a meticulous search for pathological changes specific of LCH (Vassallo *et al.*, 2003).

In patients with suggestive clinical manifestations, HRCT findings are often sufficient to establish the diagnosis, so that the need for surgical biopsy should be discussed on a case-by-case basis. A nodular and cystic pattern predominating in the upper half of the lung fields in a young asymptomatic smoker whose BAL fluid contains high macrophage counts leaves little doubt as to the diagnosis of pLCH. Conversely, in patients with systemic symptoms and cavitated pulmonary nodules, and in the rare pure nodular forms, there is a long list of differential diagnoses including mycobacterial infection, other infections, sarcoidosis, Wegener's granulomatosis, cavitated pulmonary metastases, bronchiolar-alveolar carcinoma, septic emboli, or cavitated *P. jiroveci* pneumonia. In women, pure cystic pLCH may be difficult to differentiate from lymphangioleiomyomatosis (Johnson, 1999).

In practice, a presumptive diagnosis seems appropriate during the initial work-up of patients with typical manifestations and little or no symptoms. Surgical lung biopsy can be performed during surgical pleurodesis in patients with recurrent or persistent pneumothorax. We also perform lung biopsy in women with isolated diffuse pulmonary cystic lesions, in symptomatic patients with predominant nodular lesions who are being considered for systemic corticosteroids, and in patients with atypical presentations. Finally, biopsy of an extrathoracic lesion, for instance in a bone, may provide the diagnosis when the pulmonary manifestations are consistent with LCH.

Course and prognosis

The natural history of the disease is variable and unpredictable (Tazi *et al.*, 2000; Vassallo *et al.*, 2000; Sundar *et al.*, 2003). Roughly, about 50% of patients experience a favorable outcome, either spontaneously or with glucocorticoid therapy with partial or complete clearance of the radiological abnormalities. These patients, however, can slowly develop an obstructive ventilatory defect that warrants lung function follow-up. About 10% to 20% of patients have early severe manifestations consisting in recurrent pneumothorax or progressive respiratory failure with chronic cor pulmonale. A third of patients have persistent symptoms of variable severity with conversion of radiological nodules into thick-walled then thin-walled cysts that remain stable over time. Despite the apparent quiescence of the disease in these patients, LC granulomas may be present in the pulmonary parenchyma (Soler *et al.*, 2000). Thus, long-term follow-up is mandatory and may detect exacerbation of respiratory dysfunction after many years or, rarely, a relapse with recurrent nodule formation (Tazi *et al.*, 1998).

Factors reported to predict adverse outcomes include onset of pLCH at an old age, prolonged constitutional symptoms, recurrent pneumothorax, extrathoracic lesions (except for bone involvement, which has no bearing on the prognosis), diffuse cysts on imaging studies, and severe pulmonary function abnormalities at diagnosis (particularly abnormalities in the FEV1 and FEV1/VC, $D_L CO$ and to a lesser extent in RV/TLC) (Delobbe *et al.*, 1996; Vassallo *et al.*, 2002). None of these criteria can reliably predict outcome in the individual patient. Severe pulmonary hypertension indicates a poor prognosis (Fartoukh *et al.*, 2000).

Pregnancy does not seem to influence the course of pLCH in most patients, and unless there is severe respiratory failure, LCH is not a contraindication to pregnancy. In addition to an association between LCH and lymphoma, a high rate of primary lung cancer has been reported in these patients, with continued smoking being a risk factor. Various other malignancies have also been found to occur at increased rates (Egeler *et al.*, 1993; Howarth *et al.*, 1999; Vassallo *et al.*, 2002).

Treatment

As many patients with pLCH recover spontaneously or remain stable without treatment, the effectiveness of the various treatments used in this condition is difficult to assess. In practice, no effective treatments are available, and no randomized double-blind studies have been published. As patients with minor symptoms are frequently lost to follow-up, the mortality rate is difficult to evaluate and is probably overestimated in longitudinal studies (Delobbe *et al.*, 1996; Vassallo *et al.*, 2002).

The association between pLCH and smoking suggests a causal role for cigarette smoke and smoking cessation is mandatory. Referral to a smoking cessation program should be encouraged. Resolution of the disease after smoking cessation has been observed (Mogulkoc *et al.*, 1999). Nevertheless, a few cases of recurrence despite smoking cessation have been reported (Tazi *et al.*, 1998). Smoking cessation consistently reduces the risk of primary lung cancer, cardiovascular disease, and progressive respiratory function impairment due to smoking-related chronic obstructive pulmonary disease, which commonly co-exists with pLCH.

Glucocorticoid therapy attenuates the constitutional symptoms and is advocated on empirical grounds in the treatment of recent-onset symptomatic nodular pLCH (prednisone or prednisolone in a starting dosage of 0.5–1 mg/kg/day tapered over 6–12 months) (Tazi *et al.*, 2000; Vassallo *et al.*, 2000). Although glucocorticoid therapy may be associated with resolution of symptoms and radiological abnormalities, it has not been proven to induce significant respiratory function improvement.

Glucocorticoid therapy was associated with worse outcomes in some studies, probably as a result of selection bias (Delobbe *et al.*, 1996; Vassallo *et al.*, 2002). We reserve glucocorticoid therapy for patients with symptomatic nodular disease, in the hope that this treatment may accelerate the resolution of inflammatory granulomatous lesions.

Cytotoxic agents (vinblastine and, less often, methotrexate) are indicated in combination with glucocorticoid therapy in severe multisystem LCH. There is no evidence that these agents are beneficial in adults with isolated pLCH. 2CDA has been shown to be useful in cases of refractory systemic LCH, but an improvement of lung function of patients with pLCH has not been clearly demonstrated (Saven and Burian, 1999; Goh *et al.*, 2003; Pardanani *et al.*, 2003). Whether 2CDA could be useful as a second line drug for patients with progressive pLCH remains to be evaluated.

Lower respiratory tract infections are common and should be treated promptly. Pneumothorax requires drainage. Pleurodesis may be needed (Mendez *et al.*, 2004). Pleurectomy is best avoided in these young patients who may eventually become lung transplant candidates. Patients with respiratory failure or severe pulmonary hypertension have been treated with lung transplantation, with results similar to those in patients with other patterns of diffuse infiltrating lung disease (Sulica *et al.*, 2001). However, recurrence of the disease in the transplant within the first year has been reported, with possible risk factors being resumption of smoking and extrapulmonary involvement (Sulica *et al.*, 2001).

The optimal follow-up strategy in patients with pLCH is not clear. Physical examination, a chest radiograph, and lung function tests should be obtained periodically, for instance at intervals of 3–6 months. Changes on chest radiograph should lead to HRCT scanning. Although HRCT is useful for monitoring the natural history of pLCH, the optimal frequency and the impact on management remain unclear. The severity of pulmonary abnormalities on HRCT scans is correlated with $D_L CO$, but there are no studies comparing HRCT and lung function test results over time.

Typically, obstructive lung disease is associated with worsening of the cystic lesions, which form bullous-like lesions in advanced disease. As the chest radiograph has low sensitivity for visualizing pulmonary cysts, apparent radiographic stability of the lesions, is not infrequent in patients with gradually worsening obstructive dysfunction. Doppler echocardiography should be performed in dyspneic patients to detect pulmonary hypertension.

No reliable criteria are available for assessing the activity of pLCH. HRCT is not entirely reliable for identifying inactive disease because even in patients with cysts as the only visible lesions granulomas may persist in the pulmonary parenchyma (Soler *et al.*, 2000). Recent preliminary results suggest that scintigraphy with

[111]In-pentetreotide (a somatostatin analog) may be useful for assessing lesion activity (Calming *et al.*, 2000; Weinmann *et al.*, 2000; Lastoria *et al.*, 2002).

Conclusion

Although some of the steps in the disease process that leads to pLCH are beginning to come to light, further work remains to determine the mechanisms involved according to the location and clinical expression of the disease. Improved understanding of the pathogenesis of LCH should help in the development of rational treatments for this enigmatic disease.

REFERENCES

Aicher, A., Heeschen, C., Mohaupt, M., *et al.* (2003). Nicotine strongly activates dendritic cell-mediated adaptive immunity: potential role for progression of atherosclerotic lesions. *Circulation*, **107**, 604–611.

Akbari, O., DeKruyff, R.H. and Umetsu, D.T. (2001). Pulmonary dendritic cells producing IL-10 mediate tolerance induced by respiratory exposure to antigen. *Nat Immunol*, **2**, 725–731.

Annels, N.E., Da Costa, C.E., Prins, F.A., *et al.* (2003). Aberrant chemokine receptor expression and chemokine production by Langerhans cells underlies the pathogenesis of Langerhans cell histiocytosis. *J Exp Med*, **197**, 1385–1390.

Arico, M., Haupt, R., Russotto, V.S., *et al.* (2001). Langerhans cell histiocytosis in two generations: a new family and review of the literature. *Med Pediatr Oncol*, **36**, 314–316.

Asakura, S., Colby, T.V. and Limper, A.H. (1996). Tissue localization of transforming growth factor-beta1 in pulmonary eosinophilic granuloma. *Am J Respir Crit Care Med*, **154**, 1525–1530.

Banchereau, J., Briere, F., Caux, C., *et al.* (2000). Immunobiology of dendritic cells. *Annu Rev Immunol*, **18**, 767–811.

Bernstrand, C., Cederlund, K., Sandstedt, B., *et al.* (2001). Pulmonary abnormalities at long-term follow-up of patients with Langerhans cell histiocytosis. *Med Pediatr Oncol*, **36**, 459–468.

Brabencova, E., Tazi, A., Lorenzato, M., *et al.* (1998). Langerhans cells in Langerhans cell granulomatosis are not actively proliferating cells. *Am J Pathol*, **152**, 1143–1149.

Brauner, M.W., Grenier, P., Tijani, K., *et al.* (1997). Pulmonary Langerhans cell histiocytosis: evolution of lesions on CT scans (see comments). *Radiology*, **204**, 497–502.

Burnham, K., Robb, L., Scott, C.L., *et al.* (2000). Effect of granulocyte-macrophage colony-stimulating factor on the generation of epidermal Langerhans cells. *J Interferon Cytokine Res*, **20**, 1071–1076.

Calming, U., Jacobsson, H. and Henter, J.I. (2000). Detection of Langerhans cell histiocytosis lesions with somatostatin analogue scintigraphy – a preliminary report. *Med Pediatr Oncol*, **35**, 462–467.

Caux, C., Vanbervliet, B., Massacrier, C., *et al.* (2002). Regulation of dendritic cell recruitment by chemokines. *Transplantation*, **73**, S7–S11.

Delobbe, A., Durieu, J., Duhamel, A., *et al.* (1996). Determinants of survival in pulmonary Langerhans' cell granulomatosis (histiocytosis X). Groupe d'Etude en Pathologie Interstitielle de la Societe de Pathologie Thoracique du Nord. *Eur Respir J*, **9**, 2002–2006.

Dieu-Nosjean, M.C., Massacrier, C., Homey, B., *et al.* (2000). Macrophage inflammatory protein 3alpha is expressed at inflamed epithelial surfaces and is the most potent chemokine known in attracting Langerhans cell precursors. *J Exp Med*, **192**, 705–718.

Dunzendorfer, S. and Wiedermann, C.J. (2001). Neuropeptides and the immune system: focus on dendritic cells. *Crit Rev Immunol*, **21**, 523–557.

Egeler, R.M., Neglia, J.P., Puccetti, D.M., *et al.* (1993). Association of Langerhans cell histiocytosis with malignant neoplasms. *Cancer*, **71**, 865–873.

Egeler, R.M., Favara, B.E., van Meurs, M., *et al.* (1999). Differential *in situ* cytokine profiles of Langerhans-like cells and T cells in Langerhans cell histiocytosis: abundant expression of cytokines relevant to disease and treatment. *Blood*, **94**, 4195–4201.

Egeler, R.M., Annels, N.E. and Hogendoorn, P.C. (2004). Langerhans cell histiocytosis: a pathologic combination of oncogenesis and immune dysregulation. *Pediatr Blood Cancer*, **42**, 401–403.

Epler, G., McLoud, T. and Gaensler, E. (1978). Normal chest roentgenograms in chronic diffuse infiltrative lung disease. *New Engl J Med*, **298**, 934–939.

Fartoukh, M., Humbert, M., Capron, F., *et al.* (2000). Severe pulmonary hypertension in histiocytosis X. *Am J Respir Crit Care Med*, **161**, 216–223.

Fleming, M.D., Pinkus, J.L., Alexander, S.W., *et al.* (2003). Coincident expression of the chemokine receptors CCR6 and CCR7 by pathologic Langerhans cells in Langerhans cell histiocytosis. *Blood*, **101**, 2473–2475.

Gaensler, E. and Carrington, C. (1980). Open biopsy for chronic diffuse infiltrative lung disease: clinical, reontgenographic, and physiological correlations in 502 patients. *Ann Thorac Surg*, **30**, 411–426.

Geissmann, F., Lepelletier, Y., Fraitag, S., *et al.* (2001). Differentiation of Langerhans cells in Langerhans cell histiocytosis. *Blood*, **97**, 1241–1248.

Geissmann, F., Dieu-Nosjean, M.C., Dezutter, C., *et al.* (2002). Accumulation of immature Langerhans cells in human lymph nodes draining chronically inflamed skin. *J Exp Med*, **196**, 417–430.

Glotzbecker, M.P., Carpentieri, D.F. and Dormans, J.P. (2004). Langerhans cell histiocytosis: a primary viral infection of bone? Human herpes virus 6 latent protein detected in lymphocytes from tissue of children. *J Pediatr Orthop*, **24**, 123–129.

Godefroy, S., Guironnet, G., Jacquet, C., *et al.* (2001). A combination of MIP-3alpha and TGF-beta1 is required for the attraction of human Langerhans precursor cells through a dermal – epidermal barrier. *Eur J Cell Biol*, **80**, 335–340.

Goh, N.S., McDonald, C.E., MacGregor, D.P., *et al.* (2003). Successful treatment of Langerhans cell histiocytosis with 2-chlorodeoxyadenosine. *Respirology*, **8**, 91–94.

Hamada, K., Teramoto, S., Narita, N., *et al.* (2000). Pulmonary veno-occlusive disease in pulmonary Langerhans' cell granulomatosis. *Eur Respir J*, **15**, 421–423.

Hayashi, T., Rush, W.L., Travis, W.D., *et al.* (1997). Immunohistochemical study of matrix metalloproteinases and their tissue inhibitors in pulmonary Langerhans' cell granulomatosis. *Arch Pathol Lab Med*, **121**, 930–937.

Homey, B., Dieu-Nosjean, M.C., Wiesenborn, A., *et al.* (2000). Up-regulation of macrophage inflammatory protein-3 alpha/CCL20 and CC chemokine receptor 6 in psoriasis. *J Immunol*, **164**, 6621–6632.

Houssini, I., Tomashefski, J. and Cohen, A. (1994). Transbronchial biopsy in patients with pulmonary eosinophilic granuloma. *Arch Pathol Lab Med*, **118**, 523–530.

Howarth, D.M., Gilchrist, G.S., Mullan, B.P., *et al.* (1999). Langerhans cell histiocytosis: diagnosis, natural history, management, and outcome. *Cancer*, **85**, 2278–2290.

Johnson, S. (1999). Rare diseases. 1. Lymphangioleiomyomatosis: clinical features, management and basic mechanisms. *Thorax*, **54**, 254–264.

Kambouchner, M., Basset, F., Marchal, J., *et al.* (2002). Three-dimensional characterization of pathologic lesions in pulmonary Langerhans cell histiocytosis. *Am J Respir Crit Care Med*, **166**, 1483–1490.

Knight, S.C., Burke, F. and Bedford, P.A. (2002). Dendritic cells, antigen distribution and the initiation of primary immune responses to self and non-self antigens. *Semin Cancer Biol*, **12**, 301–308.

Lambrecht, B.N. (2001). Immunologists getting nervous: neuropeptides, dendritic cells and T cell activation. *Respir Res*, **2**, 133–138.

Lastoria, S., Montella, L., Catalano, L., *et al.* (2002). Functional imaging of Langerhans cell histiocytosis by (111)In-DTPA-D-Phe(1)-octreotide scintigraphy. *Cancer*, **94**, 633–640.

Mellman, I. and Steinman, R.M. (2001). Dendritic cells: specialized and regulated antigen processing machines. *Cell*, **106**, 255–258.

Mendez, J.L., Nadrous, H.F., Vassallo, R., *et al.* (2004). Pneumothorax in pulmonary Langerhans cell histiocytosis. *Chest*, **125**, 1028–1032.

Mogulkoc, N., Veral, A., Bishop, P.W., *et al.* (1999). Pulmonary Langerhans' cell histiocytosis: radiologic resolution following smoking cessation. *Chest*, **115**, 1452–1455.

Nezelof, C. and Basset, F. (2004). An hypothesis Langerhans cell histiocytosis: the failure of the immune system to switch from an innate to an adaptive mode. *Pediatr Blood Cancer*, **42**, 398–400.

Nouri-Shirazi, M. and Guinet, E. (2003). Evidence for the immunosuppressive role of nicotine on human dendritic cell functions. *Immunology*, **109**, 365–373.

Pardanani, A., Phyliky, R.L., Li, C.Y., *et al.* (2003). 2-Chlorodeoxyadenosine therapy for disseminated Langerhans cell histiocytosis. *Mayo Clin Proc*, **78**, 301–306.

Riedl, E., Stockl, J., Majdic, O., *et al.* (2000). Ligation of E-cadherin on *in vitro* generated immature Langerhans-type dendritic cells inhibits their maturation. *Blood*, **96**, 4276–4284.

Sallusto, F. and Lanzavecchia, A. (2000). Understanding dendritic cell and T-lymphocyte traffic through the analysis of chemokine receptor expression. *Immunol Rev*, **177**, 134–140.

Saven, A. and Burian, C. (1999). Cladribine activity in adult Langerhans-cell histiocytosis. *Blood*, **93**, 4125–4130.

Schouten, B., Egeler, R.M., Leenen, P.J., *et al.* (2002). Expression of cell cycle-related gene products in Langerhans cell histiocytosis. *J Pediatr Hematol Oncol*, **24**, 727–732.

Slacmeulder, M., Geissmann, F., Lepelletier, Y., *et al.* (2002). No association between Langerhans cell histiocytosis and human herpes virus 8. *Med Pediatr Oncol*, **39**, 187–189.

Soler, P., Bergeron, A., Kambouchner, M., *et al.* (2000). Is high-resolution computed tomography a reliable tool to predict the histopathological activity of pulmonary Langerhans cell histiocytosis? *Am J Respir Crit Care Med*, **162**, 264–270.

Steinman, R.M., Hawiger, D. and Nussenzweig, M.C. (2003). Tolerogenic dendritic cells. *Annu Rev Immunol*, **21**, 685–711.

Stoitzner, P., Holzmann, S., McLellan, A.D., *et al.* (2003). Visualization and characterization of migratory Langerhans cells in murine skin and lymph nodes by antibodies against Langerin/CD207. *J Invest Dermatol*, **120**, 266–274.

Stumbles, P.A., Upham, J.W. and Holt, P.G. (2003). Airway dendritic cells: co-ordinators of immunological homeostasis and immunity in the respiratory tract. *Apmis*, **111**, 741–755.

Sulica, R., Teirstein, A. and Padilla, M.L. (2001). Lung transplantation in interstitial lung disease. *Curr Opin Pulm Med*, **7**, 314–322.

Sundar, K.M., Gosselin, M.V., Chung, H.L., *et al.* (2003). Pulmonary Langerhans cell histiocytosis: emerging concepts in pathobiology, radiology, and clinical evolution of disease. *Chest*, **123**, 1673–1683.

Tazi, A., Bouchonnet, F., Grandsaigne, M., *et al.* (1993). Evidence that granulocyte macrophage-colony-stimulating factor regulates the distribution and differentiated state of dendritic cells/Langerhans cells in human lung and lung cancers. *J Clin Invest*, **91**, 566–576.

Tazi, A., Montcelly, L., Bergeron, A., *et al.* (1998). Relapsing nodular lesions in the course of adult pulmonary Langerhans cell histiocytosis. *Am J Respir Crit Care Med*, **157**, 2007–2010.

Tazi, A., Moreau, J., Bergeron, A., *et al.* (1999). Evidence that Langerhans cells in adult pulmonary Langerhans cell histiocytosis are mature dendritic cells: importance of the cytokine microenvironment. *J Immunol*, **163**, 3511–3515.

Tazi, A., Soler, P. and Hance, A.J. (2000). Adult pulmonary Langerhans' cell histiocytosis. *Thorax*, **55**, 405–416.

Travis, W.D., Borok, Z., Roum, J.H., *et al.* (1993). Pulmonary Langerhans cell granulomatosis (histiocytosis X). A clinicopathologic study of 48 cases. *Am J Surg Pathol*, **17**, 971–986.

Trinchieri, G. (2003). Interleukin-12 and the regulation of innate resistance and adaptive immunity. *Nat Rev Immunol*, **3**, 133–146.

Unger, J., England, D. and Collins, J. (1994). Miliary nodules, Hodgkin's disease, and eosinophilic granuloma. *J Thor Imaging*, **9**, 71–73.

Valladeau, J., Duvert-Frances, V., Pin, J.J., *et al.* (1999). The monoclonal antibody DCGM4 recognizes Langerin, a protein specific of Langerhans cells, and is rapidly internalized from the cell surface. *Eur J Immunol*, **29**, 2695–2704.

Vanbervliet, B., Homey, B., Durand, I., *et al.* (2002). Sequential involvement of CCR2 and CCR6 ligands for immature dendritic cell recruitment: possible role at inflamed epithelial surfaces. *Eur J Immunol*, **32**, 231–242.

Vassallo, R., Ryu, J.H., Colby, T.V., *et al.* (2000). Pulmonary Langerhans'-cell histiocytosis. *New Engl J Med*, **342**, 1969–1978.

Vassallo, R., Ryu, J.H., Schroeder, D.R., *et al.* (2002). Clinical outcomes of pulmonary Langerhans'-cell histiocytosis in adults. *New Engl J Med*, **346**, 484–490.

Vassallo, R., Jensen, E.A., Colby, T.V., *et al.* (2003). The overlap between respiratory bronchiolitis and desquamative interstitial pneumonia in pulmonary Langerhans cell histiocytosis: high-resolution CT, histologic, and functional correlations. *Chest*, **124**, 1199–1205.

Wang, J., Snider, D.P., Hewlett, B.R., *et al.* (2000). Transgenic expression of granulocyte-macrophage colony-stimulating factor induces the differentiation and activation of a novel dendritic cell population in the lung. *Blood*, **95**, 2337–2345.

Watanabe, R., Tatsumi, K., Hashimoto, S., *et al.* (2001). Clinico-epidemiological features of pulmonary histiocytosis X. *Int Med*, **40**, 998–1003.

Weinmann, P., Crestani, B., Tazi, A., *et al.* (2000). ^{111}In-pentetreotide scintigraphy in patients with Langerhans' cell histiocytosis. *J Nucl Med*, **41**, 1808–1812.

Willman, C.L. and McClain, K.L. (1998). An update on clonality, cytokines, and viral etiology in Langerhans cell histiocytosis. *Hematol Oncol Clin North Am*, **12**, 407–416.

Youkeles, L.H., Grizzanti, J.N., Liao, Z., *et al.* (1995). Decreased tobacco-glycoprotein-induced lymphocyte proliferation *in vitro* in pulmonary eosinophilic granuloma. *Am J Respir Crit Care Med*, **151**, 145–150.

Yousem, S.A., Colby, T.V., Chen, Y.Y., *et al.* (2001). Pulmonary Langerhans' cell histiocytosis: molecular analysis of clonality. *Am J Surg Pathol*, **25**, 630–636.

Zeid, N.A. and Muller, H.K. (1995). Tobacco smoke induced lung granulomas and tumors: association with pulmonary Langerhans cells. *Pathology*, **27**, 247–254.

11

Central nervous system disease in Langerhans cell histiocytosis

Nicole Grois, Helmut Prosch, Hans Lassmann and
Daniela Prayer

Introduction

Central nervous system (CNS) involvement has been a well-known feature of Langerhans cell histiocytosis (LCH) since the early descriptions of the disease. Around the turn of the twentieth century, Hand–Schüller–Christian reported on patients with diabetes insipidus (DI), the clinical symptom of the most frequent type of CNS involvement (Schüller, 1915; Christian, 1920; Hand, 1921). Some years later, several authors described cases with 'generalized xanthomatosis of Schüller–Christian type' with cerebral involvement other than the infundibular region including isolated or multiple tumours, or demyelination, nerve cell destruction, and gliosis associated with a plethora of neurological symptoms (Chester and Kugel, 1932; Chiari, 1933; Davison, 1933; Feigin, 1956). During the last decade, in parallel to the more frequent routine use of modern imaging techniques, more and more LCH patients have been detected with CNS changes, some even in the absence of clinical symptoms (Greenwood et al., 1981; Graif and Pennock, 1986; Burn et al., 1992; Breidahl et al., 1993; Grois et al., 1993; Barthez et al., 2000). Magnetic resonance imaging (MRI) (or sometimes computed tomography, CT) is usually performed to monitor craniofacial lesions, or to evaluate patients with clinical endocrine deficiencies such as DI, growth retardation or pubertal abnormalities, or those with neurological or psychological problems.

As discussed later, histopathologically CNS involvement takes two forms, granulomas which morphologically and immunohistochemically are typical LCH lesions, and a neurodegenerative form in which no active LCH can be found. The granulomas follow a hierarchical pattern, with involvement of areas of the brain in which dendritic cells normally occur, usually outside of the blood–brain barrier (BBB) such as the hypothalamic–pituitary region (HPR), the pineal and choroid plexus. With the occurrence of inflammation however, LCH cells can infiltrate through the glia-limiting membrane and be found intraxially (within the BBB).

The incidence of HPR involvement, the commonest site of CNS involvement in LCH, has been reported to be between 10% and 15% (Gadner *et al.*, 1987; The French Langerhans Cell Histiocytosis Study Group, 1996; Willis *et al.*, 1996). The incidence of neurodegenerative LCH is not yet known, but it appears that neuro-degenerative LCH is commoner than previously believed. Recent studies estimate a frequency of 1–4% (Grois *et al.*, 1995; The French Langerhans Cell Histiocytosis Study Group, 1996; Willis *et al.*, 1996; Donadieu *et al.*, 2004). The overall frequency of CNS manifestations of LCH will remain unclear, as long as only selected LCH patients with a clinical indication undergo imaging evaluation. However, epi-demiological data evolving from large international trials will contribute to a better estimate of the frequency of CNS LCH.

The pattern and course of CNS LCH is very heterogeneous. CNS complications may be the presenting symptom, may precede the diagnosis, or develop many years after diagnosis of extracerebral LCH (Grois *et al.*, 1998). Depending on the site and type of involvement a variety of neurological symptoms may be observed in CNS LCH patients, including extrapyramidal symptoms, cerebellar signs such as tremor, gait disturbance, ataxia, reflex abnormalities, dysarthria, dysphagia, dys-functional voiding or headaches (Grois *et al.*, 1998). In addition, concern about striking psychological and behavioural problems in LCH survivors has emerged (Ransom and Murphy, 1977; Simms and Warner, 1998; Watts and Files, 2001; Nanduri *et al.*, 2003).

During the past years, due to the greater awareness of the disease and the improved international communication, an increasing number of patients have been registered on the Histocyte Society CNS LCH Study. The data deriving from this registry, has contributed to a better understanding of clinical and imaging char-acteristics of the various overlapping types of (intra)cranial LCH. Based on this experience, MRI findings in CNS LCH have been divided into four major groups: (Prayer *et al.*, 2004) (Table 11.1)

1 craniofacial bones and/or skull base and/or paranasal sinus involvement,
2 intracranial–extra-axial changes,
3 intracranial–intra-axial changes,
4 atrophy.

In the following the typical presentations of (intra)cranial LCH will be described with respect to their clinical features and course, MRI pattern, histopathology, and management.

Table 11.1 Pattern of MRI findings in LCH CNS (Prayer *et al.*, 2004)

- Craniofacial bones and/or skull base
- Intracranial–extra-axial changes
  Meninges
  Pineal gland
  Ependyma
  Choroid plexus
  HPR
- Intracranial–intra-axial changes
  Intraparenchymal disease with a vascular distribution pattern
    Dilated VR spaces
    Enhancing lesions
  Intraparenchymal neurodegenerative disease
    Grey matter changes
    Leukencephalopathy-like pattern
- Atrophy

HPR: Hypothalamopituitary region; VR: Virchow-Robin spaces.

Patterns of (intra)cranial LCH

Craniofacial bone and skull base lesions

LCH has a well-known propensity to involve craniofacial bones. Skull lesions are observed in 40–80% of patients with bone disease (Gadner *et al.*, 1987; Titgemeyer *et al.*, 2001). Otitis with otorrhea associated with temporal bone lesions, or uni- or bilateral proptosis caused by orbital lesions are key symptoms of LCH (Figure 11.1). Orbital involvement has been reported in about 15% of patients, and temporal bone with mastoid involvement in up to 40%, mostly multisystem, patients. A control study comparing MRI findings of LCH and non-LCH patients, found the paranasal sinuses (with or without clinically overt sinusitis) and mastoids significantly more frequently involved in 55% of LCH patients *versus* 20% of controls (Prayer *et al.*, 2004).

Patients with craniofacial involvement appear to have a higher risk of developing DI, often the first sign of CNS involvement (Dunger *et al.*, 1989; Grois *et al.*, 1995; The French Langerhans Cell Histiocytosis Study Group, 1996). However, the actual impact of such lesions on the risk of developing DI and other manifestations of CNS disease, can only be determined by long-term follow-up studies, including regular MRI examinations, for all LCH patients.

The appropriate therapeutic management for patients with localized craniofacial lesions remains a matter of discussion. Subtotal resection with or without intra-lesional steroid infiltration for solitary orbital lesions has been recommended (Woo and Harris, 2003). In the absence of information about the efficacy of non-steroidal anti-inflammatory drugs (NSAIDS), and bisphosphonates in preventing

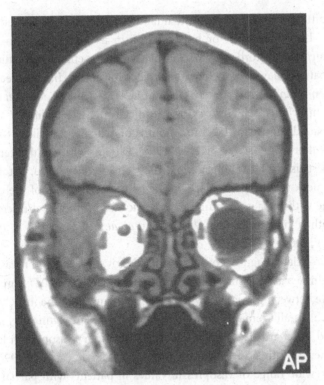

Figure 11.1   T1-weighted coronal MRI of a right-sided orbital lesion showing an expanding soft-tissue mass with destruction of the lateral wall of the orbit

DI and other CNS disease, the present recommendation for patients with extensive orbital lesions, as well as other extensive skull base lesions with intracranial extension of the soft tissue component, in whom such a local approach appears to be too risky, is for chemotherapy. The LCH III study protocol offers standard chemotherapy (LCH Study Group of the Histiocyte Society, 2001) for such cases in an attempt to accelerate healing, and possibly prevent DI and other CNS consequences. Unfortunately patient numbers preclude randomized studies, and careful and prolonged follow-up of all patients with craniofacial disease, including brain MRI scans and regular assessment of hypothalamo–pituitary axis, and neurological status, may help to resolve these important questions.

Intracranial–extra-axial disease

The extra-axial spaces include structures outside the BBB (Table 11.1).

Hypothalamic–pituitary disease

There is a well-recognized predilection of LCH for the HPR. The clinical signs and symptoms of HPR involvement include polyuria and polydipsia as manifestations of posterior pituitary dysfunction, growth failure, precocious or delayed puberty, amenorrhoea, hypothyroidism or hypocortisolism as presentations of anterior pituitary impairment. Disturbances in social behaviour, appetite, temperature regulation or sleep pattern may indicate hypothalamic involvement. In more recent studies DI has been observed in about 10–15% of LCH patients (Gadner *et al.*, 1987; The French Langerhans Cell Histiocytosis Study Group, 1996; Willis *et al.*, 1996). DI may pre-date diagnosis of LCH for months or years, and is likely to develop within 5 years after diagnosis (Grois *et al.*, 1998). Patients with multisystem disease have the highest risk of DI (Dunger *et al.*, 1989; Grois *et al.*, 1995), but disease in the head and neck region, particularly in the craniofacial bones of the orbit and temporal bone with intracranial tumour extension or proptosis, also seems to be associated with a higher frequency (Dunger *et al.*, 1989; Grois *et al.*, 1995, Donadieu *et al.*, 2004).

For the appropriate diagnosis of DI, a water deprivation test and measurement of urinary arginine vasopressin, AVP (Antidiuretic hormone, ADH) is mandatory to discriminate between partial DI, which may fluctuate spontaneously, and complete DI, which usually remains uninfluenced by treatment (Dunger *et al.*, 1989; Broadbent and Pritchard, 1997). The usefulness of urinary vasopressin levels has been questioned by other investigators, however, (Maghnie *et al.*, 1998) partly because of the wide range of vasopressin values in patients with partial DI, and repeated studies may be necessary.

The morphological changes in the HPR have been well documented by MRI during the last decade. Typical changes include lack of the posterior pituitary bright spot and pathological changes in pituitary stalk thickness (Tien *et al.*, 1991; Maghnie, 2003). Pituitary stalk thickening is observed in about 70% of patients at the time of diagnosis of DI (Grois *et al.*, 2004), and may progress to suprasellar mass lesions (Figure 11.2) (O'Sullivan *et al.*, 1991; Tabarin *et al.*, 1991). On the other hand, thread-like atrophy of the infundibulum may be seen (Grois *et al.*, 2004).

In cases of isolated DI a careful diagnostic investigation is mandatory to search for extracranial lesions, which might be more easily accessible for biopsy, to gain histological proof of LCH. If the diagnostic evaluation is negative, the major differential diagnoses of germinoma, lymphocytic infundibuloneurohypophysitis, sarcoidosis, and other granulomatous diseases like tuberculosis have to be considered. In case of an isolated hypothalamic–pituitary mass a central biopsy should be considered before the start of specific therapy (Czernichow *et al.*, 2000; Prosch *et al.*, 2004).

In LCH patients, histopathology of space-occupying lesions in the HPR demonstrated the characteristic morphology of active LCH granulomas with S100+ and CD1a+ histiocytes, intermingling with CD68+ macrophages, lymphocytes, plasma cells, and eosinophils (Favara and Jaffe, 1994; Mazal *et al.*, 1996). The findings may vary, depending on the activity stage of the lesion. In long-standing

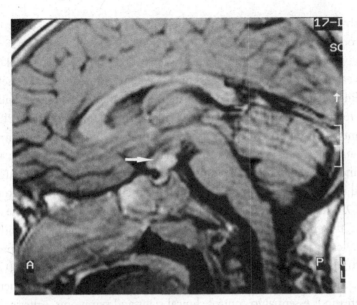

Figure 11.2 Sagittal T1-weighted contrast enhanced image. Enhancing mass lesion in the region of the median eminence (white arrow)

lesions, CD1a+ cells may no longer be detected, and some biopsies reveal a more xanthomatous or fibromatous morphology with CD68+ foamy macrophages, or a lymphocytic infiltrate only. In the hypothalamic region, CD1a+ granulomas, located in the leptomeninges can sometimes break through the glia-limiting membrane and can diffusely infiltrate brain tissue. Such granulomas are surrounded by a zone of variable size with pronounced T-cell infiltration, microglia activation, as well as degeneration of neuronal and glial elements (Grois *et al.*, 2005).

In the absence of structural changes on MRI, micro-injuries leading to vascular impairment and scarring, were postulated to cause DI (Maghnie *et al.*, 1998). Other speculation on the pathogenesis of DI includes cytokine effect from adjacent osseous lesions or an autoimmune effect (Scherbaum *et al.*, 1986; Dunger *et al.*, 1989).

The incidence of anterior pituitary deficiencies is reported to be about 10% (Sims, 1977; Dean *et al.*, 1986; Nanduri *et al.*, 2000). Patients with DI carry a risk of about 54% of developing anterior pituitary deficiencies within 10 years from DI onset (Donadieu *et al.*, 2004). Growth hormone deficiency is the most frequent endocrinopathy, followed by thyroid stimulating hormone (TSH) loss, gonadotrophic and adrenocorticotrophic hormone deficiency, and panhypopituitarism as the final stage (Nanduri *et al.*, 2000; Donadieu *et al.*, 2004).

A recent study found an alarmingly high incidence of neurodegenerative changes in 76% of DI patients studied with MRI follow-up for at least 5 years (Grois *et al.*, 2004). However, as not all DI patients undergo systematic MRI investigations, the currently available data does not allow definition of the actual risk of development of neurodegeneration after DI.

The appropriate therapeutic approaches for patients presenting with DI have been controversial, and obviously depend on the extent of disease at DI onset, and on coinciding MRI findings. The goals of therapy are the reversal of DI and prevention of further endocrine deficiencies deriving from damage to the HPR. Despite a few anecdotal reports of reversal of DI with 2-CDA, even after many months (Watts and Files, 2001; Ottaviano and Finlay, 2003), no convincing data are found in the literature that show that the majority of cases of established DI can be reversed by any treatment modality (Broadbent and Pritchard, 1997; Rosenzweig *et al.*, 1997; Kaltsas *et al.*, 2000; Ottaviano and Finlay, 2003). There is some evidence, however, that rapid start of systemic chemotherapy in multisystem disease may prevent the appearance of DI, as shown by a low incidence of DI in large prospective clinical trials administering early chemotherapy to multisystem patients (Ceci *et al.*, 1988; Gadner *et al.*, 1994; Grois *et al.*, 1995). In manifest DI, replacement therapy with desmopressin is essential to control clinical signs and symptoms. Anterior pituitary hormone deficiencies may also require hormonal substitution. It has to be noted that growth hormone replacement appears to be safe and effective in LCH patients, and is not correlated with an increased risk of disease reactivation (Howell *et al.*, 1998). In the majority of cases, DI occurs simultaneous to disease activity in other organs, which usually warrants the use of systemic chemotherapy, depending on previous therapy received by the particular patients. Controversy arises in patients with isolated DI without signs of active disease elsewhere. A cranial MRI should be read carefully looking for subtle signs of active LCH in craniofacial bones, paranasal sinuses or mastoids. Possible space-occupying lesions in the HPR and other CNS changes need to be excluded. Such additional findings might influence the choice of therapy.

Radiotherapy might be warranted in cases with isolated space-occupying hypothalamic–pituitary tumours, especially when the optic nerve is threatened. Apart from such masses, the use of radiotherapy in DI needs careful consideration in individual cases, because of the potential risks. A review of the literature failed to provide convincing evidence of a beneficial effect of irradiation on established DI (Greenberger *et al.*, 1979; Minehan *et al.*, 1992; Rosenzweig *et al.*, 1997).

The major dilemma is whether all patients with recent onset of DI, even those with isolated disease, should receive systemic chemotherapy. The chance of reversal of DI may be small if the DI is fully established, but cases have been described as late as 10 months after DI onset (Watts and Files, 2001) and theoretically early therapy to active disease with resulting reduction in cytokine activity or auto-immune response, may possibly prevent progression to anterior pituitary defects and neuropsychological defects. On the other hand, if both DI and the other defects are due to the intrinsic nature of LCH in that particular patient, then therapy will likely not effect the disease-course. A prospective study of this question with long-term follow-up is clearly needed.

Pineal gland

Changes in the pineal gland region, comprising enlargement of the gland or cyst formation have been observed in 63% of LCH patients studied by MRI, with the largest diameter reaching 24 mm (Prayer *et al.*, 2004). Interestingly, there was an association of increased pineal gland size with infundibular thickening on MRI in LCH patients (Grois *et al.*, 2004). This finding is not surprising, as both the pineal and the pituitary gland interact in the neuroendocrine network, and are both located outside the BBB. The simultaneous occurrence of pineal gland and pituitary tumours is also reported in other diseases, such as germinoma, sarcoidosis or tuberculosis (Wall *et al.*, 1985; Martin *et al.*, 1989; Benmoussa *et al.*, 1992; Dodek and Sadeghi-Nejad, 1998). The currently available data suggest a possible involvement of the pineal gland in LCH, even though biopsy proof of pineal LCH derives from single case reports only (Gizewski and Forsting, 2001).

Epidural, subdural spaces and choroid plexus

The meninges might be affected quite frequently by adjacent lesions in the craniofacial bones, but isolated focal meningeal lesions can also be rarely seen (Barthez *et al.*, 2000). They may occur as isolated (Cerda-Nicolas *et al.*, 1980; Moscinski and Kleinschmidt-DeMasters, 1985) or multifocal lesions (Goldberg *et al.*, 1987; Barthez *et al.*, 2000), and may reach an impressive size (Figure 11.3). These masses are iso- to hypointense to brain on T1-weighted with inconstant contrast enhancement, and appear hypointense on T2-weighted images. Sometimes CNS tumours are accompanied by surprisingly few neurological symptoms, but headache or other signs of raised intracranial pressure may be present (Grois *et al.*, 1998; Barthez *et al.*, 2000). Leptomeningeal involvement may also be subclinical and only detected microscopically (Rubens-Duval *et al.*, 1966).

Histological investigation of such lesions revealed different morphology, depending on the age of the lesion. These extra-axial lesions show clear borders to the CNS tissue, and are composed of histiocytes, foamy macrophages, multinucleated giant cells, as well as of lymphocytes, plasma cells, and eosinophils. As in the HPR, early lesions display typical LCH morphology, while later lesions tend to lose CD1a positivity and to exhibit CD68+ foamy histiocytes resulting in a xanthomatous appearance (Grois *et al.*, 2005).

The response to therapy might also be dependant on the lesional stage. Some lesions respond to standard chemotherapy including prednisone, vinblastine and/or etoposide, as given in the international LCH study protocols (Cerda-Nicolas *et al.*, 1980; Goldberg *et al.*, 1987; Whelan *et al.*, 1987; Barthez *et al.*, 2000).

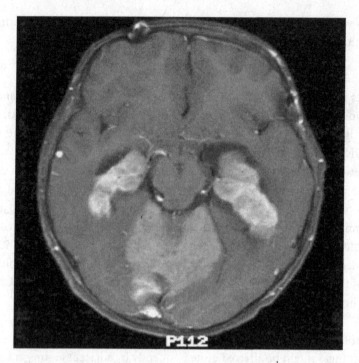

Figure 11.3 Axial T1-weighted contrast enhanced image showing bilateral enhancing masses in the choroid plexus and enhancement of an extra-axial mass originating from the tentorium

A few cases with response to 2-CDA have been reported (Watts and Files, 2001; Ottaviano and Finlay, 2003; Pardanani *et al.*, 2003), and irradiation has also been shown to be effective (Barthez *et al.*, 2000). In other cases, pronounced lesions remained more or less unchanged in spite of repeated approaches with different chemo- or immunotherapies (CNS LCH Study, unpublished observation).

Notably, over the years a high percentage of patients with meningeal or other extra-axial lesions have been detected as having neurodegenerative changes (Barthez *et al.*, 2000; CNS LCH Study, unpublished observation).

Intracranial–intraparenchymal disease

Intraparenchymal–intra-axial changes in LCH inside the BBB may involve grey and white matter. They present in different MR patterns and might be overlapping. The histopathological types comprise:

1 non-infiltrating LCH granulomas within the brain's connective tissue compartments,
2 infiltrating parenchymal granulomas,
3 neurodegenerative lesions.

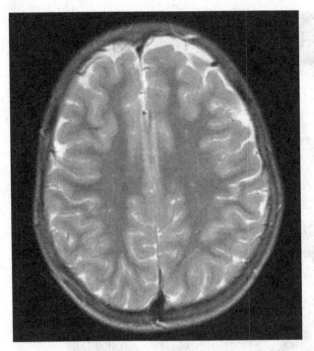

Figure 11.4 Axial T2-weighted image. Visible CSF-intense VR spaces in the deep white matter of both hemispheres

Intraparenchymal disease with a vascular distribution pattern

A vascular pattern with enlarged Virchow-Robin (VR) spaces can be seen in the deep white matter of the hemispheres on T2-weighted images. They may be barely visible, seen incidentally in neurologically asymptomatic patients (Figure 11.4). Although prominent VR spaces are not limited to patients with LCH, the incidence of this finding is significantly higher in LCH than non-LCH patients (Prayer *et al.*, 2004). The VR spaces act as lymphatic vessels of the brain, and thus present a primary site of immunological communication (Weller *et al.*, 1996). Hence the pronounced VR spaces in LCH may point towards an underlying cerebral immune process.

Small LCH granulomas may be encountered in the perivascular VR spaces and leptomeninges, and not only at intracranial sites which are devoid of a BBB, such as the dura, the circumventricular organs, and choroid plexus. In general, these granulomas are well demarcated from brain tissue by the intact superficial and perivascular glia-limiting membrane. On MRI these lesion seem to correspond to markedly enlarged and contrast-enhancing lesions, following the distribution of the perivascular spaces. Such changes can be observed in the supra- and infratentorial white matter, but also in the basal ganglia and dentate nucleus. Interestingly, such

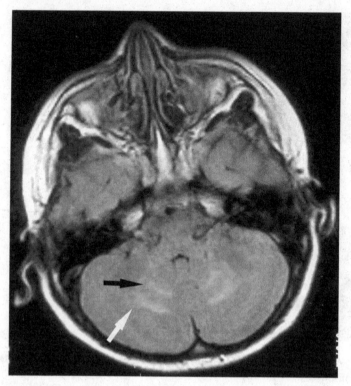

Figure 11.5 T2-weighted axial image demonstrating a hyperintensity of the dentate nucleus (black
arrow) and the surrounding white matter (white arrow)

changes were associated with neurodegenerative cerebellar or basal ganglia lesions in
all cases. Patients with such lesions were usually severely impaired.

Infiltrating parenchymal LCH granulomas

Granulomas located in the leptomeninges can penetrate the glia-limiting membrane
infiltrating the brain parenchyma. As mentioned above, this is seen in the hypothalamic region, but may also be observed in the supra- or infratentorial parenchyma. The lesions exhibit the typical LCH granuloma morphology with abundant
CD1a+ histiocytes. Importantly, these granulomas are encircled by a girdle of T-cells
and activated microglia, as well as degeneration of nerve cells, axons, and glial elements (Grois *et al.*, 2005). These microscopic infiltrations cannot be depicted on MRI.

Intraparenchymal neurodegenerative disease

The cerebellum is the most frequently involved site in CNS LCH apart from the HPR.
Cerebellar changes had already been reported prior to the era of modern imaging
(Chiari, 1933; Feigin, 1956), mostly in adolescent or adult patients, sometimes
many years after the initial diagnosis, with neurological symptoms of variable

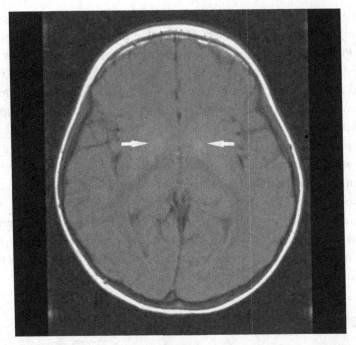

Figure 11.6 T1-weighted axial image showing bilateral symmetric hyperintense lesions in the basal ganglia

severity, including tremor, gait disturbance, ataxia, dysarthria, cognitive defects, and psychological problems. The course of the neurological changes is very heterogeneous in individual patients. Some patients show surprisingly little or even no symptoms in spite of pronounced MRI changes. Others, however, experience a rapid neurological deterioration, leading to inability to walk, tetraparesis, and profound intellectual impairment and/or behavioural changes (Barthez *et al.*, 2000).

MRI enables us to detect lesions with typical signal changes in the cerebellar dentate nucleus, the basal ganglia, and pons (Prayer *et al.*, 2004). Dentate nucleus signal changes may persist over years without neurological impairment, but it may also be followed by extension to the perinuclear white matter over months or years. In addition to the dentate nucleus (Figure 11.5), hyperintense lesions may be seen in the pallidum of the basal ganglia (Figure 11.6) (Brunberg, 1996; Saatci *et al.*, 1999; Prayer *et al.*, 2004).

A leukoencephalopathy-like pattern has been observed as symmetric patchy hyperintense areas on T2-weighted images of the cerebellar white matter, the pons or the periventricular white matter. Such white matter changes may reflect Wallerian degeneration following neuronal loss or point to an ongoing process in the white matter. All affected patients were severely neurologically impaired.

Histopathology from neurodegenerative CNS lesions, reported in a few anecdotal cases only, failed to demonstrate LCH granulomas with CD1a+ cells, but showed loss of Purkinje cells, gliosis, and demyelination (Kepes, 1979; Grois *et al.*, 1993; Barthez *et al.*, 2000). Recent findings from a neuropathology review in LCH patients revealed a pronounced inflammatory process dominated by CD8+ lymphocytes and microglial activation, expressing Class I and II major histocompatibility (MHC) molecules, as well as the phagocytic activation marker CD68. This inflammatory process supports tissue degeneration, that is, loss of nerve cells, axons, and myelin as seen in the cerebellum, the brain stem including pons and mesencephalon, and the basal ganglia. There is a profound loss of Purkinje cells, axons, and myelin, as well as reactive glial scar formation, but no primary segmental demyelination and no preferential loss of oligodendrocytes. The progressive neuronal loss in neurodegenerative LCH may lead to an overt brain atrophy which on MRI may be limited to the cerebellum and midbrain, but may involve the whole brain (Grois *et al.*, 2005) (Figure 11.7).

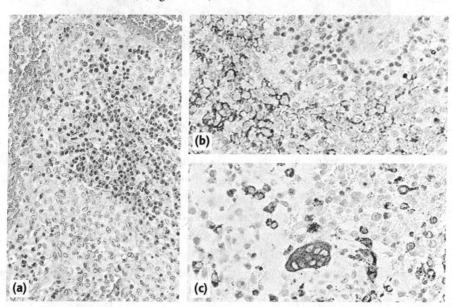

Figure 11.7 Pathological alterations present in CNS LCH: (a) Typical LCH granuloma, showing a broad mixture of different inflammatory cells, including histiocytes, macrophages, lymphocytes and (eosinophilic) granulocytes; hematoxylin and eosin ×200. (b) Many of the histiocytes within the lesion express CD1a; Immunocytochemistry ×400. (c) Besides monocytes and macrophages also multinucleated giant cells are stained with macrophage markers; Immunocytochemistry for CD68; ×400. (d) Neurodegenerative lesion in the cerebellum, showing massive loss of Purkinje cells within the cortex; only two Purkinje cells are preserved and seen at the right edge of this section; Bielschowsky silver impregnation; ×50.

(*continued on opposite page*)

The underlying pathophysiological process has been a matter of speculation. Cytokine-mediated neuroimmune activation from dendritic cells in the meningeal and perivascular spaces or the CNS parenchyma has been proposed (Grois *et al.*, 1995). Alternatively, LCH granulomas in the brain could harvest liberated brain antigens and stimulate an autoimmune response against brain tissue components or against antigens, which are shared between histiocytes and microglia (Guillemin and Brew, 2004). In this situation, the granuloma formation would trigger the autoimmune response, which may perpetuate even when all Langerhans histiocytes have been cleared from the brain lesions. The absence of Langerhans histiocytes in neurodegenerative brain lesions, which has been noted in several previous studies (Kepes, 1979; Poe *et al.*, 1994) and the similarity of the lesions to those found in paraneoplastic disease, may favour the autoimmune hypothesis.

Further basic research studies elucidating the underlying nature of CNS LCH will have an impact on future, much-needed, treatment approaches for cerebral

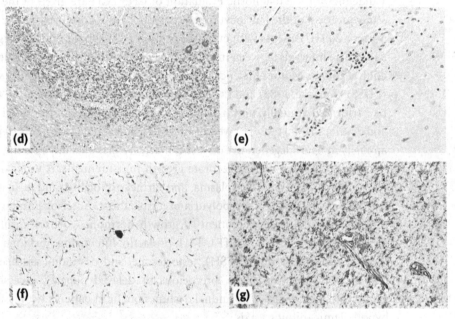

(e) This neurodegenerative process is associated with inflammation, the infiltrates mainly consist of lymphocytes and macrophages; hematoxylin and eosin; ×100. (f) In the deep white matter a massive loss of axons is found, reflected here by the scarce density of axons, immunoreactive for phosphorylated neurofilament; the large structure in the centre of this micrograph is an axonal end bulb, which develops following acute transsection of the fibre. Immunocytochemistry for phosphorylated neurofilament; ×400. (g) The inflammatory reaction within the tissue is associated with massive expression of MHC molecules, mainly on microglia cells; immunocytochemistry for Class I MHC molecules; ×100

manifestations of LCH. Various strategies including retinoic acid (Ahmed *et al.*, 2004), melatonin, different chemotherapy drugs (e.g. vinblastine, etoposide, 2-CDA, and methotrexate), or immunotherapy (e.g. prednisone, cyclosporine, and immunoglobulins) have been applied. A number of anecdotal case reports have shown the efficacy of 2-CDA against active CNS LCH, including patients who failed radiation therapy (Watts and Files, 2001; Giona F *et al.*, 2002; Ottaviano and Finlay, 2003; Pardanani *et al.*, 2003), but so far no therapeutic approach has shown to be effective in all patients (CNS LCH Study, unpublished observation). In view of the histopathology described above, long-term moderately immunosuppressive or anti-inflammatory therapies may be an option for patients with evidence of parenchymal CNS disease.

Management of patients with CNS LCH

Guidelines for the diagnostic evaluation of CNS LCH are given in the LCH CNS study protocol of the Histiocyte Society (LCH CNS Study Group of the Histiocyte Society, 2003). Patients with evidence of CNS LCH should undergo regular serial MRIs. The intervals between investigations depend on the type of changes and the clinical course. Motor efficiency tests, applying the expanded disability status scale (EDSS) (Kurtzke, 1983) and the Ataxia Rating Scale (Trouillas *et al.*, 1997), should be performed annually, and psychometric tests with age-appropriate intelligence and developmental tests, at 2-yearly intervals. Evoked potentials (BAEP) performed annually in neurodegenerative disease can detect functional impairment.

All patients need regular accurate growth measurements. A water deprivation test with measurement of plasma and urine osmolality, and urinary AVP is required in all patients with polyuria/excessive thirst. Anterior pituitary stimulation tests including measurement of growth hormone, cortisol, insulin growth factor (IGF)-I, IGFBP-3, T4, fT4, TSH, prolactin, luteinizing hormone (LH), follicle stimulating hormone (FSH), testosterone, and oestradiol are needed in all patients with growth failure, precocious or delayed puberty, excessive weight gain or other evidence of hormonal dysfunction, or in patients with lesions in the hypothalamic–pituitary axis.

Studies of cerebrospinal fluid (CSF), comprising nucleated cell count, cytospin identification, and immunohistochemistry with markers of lymphocyte subsets and histiocytes, including CD1a, should be done in patients with suspected LCH with isolated extra-axial mass lesions (HPR, choroid plexus, and meninges).

A brain biopsy is only indicated in cases with isolated extra-axial mass lesions with inconclusive CSF findings, or when combined with a curative surgical approach. In parenchymal lesions, in particular in the brain stem, stereotactic biopsies are rarely indicated, if there is a history of LCH outside the CNS.

Therapy of CNS LCH

The mode of therapy for CNS LCH depends on the type of lesions, the state of LCH outside the brain, the clinical status of the patient, and on previous therapies. Further, the efficacy of therapy may, and likely does, depend on the degree of activity of the LCH at the time therapy is given (see discussion of drugs above). It may be that early effective therapy may reduce the devastating neurodegenerative CNS manifestations whether they may be due to excess cytokine damage or an auto-immune process. A reasonable therapeutic option may therefore be a course of intensive therapy aimed at eliminating active CNS LCH, followed by long-term anti-inflammatory or immunosuppressive therapy to prevent the late and potentially devastating neurodegeneration. Proof of these concepts however, can only come from well-designed international cooperative studies.

Summary and conclusion

Clinically and by MRI, different groups of (intra)cranial LCH can be distinguished:

1 Osseous lesions in the craniofacial bones and/or skull base with/without intracranial soft tissue extension with symptoms like swelling, proptosis, aural discharge, or sinus opacification.
2 Intracranial–extra-axial disease in the HPR accompanied by DI or other endocrine deficiencies; the meninges, pineal gland, the choroid plexus or the ependyma, with or without symptoms of raised intracranial pressure.
3 Intra-axial–parenchymal disease in the grey or white matter with a striking symmetry of the lesions and a clear predominance of a neurodegenerative pattern in the cerebellum and basal ganglia.
4 Brain atrophy.

Neurodegenerative LCH frequently leads to progressive neuro-psychological deterioration over time.

These intra-cranial manifestations of LCH associated CNS disease may present in overlapping patterns or combinations. When the described clinical picture or MRI changes are found in an LCH patient, CNS LCH should be suspected, and a comprehensive diagnostic work-up, as proposed by the LCH CNS study protocol, is reasonable. The therapy of CNS LCH remains a matter of controversy, and is dependant on the type and combination of CNS changes, presence of extracranial disease, as well as on the previous treatments and on the course in the individual patients.

Pathologically two essentially different lesion types can be distinguished: LCH granulomas and a diffuse neurodegenerative process. As previously described, the CNS involvement by granulomas follows a hierarchical pattern reflecting the distribution of dendritic cells in the normal brain, but LCH cells are able under pathological (inflammatory) conditions to infiltrate areas within the BBB and the glia-limiting membrane. In contrast, in the neurodegenerative brain lesions LCH histiocytes have not been observed. Such lesions revealed a profound T-cell inflammatory process in CNS LCH, suggesting the possibility of an underlying autoimmune process.

Confirmation of these observations and further studies to elucidate the underlying nature of CNS LCH will likely have an impact on improving the success of treatment approaches of cerebral manifestations of LCH.

REFERENCES

Ahmed, I., Donadieu, J., Barthez, M.A., *et al.* (2004). Retinoic acid therapy in degenerative-like neuro-Langerhans cell histiocytosis: a prospective pilot study. *Pediatr Blood Cancer*, **43**, 55–58.

Barthez, M.A., Araujo, E. and Donadieu, J. (2000). Langerhans cell histiocytosis and the central nervous system in childhood: evolution and prognostic factors. Results of a collaborative study. *J Child Neurol*, **15**, 150–156.

Benmoussa, H., Belghmaidi, M., Tamehmacht, M., *et al.* (1992). Tuberculoma of pineal area: case report. *Neurosurg Rev*, **15**, 71–72.

Breidahl, W.H., Ives, F.J. and Khangure, M.S. (1993). Cerebral and brain stem Langerhans cell histiocytosis. *Neuroradiology*, **35**, 349–351.

Broadbent, V. and Pritchard, J. (1997). Diabetes insipidus associated with Langerhans cell histiocytosis: is it reversible? *Med Pediatr Oncol*, **28**, 289–293.

Brunberg, J.A. (1996). Hyperintense basal ganglia on T1-weighted MR in a patient with Langerhans cell histiocytosis. *Am J Neuroradiol*, **17**, 1193–1194.

Burn, D.J., Watson, J.D., Roddie, M., *et al.* (1992). Langerhans' cell histiocytosis and the nervous system. *J Neurol*, **239**, 345–350.

Ceci, A., De Terlizzi, M., Colella, R., *et al.* (1988). Etoposide in recurrent childhood Langerhans' cell histiocytosis: an Italian cooperative study. *Cancer*, **62**, 2528–2531.

Cerda-Nicolas, M., Broseta, J., Peydro-Olaya, A., *et al.* (1980). Primary eosinophilic granuloma of the frontal lobe. *Virchows Arch A Pathol Anat Histopathol*, **388**, 221–228.

Chester, W. and Kugel, V.H. (1932). Lipoidgranulomatosis (Type, Hand–Schüller–Christian): report of a case. *Arch Pathol*, **14**, 595–612.

Chiari, H. (1933). Über Veränderungen im Zentralnervensystem bei generalisierter Xanthomatose von Typus Schüller–Christian. *Virchows Arch A Pathol Pathol Anat*, **288**.

Christian, H.A. (1920). Defects in membranous bones, exophthalmos and diabetes insipidus; an unusual syndrome of dyspituitarism: a clinical study. *Med Clin North Am*, **3**, 849–871.

Czernichow, P., Garel, C. and Leger, J. (2000). Thickened pituitary stalk on magnetic resonance imaging in children with central diabetes insipidus. *Horm Res*, **53**(Suppl 3), 61–64.

Davison, C. (1933). Xanthomatosis and the central nervous system (Schüller–Christian Syndrome). *Arch Neurol*, **30**, 75–98.

Dean, H.J., Bishop, A. and Winter, J.S. (1986). Growth hormone deficiency in patients with histiocytosis X. *J Pediatr,* **109**, 615–618.

Dodek, A.B. and Sadeghi-Nejad, A. (1998). Pineal germinoma presenting as central diabetes insipidus. *Clin Pediatr (Phila),* **37**, 693–695.

Donadieu, J., Rolon, M.A., Thomas, C., *et al.* (2004). Endocrine involvement in pediatric-onset Langerhans' cell histiocytosis: a population-based study. *J Pediatr,* **144**, 344–350.

Dunger, D.B., Broadbent, V., Yeoman, E., *et al.* (1989). The frequency and natural history of diabetes insipidus in children with Langerhans-cell histiocytosis. *New Engl J Med,* **321**, 1157–1162.

Favara, B.E. and Jaffe, R. (1994). The histopathology of Langerhans cell histiocytosis. *Br J Cancer Suppl,* **23**, S17–S23.

Feigin, I. (1956). Xanthomatosis of the nervous system. *J Neuropathol Exp Neurol,* **15**, 400–416.

Gadner, H., Heitger, A., Ritter, J., *et al.* (1987). Langerhans cell histiocytosis in childhood – results of the DAL-HX 83 study. *Klin Padiatr,* **199**, 173–182.

Gadner, H., Heitger, A., Grois, N., *et al.* (1994). Treatment strategy for disseminated Langerhans cell histiocytosis. DAL HX-83 Study Group. *Med Pediatr Oncol,* **23**, 72–80.

Giona, F., Annino, L., Bongarzoni, V., *et al.* (2002). Unifocal Langerhans' cell histiocytosis involving the central nervous system successfully treated with 2-chlorodeoxyadenosine. *Med Pediatr Oncol,* **38**, 223.

Gizewski, E.R. and Forsting, M. (2001). Histiocytosis mimicking a pineal gland tumour. *Neuroradiology,* **43**, 644–646.

Goldberg, R., Han, J.S., Ganz, E., *et al.* (1987). Computed tomography demonstration of multiple parenchymal central nervous system nodules due to histiocytosis X. *Surg Neurol,* **27**, 377–380.

Graif, M. and Pennock, J.M. (1986). MR imaging of histiocytosis X in the central nervous system. *Am J Neuroradiol,* **7**, 21–23.

Greenberger, J.S., Cassady, J.R., Jaffe, N., *et al.* (1979). Radiation therapy in patients with histiocytosis: management of diabetes insipidus and bone lesions. *Int J Radiat Oncol Biol Phys,* **5**, 1749–1755.

Greenwood, S.M., Martin, J.S. and Towfighi, J. (1981). Unifocal eosinophilic granuloma of the temporal lobe. *Surg Neurol,* **17**, 441–444.

Grois, N., Barkovich, A.J., Rosenau, W., *et al.* (1993). Central nervous system disease associated with Langerhans' cell histiocytosis. *Am J Pediatr Hematol Oncol,* **15**, 245–254.

Grois, N., Flucher-Wolfram, B., Heitger, A., *et al.* (1995). Diabetes insipidus in Langerhans cell histiocytosis: results from the DAL-HX 83 study. *Med Pediatr Oncol,* **24**, 248–256.

Grois, N.G., Favara, B.E., Mostbeck, G.H., *et al.* (1998). Central nervous system disease in Langerhans cell histiocytosis. *Hematol Oncol Clin North Am,* **12**, 287–305.

Grois, N., Prayer, D., Prosch, H., *et al.* (2004). Course of diabetes insipidus in Langerhans cell histiocytosis and clinical impact of associated magnetic resonance imaging findings in diabetes insipidus associated with Langerhans cell histiocytosis. *Pediatr Blood Cancer,* **43**, 59–65.

Grois, N., Prayer, H., Prosch, H. and Lassmann, H. (2005). Neuropathology of Central Nervous System Disease in Langerhans Cell Histiocytosis. *Brain,* in press.

Guillemin, G.J. and Brew, B.J. (2004). Microglia, macrophages, perivascular macrophages, and pericytes: a review of function and identification. *J Leukoc Biol,* **75**, 388–397.

Hand, A. (1921). Defects of membraneous bones, exophthalmos and polyuria in childhood: is it dyspituitarism? *Am J Med Sci,* **162**, 509–515.

Haupt, R., Nanduri, V., Calevo, M.G., *et al.* (2004). Permanent consequences in Langerhans cell histiocytosis patients: a pilot study from the Histiocyte Society – Late Effects Study Group. *Pediatr Blood Cancer,* **42**, 438–444.

Howell, S.J, Wilton, P. and Shalet, S.M. (1998). Growth hormone replacement in patients with Langerhans cell histiocytosis. *Arch Dis Child,* **78**, 469–473.

Kaltsas, G.A., Powles, T.B., Evanson, J., *et al.* (2000). Hypothalamo–pituitary abnormalities in adult patients with Langerhans cell histiocytosis: clinical, endocrinological, and radiological features and response to treatment. *J Clin Endocrinol Metab,* **85**, 1370–1376.

Kepes, J.J. (1979). Histiocytosis X. In: Vinken, P.J. and Brujn, G.W., eds. *In Handbook of Neurology,* Vol. 38. Elsevier Publishing Company, New York, pp. 93–117.

Kurtzke, J.F. (1983). Rating neurologic impairment in multiple sclerosis: an expanded disability status scale (EDSS). *Neurology,* **33**, 1444–1452.

LCH CNS Study Group of the Histiocyte Society (2003). *LCH CNS 2003 – Registry And Diagnostic Guidelines for Central Nervous System Disease in Langerhans Cell Histiocytosis.* Protocol.

LCH Study Group of the Histiocyte Society (2001). *LCH III – Treatment Protocol of the Third International Study for Langerhans Cell Histiocytosis.* Protocol.

Maghnie, M. (2003). Diabetes insipidus. *Horm Res,* **59**(Suppl 1), 42–54.

Maghnie, M., Bossi, G., Klersy, C., *et al.* (1998). Dynamic endocrine testing and magnetic resonance imaging in the long-term follow-up of childhood Langerhans cell histiocytosis. *J Clin Endocrinol Metab,* **83**, 3089–3094.

Martin, N., Debroucker, T., Mompoint, D., *et al.* (1989). Sarcoidosis of the pineal region: CT and MR studies. *J Comput Assist Tomogr,* **13**, 110–112.

Mazal, P.R., Hainfellner, J.A., Preiser, J., *et al.* (1996). Langerhans cell histiocytosis of the hypothalamus: diagnostic value of immunohistochemistry. *Clin Neuropathol,* **15**, 87–91.

Minehan, K.J., Chen, M.G., Zimmerman, D., *et al.* (1992). Radiation therapy for diabetes insipidus caused by Langerhans cell histiocytosis. *Int J Radiat Oncol Biol Phys,* **23**, 519–524.

Moscinski, L.C. and Kleinschmidt-DeMasters, B.K. (1985). Primary eosinophilic granuloma of frontal lobe. Diagnostic use of S-100 protein. *Cancer,* **56**, 284–288.

Nanduri, V.R., Bareille, P., Pritchard, J., *et al.* (2000). Growth and endocrine disorders in multisystem Langerhans' cell histiocytosis. *Clin Endocrinol (Oxf),* **53**, 509–515.

Nanduri, V.R., Lillywhite, L., Chapman, C., *et al.* (2003). Cognitive outcome of long-term survivors of multisystem Langerhans cell histiocytosis: a single-institution, cross-sectional study. *J Clin Oncol,* **21**, 2961–2967.

O'Sullivan, R.M., Sheehan, M., Poskitt, K.J., *et al.* (1991). Langerhans cell histiocytosis of hypothalamus and optic chiasm: CT and MR studies. *J Comput Assist Tomogr,* **15**, 52–55.

Ottaviano, F. and Finlay, J.L. (2003). Diabetes insipidus and Langerhans cell histiocytosis: a case report of reversibility with 2-chlorodeoxyadenosine. *J Pediatr Hematol Oncol,* **25**, 575–577.

Pardanani, A., Phyliky, R.L., Li, C.Y., *et al.* (2003). 2-Chlorodeoxyadenosine therapy for disseminated Langerhans cell histiocytosis. *Mayo Clin Proc,* **78**, 301–306.

Poe, L.B., Dubowy, R.L., Hochhauser, L., *et al.* (1994). Demyelinating and gliotic cerebellar lesions in Langerhans cell histiocytosis. *Am J Neuroradiol*, **15**, 1921–1928.

Prayer, D., Grois, N., Prosch, H., *et al.* (2004). MR imaging presentation of intracranial disease associated with Langerhans cell histiocytosis. *Am J Neuroradiol*, **25**, 880–891.

Prosch, H., Grois, N., Prayer, D. *et al.* (2004). Central diabetes insipidus as presenting symptom of Langerhans cell histiocytosis. *Pediatr Blood Cancer*, **43**, 594–599.

Ransom, J.L. and Murphy, S.B. (1977). Histiocytosis X: abnormal cerebrospinal fluid cytology in extrahypothalamic central nervous system involvement. *South Med J*, **70**, 1367–1369.

Rosenzweig, K.E., Arceci, R.J. and Tarbell, N.J. (1997). Diabetes insipidus secondary to Langerhans' cell histiocytosis: is radiation therapy indicated? *Med Pediatr Oncol*, **29**, 36–40.

Rubens-Duval, A., Lapresle, J., Fardeau, M., *et al.* (1966). Neural determinations of Hand-Schüller–Christian disease: Study of an anatomo-clinical case. *Sem Hop*, **42**, 1425–1439.

Saatci, I., Baskan, O., Haliloglu, M., *et al.* (1999). Cerebellar and basal ganglion involvement in Langerhans cell histiocytosis. *Neuroradiology*, **41**, 443–446.

Scherbaum, W.A., Wass, J.A., Besser, G.M., *et al.* (1986). Autoimmune cranial diabetes insipidus: its association with other endocrine diseases and with histiocytosis X. *Clin Endocrinol (Oxf)*, **25**, 411–420.

Schueller, A. (1915). Über eigenartige Schädeldefekte im Jugendalter. *Fortschr Geb Rontgenstr*, **23**, 12–19.

Simms, S. and Warner, N.J. (1998). A framework for understanding and responding to the psychosocial needs of children with Langerhans cell histiocytosis and their families. *Hematol Oncol Clin North Am*, **12**, 359–367.

Sims, D.G. (1977). Histiocytosis X: follow-up of 43 cases. *Arch Dis Child*, **52**, 433–440.

Tabarin, A., Corcuff, J.B., Dautheribes, M., *et al.* (1991). Histiocytosis X of the hypothalamus. *J Endocrinol Invest*, **14**, 139–145.

The French Langerhans' Cell Histiocytosis Study Group (1996). A multicentre retrospective survey of Langerhans' cell histiocytosis: 348 cases observed between 1983 and 1993. *Arch Dis Child*, **75**, 17–24.

Tien, R., Kucharczyk, J. and Kucharczyk, W. (1991). MR imaging of the brain in patients with diabetes insipidus. *Am J Neuroradiol*, **12**, 533–542.

Titgemeyer, C., Grois, N., Minkov, M., *et al.* (2001). Pattern and course of single-system disease in Langerhans cell histiocytosis data from the DAL-HX 83- and 90-study. *Med Pediatr Oncol*, **37**, 108–114.

Trouillas, P., Takayanagi, T., Hallett, M., *et al.* (1997). International Cooperative Ataxia Rating Scale for pharmacological assessment of the cerebellar syndrome. The Ataxia Neuropharmacology Committee of the World Federation of Neurology. *J Neurol Sci*, **145**, 205–211.

Wall, M.J., Peyster, R.G., Finkelstein, S.D., *et al.* (1985). A unique case of neurosarcoidosis with pineal and suprasellar involvement: CT and pathological demonstration. *J Comput Assist Tomogr*, **9**, 381–383.

Watts, J. and Files, B. (2001). Langerhans cell histiocytosis: central nervous system involvement treated successfully with 2-chlorodeoxyadenosine. *Pediatr Hematol Oncol*, **18**, 199–204.

Weller, R.O., Engelhardt, B. and Phillips, M.J. (1996). Lymphocyte targeting of the central nervous system: a review of afferent and efferent CNS-immune pathways. *Brain Pathol*, **6**, 275–288.

Whelan, H.T., Clinton, M.E., Fogo, A., *et al.* (1987). Histiocytosis-X isolated to the cervical spinal cord. *Am J Pediatr Hematol Oncol*, **9**, 228–232.

Willis, B., Ablin, A., Weinberg, V., *et al.* (1996). Disease course and late sequelae of Langerhans' cell histiocytosis: 25-year experience at the University of California, San Francisco. *J Clin Oncol*, **14**, 2073–2082.

Woo, K.I. and Harris, G.J. (2003). Eosinophilic granuloma of the orbit: understanding the paradox of aggressive destruction responsive to minimal intervention. *Ophthal Plast Reconstr Surg*, **19**, 429–439.

12

The treatment of Langerhans cell histiocytosis

Helmut Gadner and Stephan Ladisch

INTRODUCTION

Background

The treatment of Langerhans cell histiocytosis (LCH) has varied greatly over the past century, and is still controversial. Early treatment approaches reflected contemporary views on disease pathogenesis, which included granulomatous, inflammatory or infectious origins for LCH. Consequently, children with LCH were treated with antibiotics, anti-inflammatory agents including steroids, and with radiation therapy and over the last 30–40 years with cytotoxic chemotherapy. While varying degrees of success have been reported, it remains true that only once the issues of aetiology and pathogenesis have been resolved can a definitive therapy be envisioned. Nevertheless, systematic approaches to diagnosis and treatment, which were major advances of the 1980s, have improved the outlook for children with LCH and are the main focus of this chapter.

Historical perspective

The first systematic treatment trial of children with LCH was that of Lahey (1962). In that study, children were matched for age and extent of disease, and outcome was analysed according to whether or not 'specific' treatment for LCH was given. Treatment was not controlled however, and a variety of agents, including antibiotics, steroids and cytotoxic drugs were given, making direct comparisons problematic. Nevertheless, the principal, and important, finding of this study was a significant increase in survival in the group of children receiving therapy compared to those who were untreated.

These findings led to a number of studies in which, unfortunately, the patient populations varied greatly with respect to extent of disease. This variability made interpretation of results difficult, and conclusions regarding superior treatment approaches were at best tenuous. To obtain an overview of treatment of LCH in the early 1980s, nine treatment studies, which included 433 patients and spanned the period from before 1950 to the end of the 1970s, were analysed for survival

Table 12.1 Survival in LCH

	Survival (%)			
	A	B	C	D
Oberman (1961)	61	95	44	33
Avery *et al.* (1957)	81	100	86	0
Daneshbod *et al.* (1978)	82	–	100	0
Nezelof *et al.* (1979)	52	–	59	38
Komp *et al.* (1980)	78	100	91	54
Lahey (1975)	71	–	98	33
Toogood *et al.* (1979)	80	100	90	40
Lahey *et al.* (1979)	68	100	68	–
Komp *et al.* (1977)	72	100	91	54
Total % survival	71	98	76	37

A: all LCH excluding mono-ostotic eosinophilic granuloma; B: 'mild' multifocal eosinophilic granuloma; C: soft tissue involvement (i.e. multisystem), but without oran dysfunction; D: multisystem disease with organ dysfunction.

(Ladisch, 1983). The long-term overall survival (OS) rate was 71%. When patients with mono-ostotic eosinophilic granuloma, already at that time recognized as a generally self-limited process with no mortality, were excluded, 391 patients with multifocal or multisystem disease could be classified into three groups (B, C and D; Table 12.1) according to increasing extent of disease.

Outcome was clearly related to extent and severity (presence or absence of organ dysfunction) of disease at diagnosis, and demonstrated the need to stratify patients prior to analysing response to treatment or survival. Mortality was clearly highest in patients with organ dysfunction. A disappointing conclusion from this analysis was that survival during the previous half-century had not obviously improved, particularly evident in group D (Table 12.1). It was inferred that careful stratification and ultimately randomization of patients would be essential to avoid erroneous conclusions about treatment efficacy, since this could also result from differences in the relative severity of disease in patients enrolled in the different studies. Thus, the importance of stratification for the purpose of analysis was recognized and this principle was implemented in studies initiated in the remainder of the century.

Basic issue

Ignorance of the pathogenesis of LCH and the earlier failure to establish commonly accepted diagnostic and stratification criteria were challenges for the 1980s.

As a result a number of principles were established:

1 Therapy should depend on whether patients had single- or multisystem disease.
2 The extent of disease had an important impact on morbidity and prognosis, especially in young patients with multisystem disease with organ dysfunction at presentation.
3 Chemotherapy, including cytostatic agents, likely had a beneficial, but not yet definitely proven, effect. However, no single drug or regimen had been unequivocally demonstrated to influence the unpredictable course and high mortality rate in severely affected children.
4 In a rare disease with a highly variable presentation, it is critical to use uniform clinical and histopathological criteria for diagnosis and assessment of disease extent. It is also important to distinguish LCH from other, seemingly similar forms of histiocytosis, which however behave very differently, such as haemophagocytic lymphohistiocytosis, and other histiocytic malignancies (Ladisch and Jaffe, 2002).

Thus, a concerted effort was made by the Histiocyte Society to establish generally accepted diagnostic, staging and classification systems. Previously patients were usually categorized as having localized and disseminated LCH, depending on clinical criteria. Localized disease consisted of isolated bone, lymph node or skin involvement. Disseminated disease was defined as the presence of multiple LCH lesions of any other type or combination. Using a modification (Ladisch, 1983) of a previously suggested stratification scheme (Oberman, 1961), patients with disseminated disease were categorized into two risk groups. Patients with multifocal bone involvement were distinguished from those with bone and soft tissue, or solitary soft tissue involvement, and form those with dysfunction of the liver, lungs and/or the haematopoetic system. The evaluation include specific histopathological and immunohistochemical criteria and a patient stratification based on standardized diagnostic evaluation of the extent of the disease (Writing Group of the Histiocyte Society, 1987; Broadbent et al., 1989a).

Classification and stratification systems

Taking the advantages and disadvantages of existing staging and stratification systems into account, the LCH Study Group in 1990 adopted a simple stratification system, with division of the LCH population into two overall groups: patients with 'single-system' LCH and patients with 'multisystem' LCH, defined as an involvement of two or more organs at diagnosis (Greenberger et al., 1981; Broadbent and Gadner, 1998) (Table 12.2). It should be stressed that this stratification is therapeutic-decision oriented, and further subdivision of patients according to clinical heterogeneity of the disease (i.e. different clinical patterns for the same

Table 12.2 Stratification of LCH

Single-system disease
- Single site
  - Single-bone lesion
  - Isolated skin disease
  - Solitary lymph node involvement
- Multiple site
  - Multiple bone lesions
  - Multiple lymph node involvement

Multisystem disease
- Multiple organ involvement (with or without organ dysfunction)

'Risk organs'
- Liver, lungs, haematopoetic system and spleen

'Low-risk patients'
- Over 2 years old with no risk organ involvement

'Risk patients'
- Of any age with involvement of at least one risk organ

number of involved organs) is not attempted, because these have not yet been shown to be reliable discriminating factors in predicting outcome.

Another important issue that had to be addressed before contemplating prospective clinical trials for a disease with an unpredictable course was that of establishing new definitions of disease activity, and of response to treatment. There are no morphological or immunohistochemical differences found in the lesions of good and poor responders. Even clonality is not discriminatory, as it appears that both single-system single site and multisystem disease are clonal (Willman *et al.*, 1994). Single-system disease, however, is rarely progressive and requires minimal treatment. To date, assessment of response has had to be largely subjective, depending on disease location and supported by evidence from laboratory investigations (e.g. liver function tests). According to the proposal of the LCH Study Group, response is currently defined as a measurable resolution of symptoms and signs, and prevention of permanent consequences of the disease (Ladisch and Gadner, 1994) (Table 12.3). By prospective or retrospective analysis, assessment of response at defined time points of evaluation (6 and 12 weeks after the start of therapy) has been found to be a new and very powerful, and independent predictor of outcome, allowing a rapid discrimination between responders and non-responders, and enabling the use of therapy adapted to the individual course of the disease (Gadner *et al.*, 1994; Gadner *et al.*, 2001; Minkov *et al.*, 2002b).

Table 12.3 Schematic representation of definition of disease state and response criteria

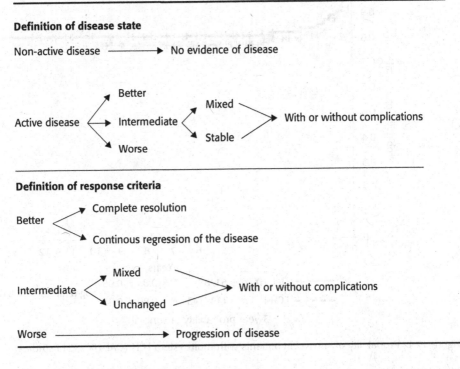

Definition of disease state

Non-active disease ⟶ No evidence of disease

Active disease ⟷ Intermediate
- Better
- Worse

Better / Worse → Mixed / Stable → With or without complications

Definition of response criteria

Better
- Complete resolution
- Continous regression of the disease

Intermediate
- Mixed
- Unchanged
→ With or without complications

Worse ⟶ Progression of disease

In the first international LCH-I study, the Histiocyte Society used the criteria of 'active' or 'non-active' disease at each response assessment, and categorized the disease into either 'better', 'intermediate' with or without complications (requirement for blood or platelet transfusions, etc.), or 'worse' (Table 12.3). Recently, a French scoring system possibly useful for objective evaluation of response and prognosis has been proposed which warrants prospective testing (Bernard *et al.*, 2003).

Large retrospective series of LCH patients have shown an overall incidence of late sequelae in the range of 50%, irrespective of whether treatment was given (Komp, 1981; Haupt *et al.*, 2004). In a series with treatment used intermittently only for exacerbations of disease, the incidence of sequelae was 67% (McLelland *et al.*, 1990). In contrast, by prospective evaluation of patients entered in therapy studies, the recent incidence decreased to 30–50%, regardless of whether 'maintenance' treatment has been continued for 2 years (Ceci *et al.*, 1993) or 1 year (Gadner *et al.*, 1994). One of the yet unanswered questions is whether late sequelae can be prevented by extending the length of treatment beyond when control of symptoms has been achieved.

Analysis of the data of the LCH-I and the Austrian-German DAL-HX 83/90 studies allowed a more detailed stratification system to be formulated, subdividing multisystem patients into a 'low-risk' group and a 'risk' group (Table 12.2). Low-risk

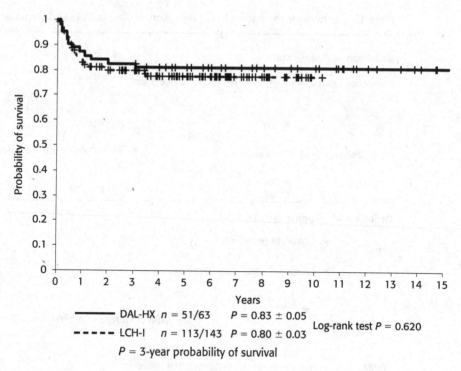

Figure 12.1 Probability of survival in patients with multisystem LCH (DAL-HX, LCH-I studies)

patients account for about 20% of all multisystem disease patients. They are characterized by freedom from involvement of 'risk organs' (liver, lungs, haematopoetic system or spleen) at diagnosis, and have an excellent prognosis. 'Risk' patients (patients of any age that have at least one or more risk organs involved (Broadbent and Gadner, 1998)) comprise about 80% of multisystem patients, and have a high probability of dying due to the disease, if they do not respond adequately to therapy (Figures 12.1 and 12.2; Table 12.4). Until recently, age under 2 years at diagnosis was believed to be independently prognostic, but the significance was lost when involvement of risk organs as a discriminatory factor was identified (preliminary LCH-II results).

Finally, patients with single-system multifocal bone disease (i.e. lesions in two or more bones and patients with localized special single sites of involvement, such as central nervous system (CNS) lesions with craniofacial, intracranial or intraspinal soft tissue extension) deserve special attention. They should be considered a subdivision of the above classification (special-site disease), and if persisting, should possibly receive systemic chemotherapy with the goal of preventing late sequelae (see Chapters 11 and 14 for a detailed discussion).

Table 12.4 Definition of organ involvement 'risk' organs

Haematopoetic involvement: with or without bone marrow involvement*	Anaemia: haemoglobin <10 g/dl, infants <9 g/dl (exclusion of iron deficiency) Leukocytopenia: leucocytes <4.0 × 10⁹/l, Thrombocytopenia: platelets <100 × 10⁹/l
Spleen involvement:	Enlargement ≥2 cm below costal margin (proven by sonography)
Liver involvement:	Enlargement >3 cm below costal margin (proven by sonography) and/or liver dysfunction (hyperbilirubinaemia, hypoproteinaemia, hypalbuminaemia, elevated γGT, alkaline phosphatase, elevated transaminases, ascites, oedema) and/or histopathological diagnosis
Lung involvement:	Typical changes on high-resolution computed tomography (HR-CT) and/or histopathological diagnosis

*Bone marrow involvement is defined as demonstration of CD1a positive cells on bone marrow smears. The clinical significance of CD1a positivity in the bone marrow remains to be proven. Hypocellularity, haemophagocytosis, myelodysplasia, and/or myelofibrosis may be regarded as secondary phenomena. Haemophagocytosis may be prominent in severe progressive cases.

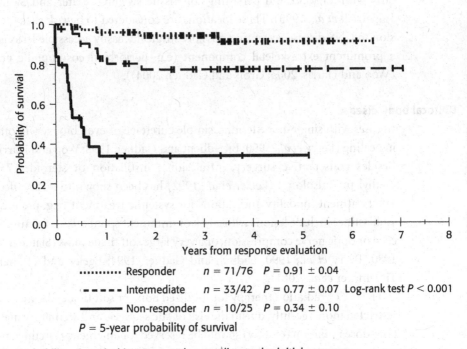

Figure 12.2 Probability of survival in LCH-I study according to the initial response

THERAPY

Single-system disease

The clinical course of LCH in patients with single-system disease is generally benign. There is a high chance of spontaneous remission and favourable outcome, over a period of months to years (Gadner and Grois, 1993; Titgemeyer et al., 2001). There is neither a general consensus, nor an ongoing clinical trial, regarding treatment of patients with single-system LCH. Various modalities are currently employed, including radiation therapy, local administration of steroids and single-agent chemotherapy (Greenberger et al., 1979; Egeler et al., 1992; Woo and Harris, 2003).

Bone and soft tissue (see also Chapter 8)

In single- as well as in multiple-site disease, the skeleton is the most frequently involved organ. Soft tissue swelling from extension of the granuloma from the bone lesion, or local oedema, is a common finding and is not considered as separate organ involvement. Only rarely is a solitary soft tissue granuloma not associated with a bone lesion (Gramatovici and D'Angio, 1988).

The skull is commonly affected, usually by cranial vault lesions. Although not as frequent, of special interest are lesions in the mastoid or petrous bone, and in craniofacial locations (including paranasal, parameningeal and periorbital), particularly with adjacent and persisting soft tissue swelling (Slater and Swarm, 1980; Kilpatrick et al., 1995). These locations are considered to be risk sites for progression to CNS disease, excepting possibly surgically easily accessible lesions without a prominent extraskeletal component (e.g. periorbital eosinophilic granuloma (Woo and Harris, 2003; Grois and Gadner, 2004)).

Unifocal bone disease

In cases with single-bone lesions, simple curettage or even biopsy will often result in healing (Berry et al., 1990; Broadbent and Gadner, 1998; Woo and Harris, 2003). Besides conservative surgery, intralesional instillation of steroids (75–150 mg methyl-prednisolone) (Egeler et al., 1992) has been shown to be an effective and safe treatment modality. Indications for systemic treatment (e.g. prednisone and vinblastine) include lesions with a risk of imminent spontaneous fracture, or spinal cord or optic nerve compression, or a very large soft tissue mass (Slater and Swarm, 1980; Berry et al., 1990; Ladisch and Gadner, 1994; Egeler and D'Angio, 1995; Titgemeyer et al., 2001).

The use of radiation therapy for localized bone or soft tissue disease has become restricted more recently, due to the risk of late sequelae and secondary malignancy. Low-dose radiation (6–8 Gy) should be reserved for emergency circumstances (e.g. optic nerve or spinal cord) (Greenberger et al., 1979; Gramatovici and D'Angio,

1988; Selch and Parker, 1990), or where curettage and/or chemotherapy are contraindicated.

Special-site involvement

Surgical curettage of lesions in the craniofacial region (skull base, temporal or zygomatical bones, mastoids, sphenoidal and ethmoidal bones, orbits, anterior and middle cranial fossa) or spinal column can be a risky and often incomplete procedure, because of a prominent intracranial or intraspinal soft tissue component. In such cases of 'special-site involvement', the risk of impairment of critical organ function by a surgical approach may instead dictate treatment with systemic chemotherapy or with low-dose (6–8 Gy) radiation therapy (Greenberger et al., 1979; Gramatovici and D'Angio, 1988; Selch and Parker, 1990). Currently, according to the LCH-III study protocol, systemic chemotherapy with prednisone and vinblastine is recommended both to induce healing and in an attempt to prevent or reduce progression to diabetes insipidus (DI) and other CNS consequences. An exception, however, is a simple periorbital osseous destruction without a significant soft tissue component as the lesion will usually regress after excholeation (Woo and Harris, 2003).

Multifocal bone disease

Over the last decades, there has been an ongoing discussion regarding the appropriate treatment of patients with multifocal bone disease. It is known that osseous lesions tend to regress spontaneously (suggesting a 'wait and see' strategy) or to respond to minimal treatment. However, bone disease also has a tendency to recur. Reactivation usually remains restricted to bone (Feldges, 1981; McLelland et al., 1990; Gadner et al., 1994; Egeler and D'Angio, 1995). Reactivation rate in single-system bone disease is up to 30% less than in multisystem disease (Berry et al., 1986; McLelland et al., 1990) but is more common in multifocal than unifocal bone LCH, as is progression to DI (Berry et al., 1986; McLelland et al., 1990; Gadner et al., 1994; Gadner et al., 2001; Titgemeyer et al., 2001).

Various systemic regimens have been used in polyostotic disease. They include corticosteroids (40 mg/m^2/day), vinblastine (6 mg/m^2/week) and etoposide. A combination of corticosteroids and vinblastine in the DAL-HX 83 study, reduced the reactivation frequency in polyostotic disease to 18%, identical to that of unifocal disease, suggesting that reduction in reactivation rates (and possibly of DI and other CNS effects) is feasible with systemic chemotherapy (Titgemeyer et al., 2001). Recently, three new approaches (indomethacin, bisphosphonates, and a combination of 6-mercaptopurine and methotrexate (MTX)) have also shown beneficial effects in small numbers of patients (Womer et al., 1995; Munn et al., 1999; Farran et al., 2001). Pending data from larger standardized clinical studies, particularly as to the efficacy in preventing progression to CNS disease, the Histiocyte Society has adopted the concept of systemic chemotherapy for multifocal bone LCH as well as special-site disease, for the ongoing LCH-III study.

Isolated skin disease

Approximately half of neonatal LCH confined to skin tends to regress spontaneously within a few months. However, progression to multisystem involvement, and sometimes to a fatal outcome, may also occur. Close observation for a long follow-up period is mandatory for this form of LCH (Hashimoto and Pritzker, 1973; Gadner and Grois, 1993; Munn and Chu, 1998). Surgical excision is the treatment of choice for isolated skin nodules. Erythematous lesions usually respond to topical corticosteroids. In severe persisting or extending skin involvement, a topical 20% solution of nitrogen mustard or psoralen with ultraviolet (PUVA) photochemotherapy may be useful, but can be recommended only for short-term therapy, due to the concern over possible carcinogenity (Neumann et al., 1988; Sheehan et al., 1991). Finally, topical application of tacrolimus or pimecrolimus ointment has recently been shown to give promising results, especially in resistant or frequently recurring cases (Egeler, personal communication). In severe resistant disease, mild systemic corticosteroid therapy, with or without vinca alkaloids, is recommended (Titgemeyer et al., 2001) (see also Chapter 7).

Lymph node involvement

For isolated lymph node involvement, excisional biopsy may be sufficient. Systemic corticosteroid therapy, with or without vinblastine, should be offered if multiple or bulky lymph nodes are present (Ladisch and Gadner, 1994; Broadbent and Gadner, 1998; Titgemeyer et al., 2001).

Lung disease

Isolated lung involvement in young children should be treated with chemotherapy using protocols for multisystem disease. In adults and in adolescents refraining from smoking is mandatory, and limiting exposure to second-hand smoke is recommended. Mild systemic therapy with corticosteroids, with or without vinblastine, can be effective in these patients (Vassallo et al., 2000; McClain, 2002; Tazi et al., 2002). In progressive disease, cyclosporine A or biphosphonates have, albeit anecdotally, shown a positive effect (Zeller et al., 2000; Brown, 2001; Egeler, 2001; Farran et al., 2001). The only successful therapy for the severe progressive lung fibrosis with respiratory failure which may occur in adults is lung transplantation (see also Chapters 10 and 13).

CNS disease

DI is often the earliest manifestation of CNS involvement.

Active CNS LCH lesions usually respond to conventional LCH chemotherapy. The choice of therapy depends on the individual case. Beneficial effects of single-drug chemotherapy (2-chlorodeoxyadenosine (2-CdA) or combination (prednisone, vinblastine, etoposide and 2-CdA) have been reported (Grois *et al.*, 1995, 1998; Watts and Files, 2001). Radiotherapy or chemotherapy, however, is usually unable to restore pituitary function if completely ablated when it becomes clinically evident. Hormone replacement therapy is usually required (Dunger *et al.*, 1989; Broadbent and Pritchard, 1997; Howell *et al.*, 1998; Donadieu *et al.*, 2004a,b), but nasal or oral vasopressin (1-desamino-8-D-arginine vasopressin, DDAVP) is well tolerated. For neurodegenerative CNS disease, no specific therapy can be recommended at present, and this remains one of the most enigmatic and devastating forms of LCH (see also Chapter 11).

Multisystem disease

Chemotherapy including cytostatic agents has been shown to have a beneficial effect in LCH. No single drug or regimen, however, has been demonstrated to unequivocally influence the unpredictable course of the young child with disseminated 'risk' disease, which is associated with a mortality rate in the range of 20% (Gadner *et al.*, 2001; Minkov *et al.*, 2002b). There is an ongoing search for new systematic therapeutic approaches using new agents in addition to the widely used and reasonably effective drugs such as vinblastine and corticosteroids (Ceci *et al.*, 1993; Egeler *et al.*, 1993; Ladisch and Gadner, 1994; Kelly and Pritchard, 1994; McCowage *et al.*, 1996; Munn *et al.*, 1999; Weitzman *et al.*, 1999; Culic *et al.*, 2001; Henter *et al.*, 2001; Minkov *et al.*, 2002a).

Throughout the last decade, two major approaches have been taken to the treatment of multisystem LCH, a conservative approach with treatment given only during disease exacerbation, and a more aggressive chemotherapy-based approach aimed at achieving a rapid decrease in disease activity, with the goal of reduction of mortality and the prevention of recurrences, chronic disease and permanent consequences.

Conservative approach

The conservative approach has been used in several institutions for many years and is based on the well-known possibility of spontaneous remission of LCH. In a large single-institutional study, cases of LCH with evidence of general symptoms (fever, pain, immobility and failure to thrive) were initially treated with prednisolone alone (McLelland *et al.*, 1990). Only in cases of disease progression and extension to vital organs were vinca alkaloids (vincristine and vinblastine) or etoposide (VP-16) added (Broadbent *et al.*, 1989b). The overall mortality rate in a selected group of patients was 14% versus 36% in children with organ dysfunction. This compares favourably to other more intensively treated groups of patients. This interesting study has never been repeated, however. In addition, the majority of survivors (67%) had permanent consequences, and DI occurred in 36% of cases (McLelland, 1990), as compared to 10% in the DAL-HX studies (see below).

Intensive chemotherapy

In the early 1980s, two large prospective multicenter trials were conducted in Italy and Germany/Austria (AIEOP-CNR-HX 83 and DAL-HX 83/90) (Ceci *et al.*, 1993; Gadner *et al.*, 1994). Newly diagnosed patients with multisystem LCH were stratified by extent of disease and presence of organ dysfunction (Lahey, 1975) and entered onto a risk-adapted protocol. These studies were designed based on the belief that LCH is a malignant process requiring relatively intensive chemotherapy. The overall mortality in both series was low, 8% and 9%, respectively. However, in the poorest prognostic group it reached 54% in the Italian study, and 38% in the DAL-HX study. The low incidence of disease reactivation seen in the DAL-HX study (overall 23%), however, provided evidence that effective treatment may beneficially influence the natural course of the disease. Disease-related permanent consequences were encountered in 48% of patients in the Italian series and in 33% of the DAL-HX study. Strikingly, DI occurred only in 20% and 10%, respectively, in contrast to the reported overall incidence of permanent consequences, which is higher than 50%, and the incidence of DI, particularly after conservative therapy, estimated to be around 36% (Komp *et al.*, 1980, 1981; Dunger *et al.*, 1989; McLelland *et al.*, 1990; Willis *et al.*, 1996).

International clinical trials

The first international randomized chemotherapy trial LCH-I for patients with multisystem disease was initiated by the Histiocyte Society in 1991. It compared two treatment arms consisting of mono-chemotherapy with either etoposide or vinblastine for 6 months (Gadner *et al.*, 2001). A single pulse of high-dose methylprednisolone (30 mg/kg i.v. for 3 days) was also given. The aim of the study was to compare response, mortality, disease reactivation and morbidity (toxicity and late sequelae) in the two arms. By August 1995, 447 patients were registered of whom 192 had multisystem disease, 136 were randomized, 72 in the vinblastine and 64 in the etoposide arm. The study showed that the two drugs were equally effective, and surprisingly, that there was no difference in the overall mortality rate compared to the earlier multiagent DAL-HX 83/90 studies (21% in LCH-I versus 17% in DAL-HX).

However, when LCH-I results were compared to the DAL-HX 83/90 with respect to initial response rate after 6 weeks of therapy (53% in LCH-I versus 79% for the DAL series), the percentage of patients showing an intermediate compared to a good response (42% versus 4%) and the rate of reactivations (56% versus

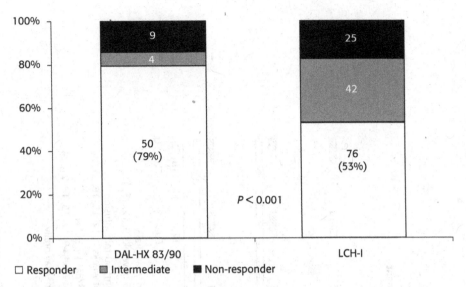

Figure 12.3　Response and degree of response at week 6 in patients included in DAL-HX and LCH-I study

29%), a clear superiority of combination therapy given for 1 year, over single-agent therapy was found (Feldges, 1981; Gadner *et al.*, 1994; Minkov *et al.*, 2002b) (Figure 12.3). Thus there appears to be strong support for the use of combination chemotherapy for multisystem disease.

These studies also revealed several previously unappreciated prognostic factors. First, despite the different intensity of therapy in the LCH-I and DAL studies, a retrospective analysis showed that all patients who died had at least one 'risk' organ involved at the time of diagnosis (Gadner *et al.*, 1994, 2001; Minkov *et al.*, 2002b). In addition, a subgroup of low-risk patients, over 2 years old and without involvement of risk organs at diagnosis, could be defined. This group includes approximately 20% of multisystem patients. They have an excellent prognosis, qualifying them for milder treatment.

The results of these studies formed the basis for the LCH-II study, which was opened in 1996 (Broadbent and Gadner, 1998). The goal of LCH-II was to compare in a randomized way the efficacy of continuous oral prednisone combined with vinblastine, to the two drugs plus etoposide, in multisystem disease patients with risk-organ involvement, or age under 2 years (risk group). As in LCH-I, continuation therapy included 6-mercaptopurine (6-MP) and was given for 24 weeks. Low-risk patients received less aggressive therapy with the two-drug arm, given for 24 weeks, without 6-MP in the continuation therapy, aimed only at shortening the disease course and reducing disease-related morbidity (Figure 12.4).

At the preliminary analysis (September, 2002), 185 patients with risk-organ involvement were randomized to one of the two treatment arms. The overall

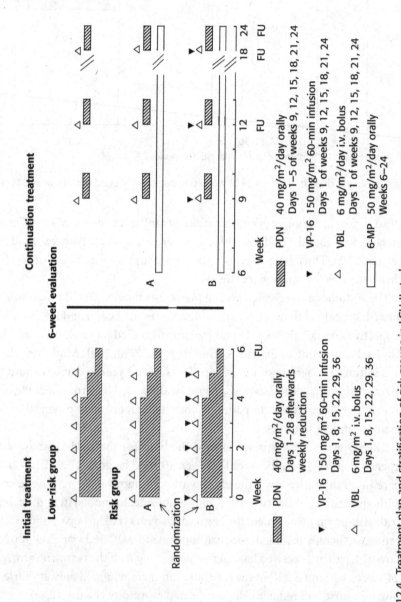

Figure 12.4 Treatment plan and stratification of risk groups in LCH-II study;
FU: follow-up evaluation; i.v.: intravenous; PDN: prednisone; VBL: vinblastine; VP-16: etoposide

probability of survival of all multisystem patients did not differ from that of the previous LCH-I and DAL-HX studies (Gadner et al., 1994, 2001) and no statistically significant difference was found between the two treatment arms. The preliminary results showed a high (88%) response rate by week 6 in the low-risk group, and no fatalities. Among the 'risk' patients, the overall response rate was superior to that in the LCH-I study and similar to that of the previous DAL studies. Among patients who did not respond at least by week 12 of treatment, and had either intermediate active or progressive disease, the probability of mortality was high (around 75%) and the probability of becoming disease free was less than 20%. In addition, as in LCH-I, all of the patients who died had involvement of at least one risk organ, while age under 2 years was no longer independently prognostic.

It therefore seems justified to regard a lack of rapid response to initial therapy in patients with risk-organ involvement, as the most important poor prognostic factor for survival. Consequently, these patients need to be switched rapidly to an alternative, efficacious salvage treatment.

The probability of reactivation after complete response to therapy (non-active disease) was around 50% in both low-risk and risk patients after 2 years. Comparison of the reactivation frequency in multisystem patients showed a similar probability of reactivation in the responders in LCH-I (54%) and LCH-II (49%) (which both had a treatment duration of only 6 months), whereas the probability of reactivation was only 29% in the DAL-HX 83/90 studies, which had a treatment duration of 12 months (Figure 12.5). As similar results were seen for low-risk and risk patients, these observations suggest a potential benefit of prolonged duration of treatment.

In the ongoing third international randomized trial LCH-III (Figure 12.6), patients are stratified into three groups:

1 Multisystem risk patients (patients with involvement of one or more risk organs).
2 Multisystem low-risk patients (patients with multiple organ involvement but without risk organ involvement).
3 Patients with single-system 'multifocal bone disease' or localized 'special-site involvement' (see earlier discussion).

Risk patients are randomized to receive or not receive MTX in addition to the standard prednisone, vinblastine and 6-MP. Initial treatment consists of one or two courses (depending on response) and is followed by continuation therapy for 12 months. Treatment of low-risk patients includes prednisone and vinblastine, with overall duration of therapy for this patient group randomly assigned to be 6 or 12 months. Patients with multifocal bone disease or special-site involvement are treated with prednisone and vinblastine for 24 weeks (Figure 12.7).

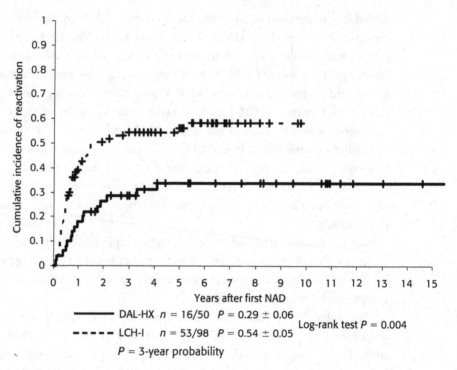

Figure 12.5 Probability of disease reactivation after non-active disease in DAL-HX and LCH-I study

In summary, the review of results of the large studies described above supports the use of combination therapy for multisystem disease as well as multifocal bone disease and special-site disease, as defined earlier. A number of chemotherapy combinations have been tried in LCH patients. Conventional first-line chemotherapy generally consists of combinations of vinca alkaloids (vinblastine or vincristine) with a corticosteroid, with or without a third drug, such as MTX. Many other chemotherapy drugs have proved to be effective in the therapy of LCH however, including cytosine-arabinoside (ara-C), alkylating agents, anthracyclines and even platinum drugs (Arceci, 1998). A protocol which is still used with some success is the combination of cytosine-arabinoside, vincristine and prednisolone (Egeler et al., 1993). Whatever the protocol, the principle underlying the choice of drugs in the LCH-III trial, namely the use of drugs which have been shown to be efficacious but have a low risk of long-term toxicity, is important.

Resistant disease

Patients who do not respond to initial treatment are considered to have a high risk of mortality (about 75% in all recent large studies). Cyclosporine A has been suggested as an alternative treatment approach. However, especially in patients with advanced chemotherapy-resistant multisystem disease, convincing data of efficacy

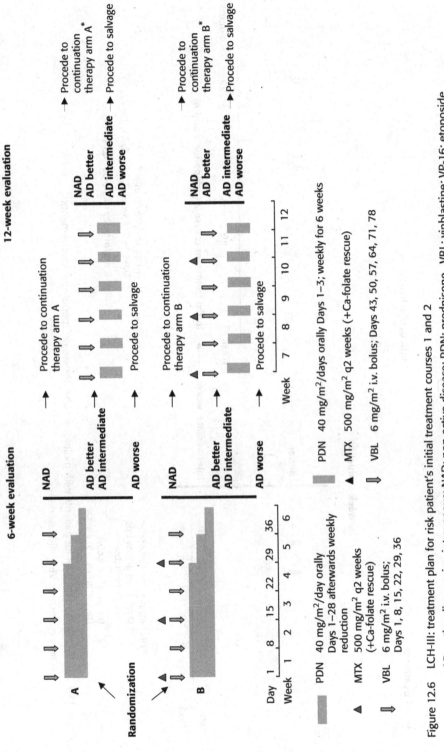

Figure 12.6 LCH-III: treatment plan for risk patient's initial treatment courses 1 and 2
AD: active disease; i.v.: intravenous; NAD: non-active disease; PDN: prednisone, VBL: vinblastine; VP-16: etoposide
* see protocol for details

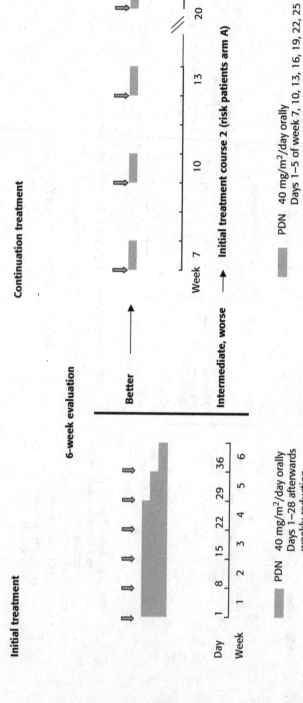

Figure 12.7 LCH-III: treatment plan for patients with multifocal bone disease or 'special-site' involvement;:
PDN: prednisone; VBL: vinblastine

are lacking (Minkov *et al.*, 1999). Many successful bone marrow transplants have been reported, but there are as yet no prospective trials and procedure-related mortality is high (Morgan, 1994). Other studies have reported success in the treatment of LCH with interferon-α (Culic *et al.*, 2001), thalidomide (Misery *et al.*, 1993), anti-CD1a (Kelly and Pritchard, 1994) and anti-tumour necrosis factor-α antibodies (Henter *et al.*, 2001). However, in each case only a few selected patients were evaluated and clearly further investigation is necessary. The use of 2-CdA and 2′-deoxycoformycin has been shown to have promise in treating refractory LCH (McCowage *et al.*, 1996; Weitzman *et al.*, 1999). Many reports suggest that 2-CdA is effective in LCH; however, preliminary results of the recently closed LCH-S-98 protocol of the Histiocyte Society suggest that it is more effective in chronically reactivating low-risk disease (Weitzman, personal communication). Accordingly the Histiocyte Society Salvage Committee will begin accrual to a follow-up study, originally planned to be used in patients who failed 2-CdA alone. This study will test the efficacy of 2-CdA in combination with cytosine-arabinoside for refractory multisystem LCH. A pilot study by The French Langerhans Cell Histiocytosis Study Group suggests that this combination may be effective in this poor prognosis group of patients (Bernard *et al.*, 2003).

A separate protocol for the prospective evaluation of reduced intensity allogeneic stem cell transplant for non-responders is also planned. The importance of using these experimental treatment approaches only as part of carefully designed clinical trials cannot be over-emphasized. Each of these approaches needs careful prospective evaluation before they can be recommended as standard for this difficult problem of non-responsive LCH (see Chapter 13 for additional discussion of salvage therapy for LCH).

Permanent consequences (see also Chapter 14)

Permanent consequences are disease-linked long-term disabilities in patients with LCH (Gadner *et al.*, 1994) and are widely variable (The French Langerhans Cell Histiocytosis Study Group, 1996; Willis *et al.*, 1996; Grois *et al.*, 1998; Donadieu *et al.*, 2004a,b; Haupt *et al.*, 2004). Their frequency and severity are related to disease extent and location, and correlate as well with a prolonged disease course, with reactivations and recurrences (Willis *et al.*, 1996; Braier *et al.*, 1999). In more than half the patients, permanent consequences are already present at the time of diagnosis of LCH. Whereas in single-system disease long-term effects are usually minimal, in survivors of multisystem disease, the overall incidence is more than 50% (Komp, 1981; Willis *et al.*, 1996). A long follow-up observation is needed to accurately estimate the incidence of late effects (Braier *et al.*, 1999; Gadner *et al.*, 2001; Haupt *et al.*, 2004). In patients with endocrine dysfunction or neurological disease, the appearance of sequelae may be hidden for years or even decades (Grois *et al.*, 1995, 1998).

A great variety of permanent consequences has been reported. They include small stature, growth hormone deficiency, hypothyroidism, DI, partial deafness, cerebellar ataxia, loss of dentition, orthopaedic problems, pulmonary fibrosis and biliary cirrhosis with portal hypertension. Of particular interest is the observation that more aggressive initial treatment protocols with prolonged continuation therapy (DAL-HX trials) resulted in a reduction in permanent consequences as compared to children treated with a conservative approach (Komp, 1980; Arceci, 1998). The assumption that intensified or prolonged treatment prevents the development of sequelae, however, has not yet been proven by prospective clinical trials, although LCH-III has the potential to answer this question. The development of a malignancy (5% in long-term survivors with LCH) is higher than expected (Greenberger *et al.*, 1981). In a recent retrospective analysis of reported cases, a high association of malignancy and LCH, even without treatment and not infrequently preceding the diagnosis of LCH, was found (Egeler *et al.*, 1998). Two distinct patterns of association were identified: acute lymphoblastic leukaemia preceding LCH suggesting that LCH is a secondary process due to immunosuppression related to leukaemia therapy, and acute myeloblastic leukaemia (AML) or solid tumours, developing after LCH treated by chemo- and/or radiotherapy, suggesting a therapy-induced event.

Although interpretation of these data is difficult, epiphyllotoxin-induced secondary AML (sAML) has been of major concern. Etoposide, which has been commonly used in the treatment of LCH (Broadbent *et al.*, 1989), has been shown to carry a risk for sAML, when used in cumulative doses greater than 4000 mg/m^2. Lower doses were used in LCH treatment, and a low (2%) incidence of sMAL was found (Ladisch *et al.*, 1994). However, a safe level of etoposide exposure is unknown and concern regarding prolonged and high-dose use of potentially carcinogenic drugs such as etoposide is warranted (Gadner *et al.*, 1994; Haupt *et al.*, 1997).

Conclusion

Recognized for over a century, LCH has only recently been subjected to rigorous uniform, and widely applied, diagnostic and stratification approaches. The international cooperation engendered by the Histiocyte Society and its members has enabled the first randomized treatment trials for this disease to be undertaken. Important knowledge regarding disease pathogenesis, clinical presentation, diagnosis, therapy and late consequences has been obtained.

Careful review of the outcome of these (and earlier) trials has resulted in an appreciation of now well-established prognostic factors. At the same time several reports detailing the permanent consequences of LCH and its therapy have served to emphasize the importance of utilizing these prognosticators in establishing risk-adjusted therapy. Thus we have learnt that therapy can safely be reduced for low-risk patients without sacrificing efficacy, but also that some low-risk patients may require systemic therapy, not only to accelerate healing, but also to prevent late effects. We have also learnt to discriminate early in their course the non-responding patients with 'risk' disease, who appear to require new and experimental approaches to improve their chance of survival.

A number of important questions with regard to the best (and least toxic) combination of drugs, as well as the optimal duration of therapy, remain to be answered and are the subject of ongoing trials. Although the aetiology remains elusive, steady progress has been made, and while far from being complete, it has allowed new hope for families and physicians of LCH patients.

REFERENCES

Arceci, R.J. (1998). Controversies and new approaches to treatment of Langerhans cell histiocytosis. *Hematol Oncol Clin North Am*, **12**, 339–357.

Avery, M.E., McAfee, J.G. and Guild, H.G. (1957). The course and prognosis of reticuloendotheliosis (eosinophilic granuloma, Schuller–Christian disease and Letterer–Siwe disease); a study of forty cases. *Am J Med*, **22**, 636–652.

Bernard, F., Thomas, C., Bertrand, Y., *et al.* (2005). Report of multicenter pilot study of 2-CdA and Ara-C combined chemotherapy in refractory Langerhans cell histiocytosis with hematological dysfunction. *Eur J Cancer* (in press) (accepted for publication Nov. 2004).

Berry, D.H., Gresik, M.V., Humphrey, B., *et al.* (1986). Natural history of histiocytosis X: a Pediatric Oncology Group Study. *Med Pediatr Oncol*, **14**, 1–5.

Berry, D.H., Gresik, M., Maybee, D., *et al.* (1990). Histiocytosis X in bone only. *Med Pediatr Oncol*, **18**, 292–294.

Braier, J., Chantada, G., Rosso, D., *et al.* (1999). Langerhans cell histiocytosis: retrospective evaluation of 123 patients at a single institution. *Pediatr Hematol Oncol*, **16**, 377–385.

Broadbent, V. and Gadner, H. (1998). Current therapy for Langerhans cell histiocytosis. *Hematol Oncol Clin North Am*, **12**, 327–338.

Broadbent, V. and Pritchard, J. (1997). Diabetes insipidus associated with Langerhans cell histiocytosis: is it reversible? *Med Pediatr Oncol*, **28**, 289–293.

Broadbent, V., Gadner, H., Komp, D., *et al.* (1989a). Histiocytosis syndromes in children II. Approach to the clinical and laboratory evaluation of children with Langerhans-cell histiocytosis. *Med Ped Oncol*, **17**, 492–495.

Broadbent, V., Pritchard, J., Yeomans, E. (1989b). Etoposide (VP16) in the treatment of multisystem Langerhans cell histiocytosis (histiocytosis X). *Med Pediatr Oncol*, **17**, 97–100.

Brown, R.E. (2001). Bisphosphonates as antialveolar macrophage therapy in pulmonary Langerhans cell histiocytosis? *Med Pediatr Oncol*, **36**, 641–643.

Ceci, A., Terlizzi, M.D., Colella, R., et al. (1993). Langerhans cell histiocytosis in childhood: results from the Italian Cooperative AIEOP-CNR-HX 83 Study. Med Pediatr Oncol, 21, 259–264.

Culic, S., Jakobson, A., Culic, V., et al. (2001). Etoposide as the basic and interferon-alpha as the maintenance therapy for Langerhans cell histiocytosis: a RTC. Pediatr Hematol Oncol, 18, 291–294.

Daneshbod, K. and Kissane, J.M. (1978). Idiopathic differentiated histiocytosis. Am J Clin Pathol, 70, 381–389.

Donadieu, J., Rolon, M.A., Pion, E.M., et al., for The French LCH Study Group. (2004a). Incidence of growth hormone deficiency in pediatric-onset Langerhans cell histiocytosis: efficacy and safety of growth hormone treatment. J Clin Endocrinol Metab, 89, 604–609.

Donadieu, J., Rolon, M.A., Thomas, C., et al., for The French LCH Study Group. (2004b). Endocrine involvement in pediatric-onset Langerhans' cell hisiotcytosis: a population-based study. J Pediatr, 144, 344–350.

Dunger, D.B., Broadbent, V., Yeoman, E., et al. (1989). The frequency and natural history of diabetes insipidus in children with Langerhans cell histiocytosis. New Engl J Med, 321, 1157–1162.

Egeler, R.M. (2001). More on pamidronate in Langerhans'-cell histiocytosis. New Engl J Med, 345, 1502–1503.

Egeler, R.M. and D'Angio, G.J. (1995). Langerhans cell histiocytosis. J Pediatr, 127, 1–11.

Egeler, R.M., de Kraker, J., Voute, P.A. (1993). Cytosine-arabinoside, vincristine, and prednisolone in the treatment of children with disseminated Langerhans cell histiocytosis with organ dysfunction: experience at a single institution. Med Pediatr Oncol, 21, 265–270.

Egeler, R.M., Neglia, J.P., Aricò, M., et al. (1998). The relation of Langerhans cell histiocytosis to acute leukemia, lymphomas, and other solid tumors. The LCH-Malignancy Study Group of the Histiocyte Society. Hematol Oncol Clin North Am, 12, 369–378.

Egeler, R.M., Thompson, R.C., Voute, P.A., et al. (1992). Intralesional infiltration of corticosteroids in localized Langerhans cell histiocytosis. J Pediatr Orthop, 12, 811–814.

Farran, R.P., Zaretski, E. and Egeler, R.M. (2001). Treatment of Langerhans cell histiocytosis with pamidronate. J Pediatr Hematol Oncol, 23, 54–56.

Feldges, A. (1981).Childhood histiocytosis X: clinical aspects and therapeutic approaches. Haematol Blood Transfusion, 27, 225–228.

Gadner, H. and Grois, N. (1993). The histiocytosis syndromes. In: Fitzpatrick, T.B., Eisen, A.Z., Wolff, K., Freedberg, I.M. and Austen, K.F., eds. Dermatology in General Medicine, Vol. II, Mc Graw-Hill, Inc., New York. pp. 2003–2017.

Gadner, H., Heitger, A., Grois, N., et al. (1994). Treatment strategy for disseminated Langerhans cell histiocytosis. Med Pediatr Oncol, 23, 72–80.

Gadner, H., Grois, N., Aricò, M., et al. (2001). A randomized trial of treatment for multisystem Langerhans' cell histiocytosis. J Pediatr, 138, 728–734.

Gramatovici, R. and D'Angio, G.J. (1988). Radiation therapy in soft-tissue lesions in histiocytosis X (Langerhans' cell histiocytosis). Med Pediatr Oncol, 16, 259–262.

Greenberger, J.S., Cassady, J.R., Jaffe, N., et al. (1979). Radiation therapy in patients with histiocytosis: management of diabetes insipidus and bone lesions. Int J Radiat Oncol Biol Phys, 5, 1749–1755.

Greenberger, J.S., Crocker, A.C., Vawter, G., *et al.* (1981). Results of treatment of 127 patients with systemic histiocytosis (Letterer–Siwe syndrome, Schuller–Christian syndrome and multifocal eosinophilic granuloma). *Medicine*, **60**, 311–338.

Grois, N., Flucher-Wolfram, B., Heitger, A., *et al.* (1995). Diabetes insipidus in Langerhans cell histiocytosis: results from the DAL-HX 83 study. *Med Pediatr Oncol*, **24**, 248–256.

Grois, N.G., Favara, B.E., Mostbeck, G.H., *et al.* (1998). Central nervous system disease in Langerhans cell histiocytosis. *Hematol Oncol Clin North Am*, **12**, 287–305.

Grois, N. and Gadner, H. (2004). Re: Is unifocal Langerhans cell histiocytosis of the orbit a 'CNS-risk' lesion? (letter to the editor) *Pediatr Blood Cancer*, **43**, 300–301.

Hashimoto, K. and Pritzker, M.S. (1973). Electron microscopic study of reticulohistiocytoma. An unusual case of congenital, self-healing reticulohistiocytosis. *Arch Dermatol*, **107**, 263–270.

Haupt, R., Fears, T.R., Heise, A., *et al.* (1997). Risk of secondary leukemia after treatment with etoposide (VP-16) for Langerhans' cell histiocytosis in Italian and Austrian–German populations. *Int J Cancer*, **71**, 9–13.

Haupt, R., Nanduri, V., Calevo, M.G., *et al.* (2004). Permanent consequences in Langerhans cell histiocytosis patients: a pilot study from the Histiocyte Society – Late Effects Study Group. *Pediatr Blood Cancer*, **42**, 438–444.

Henter, J.I., Karlen, J., Calming, U., *et al.* (2001). Successful treatment of Langerhans-cell histiocytosis with etanercept. *New Engl J Med*, **345**, 1577–1578.

Howell, S.J., Wilton, P. and Shalet, S.M. (1998). Growth hormone replacement in patients with Langerhan's cell histiocytosis. *Arch Dis Child*, **78**, 469–473.

Kelly, K.M. and Pritchard, J. (1994). Monoclonal antibody therapy in Langerhans cell histiocytosis – feasible and reasonable? *Br J Cancer*, **70**(Suppl XXIII), 54–55.

Kilpatrick, S.E., Wenger, D.E., Gilchrist, G.S., *et al.* (1995). Langerhans' cell histiocytosis (histiocytosis X) of bone. A clinicopathologic analysis of 263 pediatric and adult cases. *Cancer*, **76**, 2471–2484.

Komp, D.M. (1981). Long-term sequelae of histiocytosis X. *Am J Pediatr Hematol Oncol*, **3**, 165–168.

Komp, D.M., Vietti, T.J., Berry, D.H. *et al.* (1977). Combination chemotherapy and histiocytosis X. *Med Pediatr Oncol*, **3**, 267–273.

Komp, D.M., Mahdi, A.E., Starling, K.A., *et al.* (1980). Quality of survival in histiocytosis X: a Southwest Oncology Group Study. *Med Pediatr Oncol*, **8**, 35–40.

Ladisch, S. (1983). Histiocytosis. In: Willoughby, M.L.N. and Siegel, S.E., eds. *Butterworth's International Medical Reviews, Pediatrics Hematology*, Vol. I, Butterworth Scientific, London, pp. 95–109.

Ladisch, S. and Gadner, H. (1994). Treatment of Langerhans cell histiocytosis – evolution and current approaches. *Br J Cancer*, **70**, 41–46.

Ladisch, S. and Jaffe, E. (2002). The histiocytoses. In: Pizzo, P.A. and Poplack, D.G., eds. *Principles and Practice of Pediatric Oncology*, Lippincott, Philadelphia, pp. 733–750.

Ladisch, S., Gadner, H., Aricò, M., *et al.* (1994). LCH-I: a randomised trial of etoposide versus vinblastine in disseminated Langerhans cell histiocytosis. *Med Pediatr Oncol*, **23**, 107–110.

Lahey, E. (1975). Histiocytosis X: an analysis of prognostic factors. *J Pediatr*, **87**, 184–189.

Lahey, M.E. (1962). Prognosis in reticuloendotheliosis in children. *J Pediatr*, **60**, 664–668.

Lahey, M.E., Smith, B. and Heyn, R. (1979). Immunologic studies in histiocytosis X (meeting abstract). *Proc Am Ass Cancer Res*, **20**, 436.

LCH-III. Treatment protocol of the third international study for Langerhans cell histiocytosis (www.histio.org).

McClain, K.L., Gonzales, J., Jonkers, R., *et al.* (2002). Need for a cooperative study: Pulmonary Langerhans cell histiocytosis and its management in adults. (Position paper). *Med Pediatr Oncol*, **39**, 35–39.

McCowage, G.B., Frush, D.P. and Kurtzberg, J. (1996). Successful treatment of two children with Langerhans' cell histiocytosis with 2'-deoxycoformycin. *J Pediatr Hematol Oncol*, **18**, 154–158.

McLelland, J., Broadbent, V., Yeomans, E., *et al.* (1990). Langerhans cell histiocytosis: the case for conservative treatment. *Arch Dis Child*, **65**, 301–303.

Minkov, M., Grois, N., Broadbent, V., *et al.* (1999). Cyclosporine. A therapy for multisystem langerhans cell histiocytosis. *Med Pediatr Oncol*, **33**, 482–485.

Minkov, M., Grois, N., Braier, J., *et al.*, for the Histiocyte Society. (2002a). Immunosuppressive treatment for chemotherapy resistant multisystem Langerhans cell histiocytosis. *Med Pediatr Oncol*, **40**, 253–256.

Minkov, M., Grois, N., Heitger, A., *et al.* (2002b). Response to initial treatment: an important prognostic predictor in multisystem Langerhans cell histiocytosis. *Med Pediatr Oncol*, **39**, 581–585.

Misery, L., Larbre, B., Lyonnet, S., *et al.* (1993). Remission of Langerhans cell histiocytosis with thalidomide treatment. *Clin Exp Dermatol*, **18**, 487.

Morgan, C. (1994). Myeloablative therapy and bone marrow transplantation for Langerhans cell histiocytosis. *Br J Cancer*, **70**(Suppl XXIII), 52–53.

Munn, S. and Chu, A.C. (1998). Langerhans cell histiocytosis of the skin. *Hematol Oncol Clin North Am*, **12**, 269–286.

Munn, S.E., Olliver, L., Broadbent, V., *et al.* (1999). Use of indomethacin in Langerhans cell histiocytosis. *Med Pediatr Oncol*, **32**, 247–249.

Neumann, G., Kolde, G. and Bonsmann, G. (1988). Histiocytosis X in an elderly patient. Ultrastructure and immunochemistry after PUVA photochemotherapy. *Br J Dermat*, **19**, 385–391.

Nezelof, C., Frileux-Herbet, F. and Cronier-Sachot, J. (1979). Disseminated histiocytosis X: analysis of prognostic factors based on a retrospective study of 50 cases. *Cancer*, **44**, 1824–1838.

Oberman, H.A. (1961). Idiopathic histiocytosis. A clinicopathologic study of 40 cases and review of the literature. *Pediatrics*, **28**, 307–327.

Selch, M.T. and Parker, R.G. (1990). Radiation therapy in the management of Langerhans cell histiocytosis. *Med Pediatr Oncol*, **18**, 97–102.

Sheehan, M.P., Atherton, D.J., Broadbent, V., *et al.* (1991). Topical nitrogen mustard: an effective treatment for cutaneous Langerhans cell histiocytosis. *J Pediatr*, **119**, 317–321.

Slater, J.M. and Swarm, O.J. (1980). Eosinophilic granuloma of bone. *Med Pediatr Oncol*, **8**, 151–164.

Tazi, A., Soler, P. and Hance, A.J. (2002). Adult pulmonary Langerhans' cell histiocytosis. *Thorax*, **55**, 405–416.

The French Langerhans Cell Histiocytosis Group. (1996). A multicentric retrospective survey of Langerhans' cell histiocytosis: 348 cases observed between 1983 and 1993. *Arch Dis Child*, **75**, 17–24.

Titgemeyer, C., Grois, N., Minkov, M., *et al.* (2001). Pattern and course of single-system disease in Langerhans cell histiocytosis. *Med Pediatr Oncol*, **37**, 1–7.

Toogood, I.R., Ellis, W.M. and Ekert, H. (1979). Prognostic criteria, treatment and survival in disseminated histiocytosis X. *Aust Paediatr J*, **15**, 91–95.

Vassallo, R., Ryu, J.H., Colby, T.V., *et al.* (2000). Pulmonary Langerhans'-cell histiocytosis. *New Engl J Med*, **342**, 1969–1978.

Watts, J. and Files, B. (2001). Langerhans cell histiocytosis: central nervous system involvement treated successfully with 2-chlorodeoxyadenosine. *Pediatr Hematol Oncol*, **18**, 199–204.

Weitzman, S., Wayne, A.S., Arceci, R., *et al.* (1999). Nucleoside analogues in the therapy of Langerhans cell histiocytosis: a survey of members of the Histiocyte Society and review of the literature. *Med Pediatr Oncol*, **33**, 476–481.

Willis, B., Ablin, A., Weinberg, V., *et al.* (1996). Disease course and late sequelae of Langerhans cell histiocytosis: 25-year experience at the University of California, San Francisco. *J Clin Oncol*, **14**, 2073–2082.

Willman, C., Busque, L., Griffith, B., *et al.* (1994). Langerhans' cell histiocytosis (histiocytosis X) – a clonal proliferative disease. *New Engl J Med*, **331**, 154–160.

Woo, K.I. and Harris, G.J. (2003). Eosinophilic granuloma of the orbit – understanding the paradox of aggressive destruction responsive to minimal intervention. *Ophthal Plast Reconstr Surg*, **19**, 429–439.

Womer, R.B., Anunciato, K.R. and Chehrenama, M. (1995). Oral methotrexate and alternate-day prednisone for low-risk Langerhans cell histiocytosis. *Med Pediatr Oncol*, **25**, 70–73.

Writing Group of the Histiocyte Society. (1987). Histiocytosis syndromes in children. *Lancet*, **1**, 208–209.

Zeller, B., Storm-Mathisen, I., Smevik, B., *et al.* (2000). Multisystem Langerhans-cell histiocytosis with life-threatening pulmonary involvement – good response to cyclosporine A. *Med Pediatr Oncol*, **35**, 438–442.

13

Treatment of relapsed and/or refractory Langerhans cell histiocytosis

Sheila Weitzman, Kenneth L. McClain and Robert Arceci

The last several decades have seen enormous gains in knowledge with regard to the biology of Langerhans cell histiocytosis (LCH). However, this increased understanding has not yet translated into dramatic improvements in outcome, particularly for patients with multisystem (MS) disease whose disease is refractory to standard therapy, patients with chronic relapsing disease or those with the late chronic progressive involvement of lung, liver and central nervous system (CNS), who continue to pose a significant dilemma for treating physicians. This chapter will concentrate on the problems of therapy for patients with refractory, multiorgan disease and those with late chronic progressive disease of lung and liver. CNS neurodegenerative diseases are discussed in Chapter 10.

Refractory multiorgan disease

Early cooperative group studies have shown that patients with MS disease clearly benefit from chemotherapy. The mortality for high-risk patients with disseminated disease does not, however, appear to have changed from the early Austro-German cooperative trials, the DAL-HX 83 and 90 trials, to the later LCH-I and II studies of the Histiocyte Society. Thus, about 20% of young children with MS LCH do not respond to modern protocols and often have disease that is resistant to alternative therapies.

An important step forward has been the ability to determine which patients will have poor outcomes. Features which portend a poor outcome include involvement of 'risk' organs (such as lung, liver, spleen and hematopoietic system) and failure to respond after 6 weeks of initial therapy (Gadner *et al.*, 2001; Minkov *et al.*, 2002). 'Classic' risk factors, such as organ dysfunction and young age, are no longer considered to be independently prognostic. The probability of survival for patients who failed to respond after two courses of therapy in the LCH-I and II studies was 20–34%, and was as low as 10% after the more intensive DAL chemotherapy (Minkov *et al.*,

2002). Poor early response is now the single most important factor predicting poor survival (The French LCH Study Group, 1996).

Treatment of LCH resistant to conventional therapy has proved problematic and the outlook has been poor. The treatment ranges from alternative chemotherapy to immunomodulatory approaches, as well as stem cell transplantation (SCT).

Chemotherapy

Conventional first-line chemotherapy generally consists of combinations of vinca alkaloids (vinblastine or vincristine) plus a corticosteroid, with or without a third drug, namely cytosine arabinoside (ara-C) or methotrexate (MTX). Many chemotherapy drugs have proven to be effective in the therapy of LCH and various combinations have been tried as second-line therapies for patients with refractory disease. For more than a decade etoposide has been shown to be an effective agent in both LCH and hemophagocytic lymphohistiocytosis (HLH) (Ceci et al., 1988a; Ladisch and Gadner, 1994); however, it was not shown to be superior to vinblastine in the LCH-I randomized trial (Ladisch et al., 1994), nor when added to the 'standard drugs' in LCH-II (Gadner et al., 2001). A number of recent reports suggest that prolonged use of oral etoposide alone (Helmbold et al., 1998), or as basic therapy followed by another therapy as maintenance (Culic et al., 2001), may be efficacious. Etoposide-induced secondary leukemia remains a concern, however. The US Cancer Therapy Evaluation Program calculated the 6-year risk of leukemia to be 3.2% without an apparent dose–response effect (Felix and Blatt, 1999; Smith et al., 1999).

A number of chemotherapy combinations have been tried in patients with refractory disease, including alkylating agents, anthracyclins and platinum drugs (Arceci et al., 1998). A protocol which is still used with some success, is the combination of ara-C, vincristine and prednisolone (Egeler et al., 1993). However, neither this nor any of the other combinations which have shown efficacy in LCH, appear to improve survival in patients with refractory disease, nor have they been shown to prevent reactivations in chronically relapsing patients. New and more effective drugs or combinations are clearly needed.

Nucleoside analogs in the therapy of resistant LCH

2-Chlorodeoxyadenosine

2-Chlorodeoxyadenosine (2-CdA cladribine) is a nucleoside analog with significant activity in hairy cell leukemia, low-grade lymphoproliferative disorders and recurrent acute myeloid leukemia in children. The combined effects on DNA result in rapid inhibition of DNA replication in dividing cells (Santana et al., 1991) and failure of DNA repair causing apoptosis in resting cells. The most common toxicities are transient myelosuppression and prolonged T-cell immunosuppression.

Few serious infections have been reported in patients with LCH, although following eight courses of therapy, a child who developed disseminated Epstein–Barr virus (EBV) (Weitzman, personal communication) and another child who developed recurrent herpes zoster and cytomegalovirus (CMV) pneumonia (Joshi *et al.*, 1999) were observed. Other toxicities reported include thrombocytopenia, polyneuropathy (not described at the lower LCH doses) and skin reactions when used in combination with allopurinol (Chubar and Bennett, 2003). One patient with LCH developed chronic myelomonocytic leukemia (CMML) 38 months after 2-CdA (Saven and Burian, 1999); another developed EBV-induced lymphoproliferative disease. Assessment of the second malignancy rate in chronic lymphocytic leukemia (CLL), however, found no increase above the expected rate (Cheson *et al.*, 1999).

Since the first report by Saven *et al.*, showing 3/3 complete responses (CRs) in adults with resistant LCH (Saven *et al.*, 1994), many case reports (Dimopoulos *et al.*, 1996; Cole and Finlay, 1999; Joshi *et al.*, 1999; Goh *et al.*, 2003), and a number of case series (Stine *et al.*, 1997; Saven and Burian, 1999; Weitzman *et al.*, 1999; Rodriguez-Galindo *et al.*, 2002; Pardanani *et al.*, 2003), attest to the efficacy in both pediatric and adult LCH. Response rates range from 25% to 75%, with relatively small numbers of patients treated and a wide range of LCH system involvement. The reported responses were, however, generally durable. 2-CdA penetrates the blood–brain barrier producing cerebrospinal fluid (CSF) levels that are 25% of plasma (Liliemark, 1997). A number of reports have shown some efficacy of 2-CdA against active CNS LCH, including patients who failed radiation therapy. In two cases, 2-CdA reversed diabetes insipidus (DI) (Watts and Files, 2001; Giona *et al.*, 2002; Ottaviano and Finlay, 2003).

Early results of a Histiocyte Society study suggest that 2-CdA is more effective in patients with chronically relapsing low-risk disease. Although a minority achieved CR, less than a third of high-risk patients responded well (Weitzman *et al.*, unpublished results). The multiple effects of 2-CdA on DNA metabolism, means that it is likely to be synergistic with many cytotoxic drugs, and the combination is likely to be more effective than 2-CdA alone. The cytotoxic effect of ara-C is due to the active metabolite 5′-triphosphate, ara-CTP (Choi *et al.*, 2003). The combination of 2-CdA and ara-C results in higher intracellular concentrations and/or increased retention time of ara-CTP both *in vitro* and *in vivo* (Gandhi *et al.*, 1996). The synergistic effect of the combination has been demonstrated in acute myeloblastic leukemia (AML) (Crews *et al.*, 2002). This synergy, the efficacy of the drugs individually in LCH and the low long-term toxicity of ara-C, makes this an attractive combination. Anecdotal case reports (Choi *et al.*, 2003) and the results of a recent small series of 10 patients with progressive LCH are encouraging, despite significant pancytopenia in all patients. It is noteworthy that several patients stabilized and then achieved a delayed CR (median delay of 0.45 years) (Bernard *et al.*, 2003). Other combinations including 2-CdA and cyclophosphamide have also been tried with anecdotal responses (Robak *et al.*, 2002).

Another nucleoside inhibitor, 2′-deoxycoformycin (2′-DCF), a direct inhibitor of the adenosine deaminase enzyme, has been reported to show efficacy in refractory LCH in a limited numbers of patients (McCowage et al., 1996; Lombardi et al., 2002). The combination of 2-CdA and 2′-DCF has been reported to be synergistic in inhibiting repair of irradiation-induced DNA damage and could potentially be an interesting combination for further testing (Johnston et al., 1993).

The nucleoside analogs are drugs with demonstrated activity in LCH. It appears that used alone, 2-CdA is useful in the therapy of low-risk patients with chronic recurrent disease. In high-risk refractory patients, however, improvements to single agent 2-CdA are needed. The combination of 2-CdA with other drugs, such as ara-C, appears to be promising.

Immunomodulatory therapy

Increasing knowledge of the fundamental immune dysregulation in LCH, has led to alternative approaches to control the disease. Early attempts at immunomodulatory therapy with thymic extract (Osband et al., 1981; Ceci et al., 1988b), antithymocyte serum (ATS) or antithymocyte globulin (ATG) (Arceci et al., 1998) did not prove beneficial.

Cyclosporin (CSA)

CSA has been shown to be effective in diseases showing cytokine dysregulation, including HLH. Reports suggested it might also be efficacious in LCH, particularly if combined with other drugs (Aricò, 1991; Mahmoud et al., 1991; Körholz et al., 1997; Sako et al., 1999). Toxicity includes hypertension, hypertrichosis and anemia, but acute and chronic nephrotoxicity remains the most significant clinical problem (Burdmann et al., 2003). A retrospective review of 26 LCH-I patients, 10 switched to CSA alone and 16 to CSA in combination with other agents, found that only 4/26 (15%) of patients responded, suggesting that CSA is of limited value in high-risk patients with progressive disease (Minkov et al., 1999). Treatment of high-risk patients with immunosuppressive approaches, such as CSA, together with multiagent chemotherapy may be a rational approach, although the implications for opportunistic infections using such regimens may be significant.

Thalidomide

The potential efficacy of *thalidomide* in LCH has been ascribed to wide-ranging properties including inhibition of tumor necrosis factor alpha (TNF-α), enhancement of T-cell co-stimulatory activity and inhibition of angiogenic activity. It has shown considerable efficacy in the treatment of a number of 'cytokine-mediated' skin disorders, and has proven effect in patients with cutaneous, mucosal and vulvar LCH (Misery *et al.*, 1993; Lair *et al.*, 1998; Moraes and Russo, 2001; Claudon *et al.*, 2002). Efficacy in non-cutaneous LCH has been controversial. Two adults, one with severe systemic involvement, and another with genital, oral mucosal and a hypothalamic–hypophyseal granuloma, achieved CR with thalidomide (Claudon *et al.*, 2002; Mortazavi *et al.*, 2002). In most patients thus far reported, however, the LCH recurred within variable periods after cessation of therapy (Lair *et al.*, 1998; Moraes and Russo, 2001; Claudon *et al.*, 2002). Dramatic responses of cutaneous and ano-genital lesions to thalidomide plus interferons (IFN), have also been reported. Immunomodulating agents should be tried in LCH of the female genital tract, prior to surgery or radiation therapy (Montero *et al.*, 2003). A trial of thalidomide for treatment of LCH in 14 patients resistant to conventional therapy, showed no response in five high-risk patients, but partial or CRs in six of nine low-risk patients. However, dose-limiting toxicities, including neuropathy and neutropenia may have reduced its efficacy (McClain, submitted).

Structural analogs with improved immunomodulatory activity and toxicity profiles are being evaluated. These include selective cytokine inhibitory drugs, with improved TNF-α inhibitory activity and less toxicity (Dredge *et al.*, 2002). Early trial data suggest that these compounds may supercede thalidomide in the treatment of patients with myeloma and immune-mediated disorders.

Interferon α (INF-α)

INF-α has been used in patients with progressive LCH based on its capacity to enhance immune responses and inhibit cell proliferation (Arceci *et al.*, 1998). Some positive responses have been reported in LCH patients who received the drug over an extended period as maintenance therapy (Culic *et al.*, 2001). The successful use of intralesional INF-β in localized skin lesions was reported (Matsushima and Baba, 1991). Two adults with widespread refractory skin-only LCH achieved a CR with prolonged INF-α therapy (Kwong *et al.*, 1997; Chang *et al.*, 2002). Results in refractory MS patients have been disappointing.

The combination of *retinoic acid and INF-α* was used in two young patients with progressive disease based on the theoretical usefulness of all transretinoic acid (ATRA) in LCH, which includes increase in antigenic expression, downregulation of interleukin (IL) 1 and TNF-α production (Minkov *et al.*, 2001), induction of apoptosis of LCH cells *in vitro* (Geissmann *et al.*, 1997), and the synergistic effect of ATRA plus INF-α seen in cervical carcinoma. No clinical effect was observed (Minkov *et al.*, 2001). Another immunomodulatory experimental approach is the use of *IL-2 therapy*. To test the effect of increased CD16+ natural killer (NK)/cytotoxic activity in LCH, IL-2 therapy was used in a patient with resistant LCH with a positive clinical effect (Hirose and Kuroda, 1999).

Immunotargeted monoclonal antibody therapy

CD1a, a sialoglycoprotein member of the non-classical major histocompatibility family of proteins involved in glycolipid antigen presentation, is selectively expressed on the surface of Langerhans cells (LCs), cortical thymocytes and LCH cells (Murray *et al.*, 2000). Thymic cortical and normal LCs repopulate quickly from CD1a-negative precursors (Groh *et al.*, 1988). These features along with its ability to internalize upon antibody binding make it a potentially desirable therapeutic target. It is unclear whether the CD1a-positive LCH lesional cell arises from a CD1a-negative progenitor. This question will have to await further studies, including clinical trials to determine the potential therapeutic utility of such an antigenic target. The cytotoxic potential of unlabeled and I^{131}-radiolabeled murine anti-CD1a monoclonal antibody (MAB) (NA1/34) has been measured *in vitro* and in a xenograft model. The I^{131}-labeled-NA1/34 was shown to have greater cytotoxicity toward CD1a+ cells both *in vitro* and *in vivo* animal xenografts (Murray *et al.*, 2000).

The NA1/34 murine anti-CD1a MAB has also been used as a radiolabeled conjugate in a pilot clinical study (Kelly and Pritchard, 1994). The antibody was shown to localize to disease sites, but no therapeutic benefit was seen, although this was not the goal of this feasibility study. This approach thus has potential for immunotherapeutic targeting although several important questions will need to be studied. For example, one dose of an MAB is unlikely to be sufficient and a 'humanized' antibody is more likely to be better tolerated and less likely to produce immune reactions, including the generation of neutralizing antibodies. Issues of affinity and antigen density as well as whether unlabeled or toxin- or radiolabeled conjugates will be more effective will need to be carefully studied. The use of anti-CD1a antibodies or other monoclonal antibodies (such as Campath, an anti-CD52-specific antibody, or anti-class II-directed antibodies) will all be worth testing in the context of careful clinical trials.

Etanercept

The inflammatory cytokine TNF-α is an important cause of morbidity in LCH. TNF-α inhibitors (receptor blockers or monoclonal antibodies) have been shown to reduce circulating levels of bioactive TNF-α and to a lesser extent IL-6 and IL-1 (Charles *et al.*, 1999). Combinations of anti-TNF drugs with other therapy have been tried in LCH. Etanercept, a soluble TNF receptor: Fc fusion protein, was added to the therapy of a child with non-responsive MS LCH, with improvement in clinical symptomatology. Disease symptoms recurred when the drug was stopped after 6 months and then resolved when the therapy was restarted. Although no toxicity was observed in this single patient (Henter *et al.*, 2001), immunosuppression associated with this class of drugs may result in a variety of opportunistic infections;

furthermore, the relationship between anti-TNF agents and secondary lymphoproliferative diseases is another potential complication. For instance, one patient treated with CSA and infliximab was reported to have developed a CD30+ T-cell lymphoproliferative disorder which regressed when the treatment was stopped (Mahe *et al.*, 2003). It is possible that the addition of an anti-cytokine, such as a TNF-blocking drug may alleviate symptoms, improve the clinical condition, and allow time for other drugs to work or for bone marrow donors to be found.

Stem cell transplantation (SCT)

A number of successful SCTs have been reported in refractory LCH patients. Whether success is due to the cytotoxic effect of high-dose chemotherapy or to a graft-versus-LCH effect remains to be determined. It is known that following successful allogeneic transplantation recipient LCs are gradually replaced by donor LCs (Perreault *et al.*, 1984). A review of the literature found 35 patients transplanted for refractory LCH. Eight were found from 89 responses to a questionnaire to members of the Histiocyte Society. Of the eight, five were dead, one was alive-with-disease, one had a poor response (PR) and one achieved a CR (Broadbent and Ladisch, 1997). It is impossible to tell which of these cases were published elsewhere, and they are not included in the summary of the other 27 cases (Table 13.1). Fourteen of the 27 (52%) were alive in continuous complete remission (CCR) from 12+ to 144+ (median 25+) months at the time of reporting, 13 following allogeneic SCT and one after an autologous graft. Of the five patients receiving autologous SCT, four relapsed and three died and one was rescued with alternative chemotherapy. Of 22 allogeneic SCT, 13 (59%) are in CCR, one of whom recovered with autologous marrow. There were no major differences between survivors and those that died including age at diagnosis, time from diagnosis to SCT or type of donor (matched sibling and unrelated donors, MSD *versus* MUD, respectively). Both patients receiving haploidentical SCT died. Of 15 survivors, 7 received total body radiation (TBI) as part of their preparative regimen and 8 received chemotherapy-containing conditioning regimens. Eight of 12 patients who died received TBI. Eight toxic deaths occurred at 9–120 days post-transplant, four patients relapsed and died from 4 to 23 months post-transplant.

The majority of deaths post-allogeneic transplant are due to toxicity, while the majority of autologous recipients relapsed. A recent series from St. Jude Children's Center suggests that TBI-containing regimens are more effective than chemotherapy conditioning for histiocytic disorders (Hale *et al.*, 2003). Unfortunately, because of small numbers and the retrospective nature of reported trials, no definitive conclusions can be made regarding the optimal preparative regimen.

The question of positive-reporting bias remains a major obstacle to definitive conclusions regarding a variety of transplant-related issues and outcomes. In order to address this issue, a French study checked all cases against the French transplant database to ensure there were no unreported cases (Akkari et al., 2003). Although the numbers were small, the results were similar to those reported here and appear to confirm that allogeneic, but not autologous transplant, is potentially curative in poor-risk patients, results could be clearly improved if transplant-related mortality and morbidity could be reduced.

Pediatric patients generally have lower procedure-related mortality (Schwartz and Yeager, 2003), but are at greater risk of late complications than adult patients. Another approach to reducing treatment-related morbidity and mortality is to employ reduced intensity (RI) preparative regimens (RI-SCT). This approach has been suggested as being particularly appropriate for patients with significant organ dysfunction. The effectiveness of RI-SCT for children with immunodeficiencies (Amrolia et al., 2000) is encouraging with respect to LCH. However, the graft-versus-tumor effect with RI-SCT may occur over a significant period of time and this approach will likely benefit patients with more indolent diseases (Schwartz and Yeager, 2003). In addition, there is no evidence at this time that a graft-versus-LCH immune response has been demonstrated in any type of SCT. A single pediatric LCH patient has been reported to have died from septic shock after a non-myeloablative haploidentical transplant that followed a more traditional myeloablative SCT (Gadner et al., 2002), but two others have been successfully transplanted using RI-SCT (Webb, personal communication). The role of RI preparative regimens for pediatric LCH deserves investigation.

In summary, SCT from an allogeneic donor appears to have a role in the therapy of poor prognosis patients with MS LCH. If reduced intensity approaches are shown to be effective, either because of immunomodulation or a graft-versus-LCH effect, the success rate of transplantation in these ill children will be enhanced. Failure to respond to front-line therapy should lead to early change of therapy to more intensive treatment. One of the more promising approaches is a combination of 2-CdA along with another cytotoxic or immunosuppressive agent. A stem cell donor should be sought in patients who show a PR to initial therapy. If rapid stabilization or improvement occurs with a change to an alternative regimen, the French experience suggests that patients can be continued on therapy. Progression suggests the need to move toward SCT.

Chronic LCH involving the lung and liver

The development of chronic progressive disease in lung, liver and CNS is an uncommon but devastating complication of LCH. The initial lesion appears to be active LCH. In the lung, for example, an interaction between LCH cells, alveolar macrophages and smooth muscle actin-positive myofibroblasts has been proposed

Table 13.1 Summary of SCT patients from literature

References	Sex/age (months)	Organs pre-SCT	Therapy pre-SCT	Time from diagnosis to SCT (months)	Donor	Conditioning (GVHD prophylaxis)	Outcome (months)
1	M/21	Skin, bone, DI, liver, spleen, lung, hem, ear	VP16 (3.5 gm), 6MP, MTX, VCR, pred, dox, INF-γ, Rad, CDDP	30	MSD	Bu/CY/MEL (CSA, MTX)	34 + CCR rejected graft autorecovery
1	M/11	Skin, bone, LN, liver/spleen/lung, hem	VP16, CY, dox	47	MSD	TBI/CY/VP16, VP/CY/ACNU (CSA)	†9 days after second SCT
1	F/154	Skin, bone, hem	VBL.MTX, Pred, CSA	9	Syngeneic	CY/ATG (CSA/MTX)	49+
1	M/7	Skin, bone, LN, liver/spleen/lung, hem	VP16 (0.75 gm), ACOP, CSA, MTX	9	MSD	CY/TBI (CSA/MTX)	†9 days
2	M/132	Bone, LN, liver, lung	Rad, VBL, MTX, VCR, CLB, Pred, CY, MOPP, ara-C, VM26	110	MSD	CY/Mel/TBI, IT MTX, (CSA)	91+
3	M/180	Bone, hem, DI, lung, liver, CNS	CY, pred, VCR, 6MP, Rad	36	MSD	CY/TBI	41+
4	M/348	Bone, LN, spleen, liver, lung, hem	CHOP, splenectomy	4	MSD	CY/BCNU/TBI (MTX)	†12 relapse
4	F/18	Bone, LN, skin, liver, spleen, lung, hem	VBL, pred, 6MP, CBL, Cranial Rad	7	MSD	CY/TBI (MTX)	27+
4	F/180	LN, liver, spleen	CHOP, bleo, splenectomy	11	Autologous	CY/TBI	†0.5 relapse
4	F/540	LN, liver, spleen	MACOP-B, CY, dox, ara-C, VP16	66	Autologous	Bu/CY/TBI	54+
5	M/4	Bone, skin, lung, liver, spleen, LN	HDMPred, VBL, CY, MTX, 2-CdA, VP16	12	MSD	CY/VP16/TBI (CSA, IVIG)	16+
6	M/16	Skin, LN, liver, spleen, lung, hem	VP16, VBL, CSA, Pred	11	MSD	BU/CY/Mel (Mpred)	25+
7	M/3	Liver, spleen	ND	ND	Allogeneic	Bu/CY/VP	12+
8	ND	Refractory			Haplopbsct	CY/ATG/TBI	†12 days respiratory
8	ND	Refractory		ND	Haplopbsct	CY/ATG/TT TBI	†45 days adenovirus no LCH

Ref	Age/Sex	Sites	Therapy	No.	Donor	Conditioning	Outcome
9	M/3	Skin, liver, lung	pred, VBL, VP16, CSA, ara-C	18	Autologous	Bu/CY	Relapsed × 3 alive in CR 84 +
9	M/10	Bone, LN, skin, liver, lung, spleen, hem	pred, VBL, VP16, ara-C	7	Autologous	Bu/CY/VP	†6 relapse
9	M/8	GI, skin, liver, spleen, hem	pred, VBL, VP16, ara-C, 6MP, CSA, COPADM	18	Autologous	VP16/TBI	†4 relapse
9	F/10	Skin, LN, hem, liver, spleen	HDpred, VCR, MTX, CY/VP16, VBL, 6MP, INF-α	10	MSD	Bu/CY/VP16 (CSA)	144+ CCR liver fibrosis growth failure
9	F/5	GI, hem, lungs, skin	pred, VBL, VP16, ara-C	9	MSD	Bu/CY (CSA)	†23 sepsis relapse
9	M/8	Bone, skin	HDpred, VBL, VP16, ara-C	21	MSD	Bu/CY (CSA)	†1 month toxic
9	F/12	Bone, GI, skin, lungs, hem	HDpred, VBL, VP16 CSA	7	MSD	Bu/VP16	21+ CCR (CSA/pred)
9	M/18	Bone, skin, DI, liver, hem	pred, VBL, VP16, ara-C, 2-CdA, CSA, ATG, COPAD, ATRA	19	MUD	TBI (CSA, MMF)	†4-toxic no relapse
10	M/8	Skin, bone later liver, spleen, lung, hem	dox, VCR, CY, VP16, MTX, pred, 6MP, CSA, HD methylpred, ara-C, Mitox	9	MUD	VP16/Mel/TBI (CSA)	12 + CCR
11	F/2	Bone, skin, LN, liver, lung, hem	VBL, pred, VP16, 6MP, MTX, 2-CdA, dox	19	MUD (cord)	Bu/CY/VP16, ATG (CSA, MPred)	24+ CCR
12	M	Liver, spleen, MDS	'Refractory'	3	MUD	TBI, ara-C, CY (CSA)	†33 days
12	M	Skin, ear, liver, spleen, hem	'Refractory'	21 at SCT	MUD	TBI, ara-C, CY (CSA)	54+ CCR

GVHD: graft-versus-host disease; hem: hematopoietic system; CY: cyclophosphamide; Bu: busulfan; pred: prednisone; Mpred: methylprednisolone; HDpred: high-dose prednisone; VBL: vinblastine; VCR: vincristine; dox: doxorubicin; CBL: chlorambucil; Mel: melphalan; IVIG: IV gamma immunoglobulin; Rad: radiation therapy; †: death; GI: gastrointestinal; LN: lymph node; VP16: etoposide; IT: intrathecal; MDS: myelodysplastic syndrome; 6MP: 6 mercaptopurine; bleo: bleomycin; ACOP: adriamycin, cyclophosphamide, oncovin pred; CDDP: cisplatin; CHOP: cyclophosphamide, doxorubicin, vincristine, prednisone; COPADM: cyclophosphamide, doxorubicin, prednisolone, methotrexate, vincristine; MMF: mycophenolate mofetil; ACNU: nimustine; VM26: teniposide; ND: No details.

References: (1) Kinugawa *et al.*, 1999; (2) Ringdén *et al.*, 1987; Ringdén *et al.*, 1997; (3) Stoll *et al.*, 1990; (4) Greinix *et al.*, 1992; (5) Frost and Wiersma, 1996; (6) Conter *et al.*, 1996; (7) Ayas *et al.*, 1998; (8) Egeler *et al.*, 1998; (9) Akkari *et al.*, 2003; (10) Suminoe *et al.*, 2001; (11) Nagarajan *et al.*, 2001; (12) Hale *et al.*, 2003

to result in fibrosis (Brown, 2001). Whether through a direct effect or an associated autoimmune reaction, LCH cells likely contribute to fibrosis through generation of inflammatory cytokines and growth factors, including IL-1, IL-6, transforming growth factor (TGF)-β and platelet-derived growth factor (PDGF) (Egeler *et al.*, 1999; Debray, 2003). TGF-β in particular has been associated with progressive chronic fibrosis (Kelly *et al.*, 2003). The fibrosis around bile ducts results in chronic sclerosing cholangitis (SC) and biliary cirrhosis in the liver. Interstitial fibrosis with honeycombing in the lung characterizes chronic lung involvement. Pathology at the time of late disease shows little, if any, active LCH. Of 10 liver biopsies and five explanted livers in one series, only one biopsy showed a small number of CD1a+ cells (Braier *et al.*, 2002). A small proportion of patients present with the late fibrosis at initial presentation of LCH; in the remainder of patients, the fibrosis develops as a complication of progressive disease. In a French series, patients who presented with SC did so at a later age (median 4 years) than those presenting with liver disease as part of MS LCH (median 1.09 years) (Marti *et al.*, 2003). Most patients who present with pulmonary fibrosis are adult smokers in the third or fourth decade of life.

The clinical course of pulmonary LCH (PLCH) is unpredictable, ranging from spontaneous regression or regression after cessation of smoking or steroid therapy, to stabilization or progression to pulmonary fibrosis and respiratory failure. Around a third of the patients will succumb to their pulmonary disease (Vassallo *et al.*, 2002). Remarkable recovery can occur in children with lung involvement with LCH who respond to chemotherapy (Noseworthy *et al.*, 2003). Similarly, in patients presenting with liver disease as part of MS LCH, the development of SC after intensive or longer chemotherapy is unlikely. However, late cholestasis due to SC does not appear to improve with chemotherapy (Braier *et al.*, 2002). Thus, therapy in the early stages may be effective in controlling the disease. In the later stages, however, no effective systemic therapy is known (Debray, 2003). The prognosis of SC appears to be worse in children with LCH and is associated with more rapid progression to liver failure. The only drug that has been shown to slow the process of SC is high-dose ursodeoxycholic acid (Debray, 2003). However, a number of experimental drugs with anti-fibrotic activity may prove useful in slowing or aborting progression to end-stage fibrosis. These drugs include aerosolized heparin or urokinase, as well as IL-12 and IFN-γ, all having been shown to reduce bleomycin-induced lung fibrosis in mice. IL-12 resulted in time-dependent expression of INF-γ which correlated with the attenuation of fibrosis; prolonged IFN-γ therapy of patients with idiopathic pulmonary fibrosis has been reported to result in improved pulmonary function (Strieter, 2003). Recently, tetrathiomolybdate, a drug developed for treatment of Wilson's disease, was shown to produce a marked reduction in lung fibrosis in the murine model, possibly by reduction of copper-dependent cytokines (Brewer *et al.*, 2003).

At present, organ transplant is the only effective therapy for late lung and liver disease. A recent review of pediatric LCH patients transplanted for liver failure due to LCH found that 22 of 28 (78%) children were alive (Rajwal *et al.*, 2003) and 29% developed recurrent LCH, but only two recurrences were in the transplanted liver (Hadzic *et al.*, 2000). Similarly, five of seven adult patients receiving a lung transplant for LCH are alive and well, 15–90 months post-transplant; the other two patients recurred with PLCH after having resumed smoking (Etienne *et al.*, 1998). A third patient, who apparently did not resume smoking, recurred with PLCH, 4 years post-double lung transplant (Habib *et al.*, 1998).

An increased incidence of EBV-induced post-transplant lymphoproliferative disorder (PTLD) after liver transplant was found in one series (Newell *et al.*, 1997) and an increased incidence in severity and frequency of rejection was observed in others (Stieber *et al.*, 1990; Newell *et al.*, 1997). Addition of Basiliximab, an antibody to the alpha chain of the IL-2R, which inhibits T-cell activation, to standard anti-rejection therapy may prevent this complication (Rajwal *et al.*, 2003). Alternatively, newer anti-rejection agents such as rapamycin which exerts its effects by interference with T-cell proliferation and by increasing apoptosis of dendritic cells in a time and dose-dependent manner (Woltman *et al.*, 2001), may prove to be useful after LCH transplants.

Solid organ transplantation is effective therapy for end-stage liver and lung disease, and the outcome appears to be durable. Another challenge is the difficulty to clinically or radiographically discriminate active LCH from end-stage fibrosis (Soler *et al.*, 2000; Sundar *et al.*, 2003). Effective therapy against the proliferative phase of LCH should theoretically be able to prevent the progression to late fibrosis. An initial trial of active therapy is warranted, but failure to obtain rapid improvement should lead to early consideration of transplantation.

Conclusion

Effective therapy for refractory MS and late progressive LCH patients is available, but is still often not effective and has significant associated toxicity and cost. Improvement in the understanding of the basic biology of LCH will hopefully lead to therapies that will be more effective and available for all patients with either newly diagnosed or relapsed/refractory disease.

REFERENCES

Akkari, V., Donadieu, J., Piguet, C., *et al.* (2003). Hematopoietic stem cell transplantation in patients with Langerhans cell histiocytosis and hematological dysfunction. Experience of the French Langerhans Cell Study Group. *Bone Marrow Transplant*, **31**, 1097–1103.

Amrolia, P., Gaspar, H.B., Hassan, A., *et al.* (2000). Nonmyeloablative stem cell transplantation for congenital immunodeficiencies. *Blood*, **96**, 1239–1246.

Arceci, R.J., Brenner, M.K. and Pritchard, J. (1998). Controversies and new approaches to treatment of LCH. *Hematol Oncol Clin North Am*, **12**, 339–357.

Aricò, M. (1991). Cyclosporine therapy for refractory Langerhans cell histiocytosis. *Blood*, **78**, 3107–3110.

Ayas, M., Mustafa, M., Al-Mahr, M., *et al.* (1998). Bone marrow transplantation for refractory disseminated Langerhans histiocytosis. *Proceedings of the XIV Meeting Histiocyte Society*, Kyoto, 36.

Bernard, F., Thomas, C., Chiron, C., *et al.* (2003). Association between 2-CdA and Ara-C as a rescue for pediatric patients with LCH-hematological dysfunction and failure to standard therapy. *Proceedings of the XIX Meeting Histiocyte Society*, Philadelphia, 31.

Braier, J., Cioccca, M., Latella, A., *et al.* (2002). Cholestasis, sclerosing cholangitis, and liver transplantation in Langerhans cell histiocytosis. *Med Pediatr Oncol*, **38**, 178–182.

Brewer, G.J., Ullenbruch, M.R., Dick, R., *et al.* (2003). Tetrathiomolybdate therapy protects against bleomycin-induced pulmonary fibrosis in mice. *J Lab Clin Med*, **14**, 210–216.

Broadbent, V. and Ladisch, S. (1997). Results of the Histiocyte Society BMT salvage questionnaire. *Med Pediatr Oncol*, **31**, 45.

Brown, R.E. (2001). Bisphosphonates as antialveolar macrophage therapy in pulmonary Langerhans cell histiocytosis. *Med Pediatr Oncol*, **36**, 641–643.

Burdmann, E.A., Andoh, T.F., Yu, L., *et al.* (2003). Cyclosporine nephrotoxicity. *Semin Nephrol*, **23**, 465–476.

Ceci, A., de Terlizzi, M., Colella, R., *et al.* (1988a). Etoposide in recurrent childhood Langerhans' cell histiocytosis: an Italian cooperative study. *Cancer*, **62**, 2528–2531.

Ceci, A., de Terlizzi, M., Toma, M.G., *et al.* (1988b). Heterogeneity of immunological patterns in Langerhans cell histiocytosis and response to crude thymic extract in 11 patients. *Med Pediatr Oncol*, **16**, 111–115.

Chang, S.E., Koh, G.J., Choi, J.H., *et al.* (2002). Widespread skin-limited adult Langerhans cell histiocytosis: long term follow up with good response to interferon alpha. *Clin Exp Dermatol*, **27**, 135–137.

Charles, P., Elliot, M.J., Davis, D., *et al.* (1999). Regulation of cytokines, cytokine inhibitors and acute phase proteins following anti-TNFα therapy in rheumatoid arthritis. *J Immunol*, **163**, 1521–1528.

Cheson, B., Vena, D.A., Barrett, J., *et al.* (1999). Second malignancies as a consequence of nucleoside analog therapy for chronic lymphoid leukemia. *J Clin Oncol*, **13**, 2454–2464.

Choi, S.W., Bangaru, B.S., Wu, C.D., *et al.* (2003). Gastrointestinal involvement in disseminated Langerhans cell histiocytosis (LCH) with durable complete response to 2-chlorodeoxyadenosine and high-dose cytarabine. *J Pediatr Hematol Oncol*, **25**, 503–506.

Chubar, Y. and Bennett, M. (2003). Cutaneous reactions in hairy cell leukaemia treated with 2-chlorodeoxyadenosine and allopurinol. *Br J Haematol*, **122**, 768–770.

Claudon, A., Dietamann, J.L., Hamman, D.C.A., *et al.* (2002). Interest in thalidomide in cutaneomucous and hypothalamo–hypophyseal involvement of Langerhans cell histiocytosis. *Rev Med Interne*, **23**, 651–656.

Cole, S. and Finlay, J. (1999). 2-Chlorodeoxyadenosine for adults with multi-system Langerhans cell histiocytosis. *Med Pediatr Oncol*, **33**, 512.

Conter, V., Reciputo, A., Arrigo, C., et al. (1996). Bone marrow transplantation for refractory Langerhans cell histiocytosis. *Hematologica*, **81**, 468–471.

Crews, K.R., Gandhi, V., Srivastava, D.K., et al. (2002). Interim comparison of a continuous infusion versus a short daily infusion of cytarabine given in combination with cladribine for pediatric acute myeloid leukemia. *J Clin Oncol*, **20**, 4217–4224.

Culic, S., Jakobson, Ä., Culik, V., et al. (2001). Etoposide as the basic and interferon – as the maintenance therapy for Langerhans cell histiocytosis: a RTC. *Pediatr Hematol Oncol*, **18**, 291–294.

Debray, D. (2003). Sclerosing cholangitis in children: an overview. *Proceeding of XIX Meeting Histiocyte Society*, Philadelphia, 17.

Dimopoulos, M.A., Theodorakis, M., Kostis, E., et al. (1996). Treatment of Langerhans cell histiocytosis with 2 chlorodeoxyadenosine. *Leukemia lymphoma*, **25**, 187–189.

Dredge, K., Marriott, J.B. and Dalgleish, A.G. (2002). Immunological effects of thalidomide and its chemical and functional analogs. *Crit Rev Immunol*, **22**, 425–437.

Egeler, R.M., de Kraker, J. and Voûte, P.A. (1993). Cytosine–arabinoside, vincristine, and prednisolone in the treatment of children with disseminated Langerhans cell histiocytosis with organ dysfunction: experience at a single institution. *Med Pediatr Oncol*, **21**, 265–270.

Egeler, R.M., Anderson, R.A., Wolff, J.E.A., et al. (1998). Allogeneic peripheral blood stem cell transplantation in Langerhans cell histiocytosis. *Proceeding of XIVth Meeting Histiocyte Society*, Kyoto, Japan, 34.

Egeler, R.M., Favara, B.E., van Meurs, M., et al. (1999). Differential *in situ* cytokine profiles of Langerhans-like cells and T cells in Langerhans cell histiocytosis: Abundant expression of cytokines relevant to disease and treament. *Blood*, **94**, 4195–4201.

Etienne, B., Bertocchi, M., Gamondes, J.-P., et al. (1998). Relapsing pulmonary Langerhans cell histiocytosis after lung transplantation. *Am J Resp Crit Care Med*, **157**, 288–291.

Felix, C.A. and Blatt, J. (1999). Etoposide and Langerhans cell histiocytosis: second malignancies, a second look. *Pediatr Hematol Oncol*, **16**, 183–185.

Frost, J.D. and Wiersma, S.R. (1996). Langerhans cell histiocytosis in an infant with Klinefelters syndrome successfully treated with allogeneic bone marrow transplantation. *J Pediatr Hematol Oncol*, **18**, 396–400.

Gadner, H., Grois, N., Arico, M., et al. (2001). A randomized trial of treatment for multisystem Langerhans' cell histiocytosis. *J Pediatr*, **138**, 728–734.

Gadner, H., Matthes-Martin, S., Grois, N., et al. (2002). Stem cell transplantation (SCT) with reduced intensity conditioning – a possible salvage strategy for high risk Langerhans cell histiocytosis. *Med Pediatr Oncol*, **38**, 222.

Gandhi, V., Estey, E., Keating, M.J., et al. (1996). Chlorodeoxyadenosine and arabinosylcytosine in patients with acute myelogenous leukemia: pharmacokinetic, pharmacodynamic and molecular interactions. *Blood*, **87**, 256–264.

Geissmann, F., Landman-Parker, J., Thomas, C., et al. (1997). *In vitro* effects of retinoic acid on Langerhans cell histiocytosis cells and normal dendritic cells. *Med Pediatr Oncol*, **31**, 49.

Giona, F., Annino, L., Bongarzoni, V., et al. (2002). Unifocal Langerhans' cell histiocytosis involving the central nervous system successfully treated with 2-chlorodeoxyadenosine. *Med Pediatr Oncol*, **38**, 223.

Goh, N.S., McDonald, C.E., Macgregor, D.P., *et al.* (2003). Successful treatment of Langerhans cell histiocytosis with 2-chlorodeoxyadenosine. *Respirology*, **8**, 91–94.

Greinix, H.T., Storb, R., Sanders, J.E., *et al.* (1992). Marrow transplantation for treatment of multisystem progressive Langerhans cell histiocytosis. *Bone Marrow Transplant*, **10**, 39–44.

Groh, V., Gadner, H., Radaszkiewicz, T., *et al.* (1988). The phenotypic spectrum of histiocytosis X cells. *J Invest Dermatol*, **90**, 441–447.

Habib, S.B., Congleton, J., Carr, D., *et al.* (1998). Recurrence of recipient Langerhans cell histiocytosis following bilateral lung transplantation. *Thorax*, **53**, 323–325.

Hadzic, N., Pritchard, J., Webb, D., *et al.* (2000). Recurrence of Langerhans cell histiocytosis in the graft after pediatric liver transplantation. *Transplantation*, **15**, 815–819.

Hale, G.A., Bowman, L.C., Woodard, J.P., *et al.* (2003). Allogeneic bone marrow transplantation for children with histiocytic disorders: use of TBI and omission of etoposide in the conditioning regimen. *Bone Marrow Transplant*, **31**, 981–986.

Helmbold, P., Hegemann, B., Holzhausen, H.-J., *et al.* (1998). Low dose oral etoposide monotherapy in adult Langerhans cell histiocytosis. *Arch Dermatol*, **134**, 1275–1278.

Henter, J.-I., Karlén, J., Calming, U., *et al.* (2001). Successful treatment of Langerhans'-cell histiocytosis with Etanercept. *New Engl J Med*, **345**, 1577–1578.

Hirose, M. and Kuroda, Y. (1999). Successful induction therapy of natural killer/cytotoxic T-lymphocyte cells in the treatment of Langerhans' cell histiocytosis. *Int J Hematol*, **69**, 272–273.

Johnston, J.B., Williams, M., Verburg, L., *et al.* (1993). Combined therapy with deoxyadenosine plus 2'-deoxycoformycin and alkylating agents. *Proc Annu Meet AACR*, **34**, A1765.

Joshi, S., Parisi, M., Smogorzevska, E., *et al.* (1999). Long term immune deficiency in a patient with Langerhans cell histiocytosis treated with 2 chlorodeoxyadenosine. *Med Pediatr Oncol*, **33**, 523.

Kelly, K.M. and Pritchard, J. (1994). Monoclonal antibody therapy in Langerhans cell histiocytosis-feasible and reasonable? *Br J Cancer*, **23**(Suppl), S54–S55.

Kelly, M., Kolb, M., Bonniaud, *et al.* (2003). Re-evaluation of fibrogenic cytokines in lung fibrosis. *Current Pharm Design*, **9**, 39–49.

Kinugawa, N., Imashuku, S., Hirota, Y., *et al.* (1999). Hematopoietic stem cell transplantation (HSCT) for Langerhans cell histiocytosis (LCH) in Japan. *Bone Marrow Transplant*, **24**, 935–938.

Körholz, D., Janssen, G. and Göbel, U. (1997). Treatment of relapsed Langerhans cell histiocytosis by cyclosporin A combined with etoposide and prednisone. *Pediatr Hematol Oncol*, **14**, 443–449.

Kwong, Y.L., Chan, A.C.L. and Chan, T.K. (1997). Widespread skin-limited Langerhans cell histiocytosis: complete remission with interferon alfa. *J Am Acad Dermatol*, **36**, 628–629.

Ladisch, S. and Gadner, H. (1994). Treatment of Langerhans cell histiocytosis – evolution and current approaches. *Br J Cancer*, **70**(Suppl XXIII), S41–S46.

Ladisch, S., Gadner, H., Aricó, M., *et al.* (1994). A randomized trial of etoposide vs. vinblastine in disseminated Langerhans cell histiocytosis. *Med Pediatr Oncol*, **23**, 107–110.

Lair, G., Marie, I., Cailleux, N., *et al.* (1998). Langerhans cell histiocytosis in adults: cutaneous and mucous lesion regression after treatment with thalidomide. *Rev Med Interne*, **19**, 196–198.

Liliemark, J. (1997). The clinical pharmacokinetics of cladribine. *Clin Pharmacokinet*, **32**, 120–131.

Lombardi, A., Caniglia, M., Longo, D., *et al.* (2002). Treatment of severe Langerhans cell histiocytosis with 2' deoxycoformycin (2'-DCF). *Hematol J*, **3**, 118–119.

Mahe, E., Descamps, V., Grossin, M., *et al.* (2003). CD30+ T-cell lymphoma in a patient with psoriasis treated with cyclosporin and infliximab. *Br J Dermatol*, **149**, 170–173.

Mahmoud, H., Wang, W. and Murphy, S. (1991). Cyclosporine therapy for advanced Langerhans cell histiocytosis. *Blood*, **77**, 721–725.

Marti, L., Thomas, C., Emilé, J.F., *et al.* (2003). Liver involvement in LCH. The French experience. *Proceedings of the XIX Meeting Histiocyte Society*, Philadelphia, 20.

Matsushima, Y. and Baba, T. (1991). Resolution of cutaneous lesions of histiocytosis-X by intralesional injections of interferon-beta. *Int J Dermatol*, **30**, 373–374.

McCowage, G.B., Frush, D.P. and Kurtzberg, J. (1996). Successful treatment of two children with Langerhans cell histiocytosis with 2′-deoxycoformycin. *J Pediatr Hematol Oncol*, **18**, 154–158.

Minkov, M., Grois, N., Broadbent, V., *et al.* (1999). Cyclosporine A therapy for multisystem Langerhans cell histiocytosis. *Med Pediatr Oncol*, **33**, 482–485.

Minkov, M.L., Novichkova, L.A., Maschan, A.A., *et al.* (2001). Retinoic acid and alfa-interferon in poor prognosis Langerhans cell histiocytosis (LCH). *Med Pediatr Oncol*, **31**, 46.

Minkov, M., Grois, N., Heitger, A., *et al.* (2002). Response to initial treatment of multisystem Langerhans cell histiocytosis: an important prognostic indicator. *Med Pediatr Oncol*, **39**, 581–585.

Misery, L., Larbre, B., Lyonnet, S., *et al.* (1993). Remission of Langerhans cell histiocytosis with thalidomide treatment. *Clin Exp Dermatol*, **18**, 487.

Montero, A.J., Diaz-Montero, C.M., Malpica, A., *et al.* (2003). Langerhans cell histiocytosis of the female genital tract: a literature review. *Int J Gynecol Cancer*, **13**, 381–388.

Moraes, M. and Russo, G. (2001). Thalidomide and it's dermatologic uses. *Am J Med Sci*, **321**, 321–326.

Mortazavi, H., Ehsani, A., Namazi, M.R., *et al.* (2002). Langerhans' cell histiocytosis. *Dermatol Online J*, **8**, 18.

Murray, S., Rowlinson-Busza, G., Morris, J.F., *et al.* (2000). Diagnostic and therapeutic evaluation of an anti-Langerhans cell histiocytosis monoclonal antibody (NA1/34) in a new xenograft model. *J Invest Dermatol*, **114**, 127–134.

Nagarajan, R., Neglia, J., Ramsay, N., *et al.* (2001). Successful treatment of refractory Langerhans cell histiocytosis with unrelated cord blood transplantation. *J Pediatr Hematol Oncol*, **23**, 629–632.

Newell, K.A., Alonso, E.M., Kelly, S.M., *et al.* (1997). Association between liver transplantation for Langerhans cell histiocytosis, rejection and development of posttransplantation lymphoproliferative disease in children. *J Pediatr*, **131**, 98–104.

Noseworthy, M., Odame, I., Doda, W., *et al.* (2003). Pulmonary Langerhans cell histiocytosis – a variable disease in childhood. *Med Pediatr Oncol*, **40**, 180.

Osband, M.E., Lipton, J.M., Lavin, O., *et al.* (1981). Histiocytosis X: demonstration of abnormal immunity, T-cell histamine H2 receptor deficiency, and successful treatment with thymic extract. *New Engl J Med*, **304**, 146–153.

Ottaviano, F. and Finlay, J.L. (2003). Diabetes insipidus and Langerhans cell histiocytosis: a case report of reversibility with 2-chlorodeoxyadenosine. *J Pediatr Hematol Oncol*, **25**, 575–577.

Pardanani, A., Phyliky, R.L., Li, C.-Y., *et al.* (2003). 2-Chloro-deoxyadenosine therapy for disseminated Langerhans cell histiocytosis. *Mayo Clin Proc*, **78**, 301–306.

Perreault, C., Pelletier, M., Landry, D., *et al.* (1984). Study of Langerhans cells after allogeneic bone marrow transplantation. *Blood*, **63**, 807–811.

Rajwal, S.R., Stringer, M.D., Davison, S.M., *et al.* (2003). Use of basiliximab in pediatric liver transplantation for Langerhans cell histiocytosis. *Pediatr Transplant*, 7, 247–251.

Ringdén, O., Åhström, L., Lönnqvist, B., *et al.* (1987). Allogeneic bone marrow transplantation in a patient with chemotherapy resistant progressive histiocytosis-X. *New Engl J Med*, 316, 733–735.

Ringdén, O., Lonnqvist, B. and Holst, M. (1997). 12-year follow-up of allogeneic bone-marrow transplant for Langerhans' cell histiocytosis. *Lancet*, 349, 476.

Robak, T., Blonski, J.Z., Kasznicki, M., *et al.* (2002). Cladribine combined with cyclophosphamide is highly effective in the treatment of chronic lymphocytic leukemia. *Hematol J*, 244–250.

Rodriguez-Galindo, C., Kelly, P., Jeng, M., *et al.* (2002). Treatment of children with Langerhans cell histiocytosis with 2-chlorodeoxyadenosine. *Am J Hematol*, 69, 179–184.

Sako, M., Hosoi, G., Ikemiya, M., *et al.* (1999). Successful remission induction in a case of disseminated and refractory Langerhans cell histiocytosis (LCH) with a combination of cyclosporin (CSA) plus multiagent chemotherapy (ACOP). *Med Pediatr Oncol*, 33, 521.

Santana, V.M., Mirro, J., Harwood, F.C., *et al.* (1991). A phase 1 clinical trial of 2-chlorodeoxyadenosine in pediatric patients with acute leukemia. *J Clin Oncol*, 9, 416–422.

Saven, A. and Burian, C. (1999). Cladribine activity in adult Langerhans cell histiocytosis. *Blood*, 93, 4125–4130.

Saven, A., Foon, K. and Piro, L. (1994). 2-Chlorodeoxyadenosine induced complete remissions in Langerhans cell histiocytosis. *Ann Intern Med*, 21, 430–432.

Schwartz, J.E. and Yeager, A.M. (2003). Reduced-intensity allogeneic hematopoietic cell transplantation: graft versus tumor effects with decreased toxicity. *Pediatr Transplant*, 7, 168–178.

Smith, M.A., Rubenstein, L., Anderson, J.R., *et al.* (1999). Secondary leukemia or myelodysplastic syndrome after treatment with epipodophyllotoxins. *J Clin Oncol*, 17, 569–577.

Soler, P., Bergeron, A., Kambouchner, M., *et al.* (2000). Is high resolution computed tomography a reliable tool to predict the histopathological activity of pulmonary Langerhans cell histiocytosis. *Am J Resp Crit Care Med*, 162, 264–270.

Stieber, A.C., Sever, C. and Starzl, T.E. (1990). Liver transplantation in patients with Langerhans' cell histiocytosis. *Transplantation*, 50, 338–340.

Stine, K.C., Saylors, R.L., Willimas, L.L., *et al.* (1997). 2-Chlorodeoxyadenosine (2-CdA) for the treatment of refractory or recurrent Langerhans cell histiocytosis (LCH) in pediatric patients. *Med Pediatr Oncol*, 29, 288–292.

Stoll, M., Freund, M., Schmid, H., *et al.* (1990). Allogeneic bone marrow transplantation for Langerhans cell histiocytosis. *Cancer*, 66, 284–288.

Strieter, R.M. (2003). Mechanisms of pulmonary fibrosis – conference summary. *Chest*, 120(Suppl), 77S–85S.

Suminoe, A., Matsuzaki, A., Hattori, H., *et al.* (2001). Unrelated cord blood transplantation for an infant with chemotherapy resistant progressive Langerhans cell histiocytosis. *J Pediatr Hematol Oncol*, 23, 633–666.

Sundar, K.M., Gosselin, M.V., Chung, H.L., *et al.* (2003). Pulmonary Langerhans cell histiocytosis. Emerging concepts in pathobiology, radiology, and clinical evolution of disease. *Chest*, 123, 1673–1683.

The French LCH Study Group (1996). A multicentre retrospective survey of LCH: 348 cases observed between 1983 and 1993. *Arch Dis Child*, **75**, 17–24.

Vassallo, R., Ryu, J.H., Schroeder, D.R., *et al.* (2002). Clinical outcomes of pulmonary Langerhans'-cell histiocytosis in adults. *New Engl J Med*, **346**, 484–490.

Watts, J. and Files, B. (2001). Langerhans cell histiocytosis: central nervous system involvement treated successfully with 2-chlorodeoxyadenosine. *Pediatr Hematol Oncol*, **18**, 199–204.

Weitzman, S., Wayne, A.S., Arceci, R., *et al.* (1999). Nucleoside analogues in the therapy of Langerhans cell histiocytosis: a survey of members of the Histiocyte Society and review of the literature. *Med Pediatr Oncol*, **33**, 476–481.

Woltman, A.M., de Fijter, J.W., Kamerling, S.W.A., *et al.* (2001). Rapamycin induces apoptosis in monocyte- and CD34-derived dendritic cells but not in monocytes and macrophages. *Blood*, **98**, 174–180.

14

Late effects of Langerhans cell histiocytosis and its association with malignancy

Riccardo Haupt, Vasanta Nanduri and R. Maarten Egeler

Introduction

Langerhans cell histiocytosis (LCH), although considered a benign and treatable condition, can result in sequelae in the various tissues involved. Some of the problems, such as diabetes insipidus (DI), can arise at the time of diagnosis of LCH or even before. It has therefore been suggested that the term 'permanent consequences' might be better than the term 'late effects' when describing these disabilities (Gadner *et al.*, 1994).

It was recognized decades ago that up to half the survivors of LCH may have residual disabilities which impact on the quality of survival (Komp *et al.*, 1980; Komp, 1980). There have since been reports from single institutions and from co-operative national groups describing long-term complications in LCH patients (Sims, 1977; Ceci *et al.*, 1993; Gadner *et al.*, 1994; French LCH Study Group, 1996; Willis *et al.*, 1996; Haupt *et al.*, 2004). However, there are considerable differences in the reported incidence and prevalence of sequelae, ranging from 20% to 70%, in the various studies. This discrepancy may be due to several different factors including the study size, selection of patient cohorts, treatments used, definitions for diagnosis of sequelae, referral bias to institutions and methods used for follow-up assessment (telephone interviews, questionnaire-based studies and clinical examination) (Table 14.1).

Most of the published literature on permanent consequences are follow-up studies in subjects who had LCH during childhood. Children are more at risk of sequelae because the disease may interfere with growth and development during childhood and adolescence, and because late effects have a longer time to become manifest.

In the following sections, we will describe the relevant permanent consequences in various systems, collated from evidence from published reports and personal communications from researchers in the field.

Table 14.1 Published comprehensive studies of clinical outcome in LCH

Author (year)	No. of long term survivors	Mean length of follow up (years)	Prevalence of sequelae (%)	DI (%)	Short stature/ GHD (%)	Other endocrine (%)	Orthopaedic (%)	Dental (%)	Liver (%)	Pulmonary (%)	Hearing (%)	CNS (%)	Low IQ (%)	Psycho (%)	Type of assessment at follow up
Sims (1977)	29		52	50	17		3			27 3/11 tests	NA	NA	10	NA	Questionnaire and examination
Komp (1980)	60	>5	47	20	10	1.6	15			13	5	12	8	6	Case note review, examination
Ceci (1993)	90		48	20	5		15	3	3						Co-operative national study
Gadner (1994)	96*	6	33**	15	7	8	11	2	3	2	5	1	–	–	Questionnaires to participating institutions
French LCH Study Group (1996)	320	3.3	22	17	5	3	3	1	1	1	3	4	–	–	Co-operative national study
Willis (1996)	71	8.1	64	25	20	16	42	30	2	8	16	14			Case note review, mail, telephone questionnaire
Braier (1999)	123	3	28	14	2		9		5	5	11				Case note review, single institution
Kusumakumary (2000)	41	7.1	29	17	19		–	15	–	–	5	–	5	–	Single institution examination
Haupt (2004)	182	8.8	52	24	9		20	7	0	4	13	4	7	–	Retrospective, international institutions

*Survivors out of 106 total patients; **reported in 106 patients.

GHD, growth hormone deficiency; IQ, intellectual quotient; NA, not applicable

Orthopaedic disabilities

The skeleton is the commonest site affected by LCH. In children there is often reconstitution and remodelling of bones, but residual problems, when present, may be more severe than in adult patients because of damage to a growing skeleton. Sequelae might also be a consequence of treatment such as radiation, which can cause permanent damage and loss of growth. In some studies, orthopaedic disabilities are the most commonly reported consequences with 42% of long-term survivors affected, and include pathological fractures, malformation, scoliosis and vertebra plana (Willis *et al.*, 1996). However, other studies have reported a much lower incidence ranging from 2.5% (French LCH Study Group, 1996) to 15% (Komp *et al.*, 1980; Ceci *et al.*, 1993) to 20% (Haupt *et al.*, 2004). In a study on single-system bone disease, 26% of subjects were reported to suffer from permanent orthopaedic consequences (Titgemeyer *et al.*, 2001). These differences may reflect the fact that different groups of patients have been studied (multisystem/single system), that follow-up was short in some cases, and methods used for assessment differed (Table 14.1). It is clear that final assessment of orthopaedic deformities should be made after completion of growth, as some problems might only manifest during periods of rapid growth such as puberty.

Since the skull and facial bones are frequent sites of localization of LCH, abnormalities of the face are often described and may affect 'body image' resulting in an impact on the quality of life of the patient. Residual proptosis is common (Figure 14.1) and may be asymmetrical. Facial asymmetry may become manifest as the child

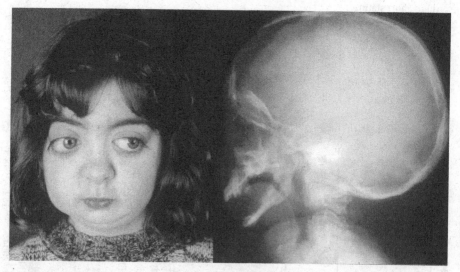

Figure 14.1   Severe proptosis, facial asymmetry, jaw hypoplasia, loss of teeth and DI following single system, multifocal bone LCH diagnosed at 18 months

grows, and in severe deformity major reconstructive surgery may be required. Loss of teeth may be permanent, resulting either directly from LCH affecting the jaw, or secondary to treatment such as curettage or radiotherapy. There may also be reduced or asymmetrical growth of the jaw requiring corrective orthodontic surgery.

LCH of the spine can result in vertebral body compression, resulting in *vertebra plana*, and as growth progresses scoliosis may become apparent (Figure 14.2). In some patients complete reconstitution of the spine has been reported (Nesbit *et al.*, 1969).

Involvement of the long bones may result in shortening of one limb with asymmetry. However, limb deformities are infrequent and have not been reported to cause significant morbidity.

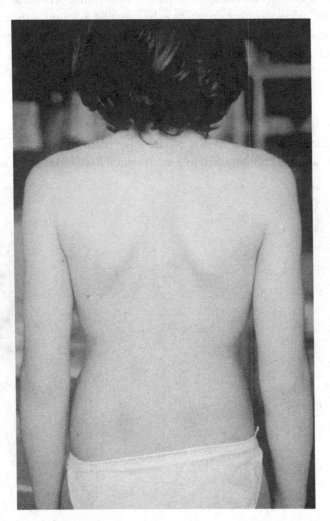

Figure 14.2 Scoliosis following single system, single bone vertebral LCH at age 6 years

Ears

Mastoid lesions can cause permanent damage and hearing loss with an incidence ranging from 3% to 16% (Komp *et al.*, 1980; Ceci *et al.*, 1993; Gadner *et al.*, 1994; French LCH Study Group, 1996; Braier *et al.*, 1999). Although deafness is often conductive, damage to the inner ear and bony labyrinth may result in permanent sensorineural hearing loss (Nanduri *et al.*, 1998). Involvement of the vestibular region is rare, but may present with loss of balance in addition to hearing loss. Damage to the bony structures of the inner ear is best seen on computed tomography (CT) scan of petrous temporal bones. All children with hearing loss or other symptoms of inner ear involvement should have appropriate imaging performed.

Hearing loss may go undiagnosed resulting in learning problems (see later). Children with ear involvement should thus be carefully followed with audiometry and assessment throughout childhood, as early diagnosis and interventional strategies such as hearing aids can significantly improve outcome.

Skin

Scarring can be seen at sites of previous skin involvement, and from surgical procedures. Deposition of fat in skin lesions may result in xanthomatous areas (Figure 14.3) and concomitant juvenile xanthogranuloma (Hoeger *et al.*, 2001).

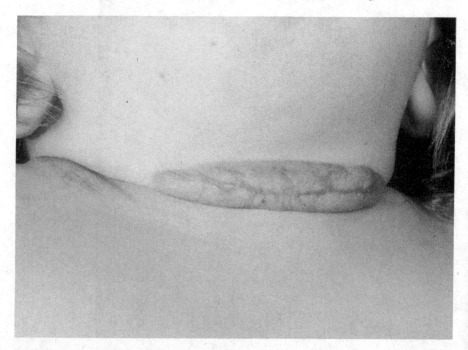

Figure 14.3 Xanthogranuloma in the area of a previous LCH rash

Treatment of LCH skin lesions with topical mustine hydrochloride appears to be safe and no long-term sequelae have been identified (Hoeger *et al.*, 2000). However, radiation to the area may result in secondary basal cell carcinoma or melanoma or precancerous lesions which need careful follow-up (see later).

Endocrine sequelae

Diabetes insipidus

LCH has a special predilection for the posterior pituitary gland and DI can either precede the diagnosis of LCH by many years, or become manifest after LCH is diagnosed. The reported incidence of DI ranges from 15% to 50% (Gadner *et al.*, 1994; French LCH Study Group, 1996; Willis *et al.*, 1996; Nanduri *et al.*, 2000), while the reported long-term cumulative risk of developing DI varies between 26% (Haupt *et al.*, 2004) and 42% (Dunger *et al.*, 1989). The variations in reported incidence may be a reflection of factors such as the referral bias to institutions, different criteria for establishing the diagnosis, ranging from a clinical history of polyuria and polydipsia, measurement of early morning plasma and/or urine osmolality, to the ideal investigation – a water deprivation test with measurement of urinary arginine vasopressin (AVP) levels (Dunger *et al.*, 1988). The risk factors for development of DI include multisystem disease and involvement of craniofacial bones, especially the orbit and base of skull (Grois *et al.*, 1998).

DI is usually permanent (Broadbent and Pritchard, 1997; Rosenzweig *et al.*, 1997), but there have been a few reports of reversibility with treatment (Greenberger *et al.*, 1979; Ottaviano and Finlay, 2003). It is possible that some of these patients might have had partial DI with higher AVP levels and this needs to be fully assessed with appropriate investigations before a conclusive diagnosis is made. There has been a suggestion that the use of intensive chemotherapy at onset of LCH, can reduce the development of DI (Ceci *et al.*, 1993; Grois *et al.*, 1995). This too needs further study.

Anterior pituitary dysfunction

Growth hormone deficiency (GHD) is the next most common endocrine abnormality, occurring in up to 20% of subjects, with secondary hypothyroidism, gonadotrophin-deficiency and corticotrophin-deficiency occurring less frequently. Pituitary irradiation as therapy for DI does not ameliorate the condition, and may in fact result in anterior pituitary damage and hormone deficiency, and should be avoided.

All children with DI, short stature and poor growth, or delayed puberty, should have anterior pituitary hormone function measured. It should be noted however, that growth may be affected due to a combination of factors, including hormone deficiency, bony involvement, chronic steroid therapy and the effects of the chronic disease itself, resulting in a compromised final height (Nanduri *et al.*, 2000).

Children with hypothalamic damage may have not only pituitary endocrinopathies, but may also develop behavioural problems, the 'hypothalamic syndrome'. Features of this include aggressive behaviour, eating disorders, obesity and temperature instability.

Rarely, the thyroid gland may be directly affected by LCH resulting in primary hypothyroidism. This has been described predominantly in adults, although there are a few reports in children (Rami *et al.*, 1998).

Lungs

Lung involvement may occur during the acute phase of the disease in up to 50% of children with multisystem LCH. However, permanent lung damage is less common in children, ranging between 1% and 8% in different reports, possibly due to the ability to repair alveoli in the young child. Lung disease appears to be predominantly a disease of young adults, particularly in smokers (Bernstrand *et al.*, 2001). In this long-term follow-up study, 24% of patients, including some in whom LCH was diagnosed during childhood, had radiological lung abnormalities, and 70% of these were or had been smokers. However, only 20% of these patients were symptomatic and the natural history of pulmonary disease is still unknown. Some patients with severe lung fibrosis and emphysema (Figure 14.4) and significant restriction of activity may require lung transplantation.

As smoking has been shown by several groups to be the most important risk factor for worsening lung disease, patients with LCH should be strongly recommended to refrain from smoking. In addition, all patients who smoke should have long-term pulmonary follow-up as there is a known association between LCH and lung cancer in patients who smoke (Howarth *et al.*, 1999).

Brain

Neurological problems such as cerebellar ataxia, psychological problems and learning difficulties can develop concurrently with, or more commonly, several years after diagnosis of LCH. The natural history of LCH central nervous system (CNS) disease is unclear and the abnormalities may remain stable or progress, resulting in severe disability. The prevalence of CNS disease varies in different reports depending on the mode of assessment and the depth of investigation.

Cerebellar damage may be seen in up to 12% of all patients with LCH (Willis *et al.*, 1996), but this increases to 60% in patients with recognized CNS involvement (Grois *et al.*, 1998).

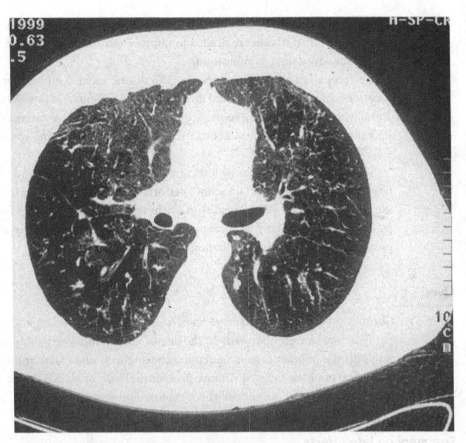

Figure 14.4 Chest CT scan showing pulmonary sequelae of LCH

Learning difficulties have been reported in patients with LCH, but there are few comprehensive studies. Neuropsychological sequelae of LCH include intellectual loss, learning deficits, poor school performance, and emotional disturbances. Detailed testing has shown global deficits in functioning with a drop in intelligent quotient (IQ) (Whitsett *et al.*, 1999) and significant cognitive impairment in up to 40% of patients with multisystem disease (Nanduri *et al.*, 2003). CNS involvement in LCH seems to affect general cognitive development – both verbal and non-verbal. Patients have been shown to have problems with immediate auditory verbal memory span, and immediate recall of geometric designs. Similarly, the patients also showed increased vulnerability to distraction during learning. Deficits in memory can further affect the ability to retain information and learn.

Abnormalities on magnetic resonance imaging (MRI) scan of the brain may be seen and include bilateral cerebellar signal change. However, there is still not enough evidence to correlate MRI abnormalities and clinical findings, and there may be a discrepancy between the MRI findings and the severity of clinical symptoms. The natural history and course of CNS disease in LCH is unknown, and more long-term co-operative studies are needed to improve our understanding of this infrequent, but devastating complication.

It is recognized that 'risk factors' for CNS disease include multisystem involvement, craniofacial bone lesions and the presence of DI (Grois *et al.*, 1998; Haupt *et al.*, 2004). Patients who belong to these groups should have more careful follow-up, including MRI of brain and neuropsychometric studies, looking specifically for CNS damage.

Neurological damage may be less common than other sequelae and may be less obvious. Due to the impact on school performance, ability to lead an independent life and the effect on overall quality of life however, it is important to assess every patient in detail regularly, so that abnormalities can be picked up early and appropriate intervention and rehabilitation can be planned.

Liver

Chronic, progressive liver damage may result in sclerosing cholangitis and cirrhosis. This may be seen quite early in the disease course and may be associated with active disease in other organs. Sclerosing cholangitis is often fatal, and liver transplantation might be the only curative procedure (Braier *et al.*, 2002). Recurrence of LCH in the graft has occasionally been reported however (Hadzic *et al.*, 2000).

Summary on late effects

Single-institution studies have shown that overall morbidity can be significant, resulting in disability and handicap in over half of the survivors of multisystem LCH. Health-related quality of life, which assesses the patient's perspective of the burden of disease, has also been studied in the same patients and found to correlate closely with the morbidity as measured by professionals. Both parameters were especially affected by the presence of CNS and lung involvement with inability to lead independent lives in the most severely affected patients (Nanduri, personal communication).

While permanent consequences are commoner in growing children, adults too suffer significant late consequences, described in Chapter 9.

LCH and malignancies

The association of LCH with malignancy has been described in many reports (Egeler *et al.*, 1994, 1998; Haupt *et al.*, 1997; Kager *et al.*, 1999; Lopes and de Camargo, 1999; Wu *et al.*, 1999; Chiles *et al.*, 2001; Raj *et al.*, 2001; Macedo Silva *et al.*, 2002),

Table 14.2 Number of malignancies reported in subjects with LCH

	Age (years) at LCH diagnosis		
	≤18	>18	Total
	n (%)	*n* (%)	*n* (%)
Solid tumours	27 (37)	34 (41)	61 (39)
Lymphomas	7 (10)	37 (44)	44 (28)
AnLL	23 (31)	12 (14)	35 (22)
ALL	16 (22)	1 (1)	17 (11)
Total	73 (100)	84 (100)	157 (100)

ALL: acute lymphoblastic leukaemia; AnLL: acute non-lymphoblastic leukaemia.

and it is clear that the frequency is greater than could be expected by chance alone. In 1991, members of the Histiocyte Society (HS) formed the LCH – Malignancy Registry with the goal of defining the patterns of occurrence of malignancy and LCH in the same individual. Information on timing of the two diagnoses (synchronous or asynchronous), the type of malignancy, and the treatments given for the first disease, were sought, so that hypotheses could be generated for investigation of possible linkages between the two diseases. The Registry is updated through periodic literature review and registration of cases by HS members. Two reports have been published (Egeler *et al.*, 1994, 1998), and this chapter will discuss the cases observed to date in subjects in whom LCH occurred either in childhood or during adulthood.

At the last update, 157 LCH – malignancy cases had been registered: 73 subjects had LCH diagnosed during childhood, while the remaining 84 were diagnosed as adults (Table 14.2). Solid tumours, followed by acute non-lymphoblastic leukaemia (AnLL) are the most frequently reported malignancies among children with LCH; while lymphomas, followed by solid tumours are more frequently reported among adults (Tables 14.3–14.5).

In the subjects diagnosed with LCH before age 18, solid tumours were most frequent (27 cases reported), followed by AnLL (23 cases), acute lymphoblastic leukaemias (ALL, 16 cases) and lymphomas (7 cases) (Tables 14.3–14.5). In general, there appear to be two patterns of association of LCH and malignancy: ALL usually precedes LCH, whilst AnLL and solid tumours develop after LCH.

LCH and solid tumours

LCH was associated with a solid tumour in 27 patients who had LCH during childhood (Table 14.3). LCH preceded the tumour in 16 cases, in four it was concurrent, in the remaining seven patients it followed the malignancy. Of the 16 patients

Table 14.3 Association of LCH with solid tumours by age (years) at LCH diagnosis

	≤18				>18			
	Precedes ([a])	Concurrent	Follows	Total	Precedes	Concurrent	Follows	Total
CNS	3 (3)	1	3	7	–	–	–	–
Retinoblastoma	1 (1)	1	2	4	–	–	–	–
Neuroblastoma	–	2	1	3				
Skin	3 (3)	–	–	3	–	1	1	2
Bone	3 (1)	–	–	3	–	–	–	–
Ewing/PNET	1 (0)	–	1	2	–	–	–	–
Breast	1 (0)	–	–	1	–	–	3	3*
Hepatic	1 (0)	–	–	1	–	–	–	–
Thyroid	1 (1)	–	–	1	–	3	3	6
Lung	1 (0)	–	–	1	7	5	2	14*
Colon cancer	–	–	–	–	–	1	1	2
Parotid	–	–	–	–	–	1	–	1
Testicular	–	–	–	–	–	–	1	1
Gastric	–	–	–	–	–	1	–	1
Dysgerminoma	1 (1)	–	–	1	–	–	1	1
Bladder	–	–	–	–	–	–	1	1
Undefined	–	–	–	–	2	–	–	2*
Total	16 (10)	4	7	27	9	12	13	34*

* Thirty-four solid tumours in 33 subjects: 1 with lung and breast cancer; 1 with an histologically undefined cancer and a non-Hodgkin's lymphoma.
[a] Cases within irradiation field.

in whom LCH preceded the malignancy, 14 had received radiotherapy as treatment for LCH, in 10 the malignancy arose within the radiation field. In particular, this association was seen in all three cases who developed skin cancer, and the single case of thyroid cancer. With regard to CNS tumours ($n = 7$), three preceded the LCH, one occurred concurrently, the remaining three followed LCH and arose within the radiation field.

The development of solid tumours within the radiation field used for LCH treatment suggests that radiotherapy is the oncogenic stimulus in these patients. It is possible that the frequency of this observation will be reduced in future since radiotherapy is now rarely used for treatment of LCH.

Other interesting findings that might deserve further investigation are four cases of retinoblastoma and three cases of neuroblastoma reported in association with LCH.

Table 14.4 Association of LCH with leukaemias by age (years) at LCH diagnosis

		≤18				>18			
		Precedes	Concurrent	Follows	Total	Precedes	Concurrent	Follows	Total
ALL	T-ALL	3	–	6	9	–	–	–	–
	B-ALL	2	–	3	5	–	–	1	1
	Unspecified	1	–	1	2	–	–	–	–
AnLL	FAB M1	4	–	–	4	–	–	–	–
	FAB M2	2	–	–	2	1	–	–	1
	FAB M3	9	–	–	9	–	–	–	–
	FAB M4	2	1	–	3	2	–	–	2
	FAB M5	2	–	–	2	4	–	–	4
	FAB M7	1	–	–	1	–	–	–	–
	Unspecified	–	–	–	–	1	–	–	1
Other	MDS	1	–	–	1	–	–	–	–
	JCML	1	–	–	1	–	–	–	–
	CMML	–	–	–	–	2	1	–	3
	CLL	–	–	–	–	1	–	–	1
	Total	28	1	10	39	11	1	1	13

CLL: chronic lymphocytic leukaemia; CMML: chronic myelomonocytic leukaemia; JCML: juvenile chronic myelocytic leukaemia; MDS: myelodysplastic syndrome.

LCH and acute leukaemia

Thirty-nine patients had LCH in association with acute leukaemia. Most of the leukaemias reported are AnLL ($n = 21$) (Table 14.4). In all except one, who was diagnosed concurrently with LCH, the leukaemia followed LCH, with an interval ranging from 0.7 to 24.9 years (median 4.3 years) (Table 14.5). The distribution of the different subtypes is not similar to what is expected in *de novo* leukaemia; in particular nine cases of FAB-M3 (promyelocytic) leukaemia have been reported. Most of these cases occurred in subjects of either Latino or Japanese origin and ethnicity has been hypothesized to play a role (Haupt *et al.*, 1997). Another interesting observation comes from cytogenetic analysis of available cases; besides the classical t(15;17), chromosome 7 abnormalities were reported in an apparently non-random fashion.

It is likely that most of the AnLL were secondary to treatment given for LCH (Table 14.5). All cases, except one who was diagnosed 24 years after LCH, were previously treated with chemotherapy or radiotherapy or both. Etoposide or other intercalating agents were part of treatment regimens in 13 cases, two received alkylating agents, while the remaining four received chemotherapy not described as leukaemogenic. These observations, together with the evidence of a minor role for etoposide in multisystem LCH, led to the exclusion of this drug from standard

Table 14.5 Association of LCH and non-lymphoblastic leukaemias in subjects with LCH diagnosed

UPN	Sex	Age LCH (years)	Extent of LCH	Age at malignancy (years)	Morphology	Cytogenetics	Interval (years) malignancy – LCH
11	M	11.5	Single-S/SS	36.4	FAB M2	Not done/available	24.9
5	M	17.1	Multi-S	31.2	FAB M5	Not done/available	14.0
6	M	0.3	Multi-S	9.6	FAB M1	46 XY, t(7;21)	9.3
10	F	0.4	Multi-S	9.3	FAB M3	Not done/available	8.9
63	F	0.4	Multi-S	8.0	FAB M4/M5	Not done	7.6
104	M	1.8	Multi-S	6.9	FAB M1/M2	Not specified	5.2
19	F	2.4	Multi-S	7.5	FAB M3	46 XY, t(15;17), (q22; q21)	5.1
65	M	3.9	Multi-S	8.5	FAB M3	46 XY t(1,3)(p36; q21); del17p, del18p, iso16q	4.6
13	F	0.3	Multi-S	4.9	FAB M1	45 XX, −7, t(3;3)	4.6
15	F	1.7	Multi-S	6.2	FAB M3	46 XX, 11p−, 14q+, t(15;17)	4.5
3	M	1.0	Multi-S	5.2	FAB M1	46 XY	4.2
16	M	1.7	Multi-S	5.7	FAB M7	Not done/available	4.0
2	F	7.7	Single-S/MS	11.6	FAB M3	46 XX, del(20) (q11; q13) (at relapse)	3.9
18	M	1.5	Multi-S	4.9	FAB M3	46 XY, t(15;17)	3.4
12	F	0.4	Multi-S	3.4	FAB M3	46 XX, t(15;17), (q22; q12)	3.0
14	F	5.6	Single-S/MS	8.4	FAB M3	46 XX, t(15;17), (q22; q21)	2.8
1	F	8.6	Single-S/MS	11.1	FAB M3	46 XX, −6?, −10?, +mar, +ring	2.4
115	M	4.0	Multi-S	6.2	FAB M4	46 XY, t(11;11) (p13–p15;q23)	2.2
73	M	0.3	Multi-S	1.6	FAB M5	Not done/available	1.3
4	M	0.0	Multi-S	0.7	FAB M2	46 XY, t(5;6) (q31; q22)	0.7
17	M	3.2	Multi-S	3.3	FAB M4	45 XY, del(6)(q12; q25) −7, 22S+	0.0
64	F	1.0	Multi-S	6.7	RAEB-t	46 XX	5.7
113	?	0.3	Multi-S	4.3	JCML	Not done/available	4.0

*Positive values: LCH preceded the malignancy; negative values: LCH followed the malignancy; 0.0: LCH
Multi-S: multiple site; Single-S/MS: single system/multiple site; Single-S/SS: single system/single site.

≤18 years of age

RT LCH	Chemo LCH	VP16	Other Chemo	Specify Other Chemo	Did the malignancy occur within previous radiation port?	Status	Cause of death
No	No	No	No		Not irradiated	Dead	Malignancy, Aspergillosis post BMT
Yes	No	No	No		Yes	Dead	Malignancy
Yes	Yes	Yes	No		No	Dead	Malignancy
No	Yes	Yes	Yes	ADR	Not irradiated	Alive	
Yes	Yes	Yes	Yes	6MP	No	Dead	Malignancy
Not specified	Not specified	No	No		Not irradiated	Dead	Malignancy
No	Yes	Yes	No		Not irradiated	Alive	
No	Yes	Yes	No		Not irradiated	Dead	Malignancy
No	Yes	No	No		Not irradiated	Dead	Malignancy
No	Yes	Yes	No		Not irradiated	Alive	
No	Yes	Yes	Yes	CTX, 6MP	Not irradiated	Dead	Malignancy
Yes	Yes	Yes	Yes	ARA-C	Not irradiated	Dead	Malignancy
No	Yes	Yes	No		Not irradiated	Dead	Malignancy
No	Yes	Yes	No		Not irradiated	Dead	Malignancy
No	Yes	Yes	Yes	CTX	Not irradiated	Dead	Malignancy
No	Yes	Yes	No		Not irradiated	Alive	
No	Yes	Yes	No		Not irradiated	Alive	
No	Yes	Yes	No		Not irradiated	Dead	Malignancy
No	Yes	Yes	No		Not irradiated	Dead	Malignancy
No	Yes	No	Yes	6MP	Not irradiated	Dead	LCH and malignancy
No	Yes	No	Yes	AML BFM 87	Not irradiated	Dead	Malignancy
No	Yes	Yes	Yes	IFO, ADR, 6MP	Not irradiated	Alive	
No	Yes	Yes	No		Not specified	Dead	Malignancy

concurrent with malignancy.

Table 14.6 Association of LCH and ALL in subjects with LCH diagnosed ⩽18 years of age

UPN	Sex	Age LCH (years)	Extent of LCH	Age at malignancy (years)	Immunology	Cytogenetics	Interval (years) malignancy- LCH*
46	M	9.7	Multi-S	16.9	B-ALL	46 XY, t(9;22) (q34;q11)	7.2
66	F	1.2	Single-S/SS	7.6	B-ALL	46 XX	6.4
72	M	3.7	Single-S/MS	9.7	T-ALL	Not done/ available	6.0
43	M	3.5	Single-S/MS	9.0	T-ALL	Not done/ available	5.5
47	F	2.2	Multi-S	6.0	Not done	Not done	3.8
50	F	4.1	Single-S/MS	7.8	T-ALL	Not done/ available	3.7
89	M	4.2	Single-S/MS	3.9	T-ALL	Not done/ available	−0.3
49	M	9.6	Multi-S	9.2	B-ALL	Not done/ available	−0.4
55	M	14.0	Single-S/MS	13.4	B-ALL	Not done/ available	−0.5
82	M	5.0	Multi-S	4.4	T-ALL	Not done/ available	−0.6
42	M	6.7	Multi-S	6.0	T-ALL	Not done/ available	−0.7
44	F	5.8	Multi-S	4.8	T-ALL	Not done/ available	−1.0
41	M	4.8	Single-S/SS	3.8	T-ALL	46 XY; del(9)(p−)	−1.0
45	M	10.8	Multi-S	9.8	T-ALL	Not done/ available	−1.0
48	M	4.1	Multi-S	2.8	ND	Not done	−1.3
81	M	7.0	Single-S/MS	2.0	B-ALL	46 XY	−5.0

*Positive values: LCH preceded the malignancy; negative values: LCH followed the malignancy; 0.0: LCH
multi-S: multiple site; single-S/MS: single system/multiple site; Single-S/SS: single system/single site.

front-line treatment. However, even if most of the LCH-associated AnLL are probably treatment related, LCH patients seem to behave differently from other patients who develop secondary AnLL in whom FAB M5 subtypes seem to occur more frequently (Hawkins, 1992; Haupt *et al.*, 1997).

Acute lymphoblastic leukemia (ALL) has been reported in association with LCH in 16 cases; in six it preceded the diagnosis of LCH by 0.3–5 years, while in the remaining

RT LCH	Chemo LCH	VP16	Others chemo	Specify others chemo	Did the malignancy occur within previous radiation port?	Status	Cause of death
Yes	Yes	No	Yes	6MP	Yes	Dead	Malignancy
No	Yes	No	Yes	6MP	Not irradiated	Alive	
?	?	No	No		No	Alive	
No	No	No	No		Not irradiated	Alive	
Yes	Yes	No	No		Yes	Dead	Malignancy and pneumonia
No	Yes	No	No		Not irradiated	Dead	Malignancy
No	No	No	Yes	Treatment for ALL	Not applicable	Alive	
No	Yes	No	Yes	Treatment for ALL	Not applicable	Dead	Malignancy
No	Yes	Yes	No		Not applicable	Alive	
No	Yes	Yes	Yes	Topical mustard	Not applicable	Dead	LCH
No	Yes	Yes	Yes	CTX, C-ARA, ADR	Not applicable	Alive	
No	Yes	Yes	No		Not applicable	Dead	LCH
Yes	No	No	No		Not applicable	Alive	
No	Yes	Yes	Yes	CTX, Vindesine	Not applicable	Dead	LCH and pneumonia
No	Yes	Yes	No		Not applicable	Dead	LCH
No	No	No	No		Not applicable	Alive	

concurrent with malignancy.

10 patients ALL occurred between 3.5 and 7 years after LCH (Tables 14.4–14.6). Again the distribution of subtypes is not what one would expect in *de novo* ALL; with T-cell leukaemias (nine cases, 56%) being the commonest immunophenotype, and in general occurring close to LCH diagnosis (between 1 year before and 6 years after LCH, median 0.6 years) (Table 14.6). The review of biological material of these and other similar cases might possibly lead to the identification of a common pathway

between the two diseases. As most patients with ALL rapidly attain remission on starting treatment, it is felt to be less likely that LCH develops as a 'reaction' to the leukaemia. Another hypothesis to explain the few cases in which LCH followed ALL, is that chemotherapy-induced immunosuppression may play a role in the development of at least some cases of LCH. In view of the rather high incidence of patients with associated LCH and T-cell ALL, one of us (RME) always speculated the possible clonal relation between these two disorders. Through the Registry these kind of observations can be made and appropriate research could be developed.

LCH and lymphomas

Lymphomas (as lung cancer) are more frequently reported among adults with LCH (Egeler, 1998) and often the two diagnoses are almost concurrent (Table 14.2). This suggests that in these cases LCH represents a reaction to the lymphoma or lung cancer. Lymphomas have been reported in only seven children with LCH: in four cases Hodgkin's disease and in three non-Hodgkin's lymphoma.

Conclusions

There is a considerable variation in the reported incidence and prevalence of permanent consequences after LCH, according to available sources. Some of these discrepancies may relate to the widely varying treatment approaches used in the past. Methods of collection of data and criteria for definition of each of the late effects have also varied in different studies, leading to a lack of homogeneous data. It is therefore difficult to draw conclusions regarding risk factors for development of sequelae, and the association of treatment with outcome.

In the past, patients who had LCH were often lost to follow-up, as LCH was considered a benign condition, and the potential risk for late effects was underestimated. As more is now known regarding long-term problems, it is important that all patients and their families are counselled regarding the possibility of developing late consequences, especially when the risk factors mentioned above are present.

In a recent multicentre study sponsored by the HS, it was clearly shown that a significant proportion of subjects are lost to follow-up and that among subjects still in follow-up, non-homogeneous criteria are used in the different institutions to assess permanent consequences. It is important to use a 'common language' to define late effects/permanent consequences and to develop a consensus for the method of investigation and selection of patients who need specific tests performed. In Table 14.7 we propose a simple outline for standardized, multidisciplinary follow-up of long-term survivors of LCH.

The consequences reported in the literature relate to patients who were treated on older regimens, and some modalities, such as radiotherapy, etoposide, high

Table 14.7 Proposal for standardized follow-up for permanent consequences in LCH patients

System involvement	Test	Frequency	Notes
All patients	Clinical assessment, height, weight, pubertal status Neurological assessment History of thirst, polyuria	End of therapy Every 6 months for 2 years Annually for 10 years	If thirst or polyuria: water deprivation test with measurement of plasma and urinary osmolality +/− urinary AVP If poor growth, delayed puberty or DI: growth hormone and other pituitary hormone secretion tests
Bone – axial skeleton and/or limbs	Orthopaedic assessment	End of therapy Annually until completion of pubertal growth	
Ear, mastoid and skull base	Audiometry or audiometry evoked responses in younger children	End of therapy Before entering school If symptoms develop	If hearing loss: CT scan of petrous temporal bone
Oral tissue and jaw	Dental assessment	Annually	
CNS or skull base. Orbital lesions, DI, anterior pituitary deficiency	Neuropsychometric assessment	End of therapy Every 1–2 years	
CNS or skull base. Orbital lesions, DI, anterior pituitary deficiency	Cerebral MRI	End of therapy	If mass lesion present, scan every 6 months until resolution or stable
Lungs	Spirometry	End of therapy Every 6 months for 2 years Annually for 10 years	Dangers of smoking should be explained and smoking avoided if possible. If spirometry is abnormal or chest symptoms: chest X ray and high resolution CT scan
Liver	Sonography, bilirubin, gammaglutamyl peptidase, alkaline phosphatase	End of therapy	Repeat if abnormal

For disease-specific monitoring, follow guidelines of the new LCH-III protocol.

dose alkylating agents and mutilating surgery, are now used less often for treatment. It is possible that this may reduce the long-term problems, such as development of secondary malignancies following treatment.

REFERENCES

Bernstrand, C., Cederlund, K., Sandstedt, B., et al. (2001). Pulmonary abnormalities at long-term follow-up of patients with Langerhans cell histiocytosis. *Med Pediatr Oncol*, **36**, 459–468.

Braier, J., Chantada, G., Rosso, D., et al. (1999). Langerhans cell histiocytosis: retrospective evaluation of 123 patients at a single institution. *Pediatr Hematol Oncol*, **16**, 377–385.

Braier, J., Ciocca, M., Latella, A., et al. (2002). Cholestasis, sclerosing cholangitis, and liver transplantation in Langerhans cell histiocytosis. *Med Pediatr Oncol*, **38**, 178–182.

Broadbent, V. and Pritchard, J. (1997). Diabetes insipidus associated with Langerhans cell histiocytosis: is it reversible? *Med Pediatr Oncol*, **28**, 289–293.

Ceci, A., Terlizzi, M.D., Colella, R., et al. (1993). Langerhans cell histiocytosis in childhood: results from the Italian Cooperative AIEOP-CNR-H.X '83 Study. *Med Pediatr Oncol*, **21**, 259–264.

Chiles, L.R., Christian, M.M., McCoy, D.K., et al. (2001). Langerhans cell histiocytosis in a child while in remission for acute lymphocytic leukemia. *J Am Acad Dermatol*, **45**, S233–S234.

Dunger, D.B., Seckl, J.R., Grant, D.B., et al. (1988). A short water deprivation test incorporating urinary arginine vasopressin estimations for the investigation of posterior pituitary function in children. *Acta Endocrinol*, **117**, 13–18.

Dunger, D.B., Broadbent, V., Yeoman, E., et al. (1989). The frequency and natural history of diabetes insipidus in children with Langerhans-cell histiocytosis. *New Engl J Med*, **321**, 1157–1162.

Egeler, R.M., Neglia, J.P., Arico, M., et al. (1994). Acute leukemia in association with Langerhans cell histiocytosis. *Med Pediatr Oncol*, **2**, 381–385.

Egeler, R.M., Neglia, J.P., Arico, M., et al. (1998). The relation of Langerhans cell histiocytosis to acute leukemia, lymphomas, and other solid tumors. The Histiocyte Society LCH – Malignancy Study Group. *Hematol Oncol Clin North Am*, **12**, 369–378.

Gadner, H., Heitger, A., Grois, N., et al. (1994). Treatment strategy for disseminated Langerhans cell histiocytosis. *Med Pediatr Oncol*, **23**, 72–80.

Greenberger, J.S., Cassady, J.R., Jaffe, N., et al. (1979). Radiation therapy in patients with histiocytosis: management of diabetes insipidus and bone lesions. *Int J Radiat Oncol Biol Phys*, **5**, 1749–1755.

Grois, N., Flucher Wolfram, B., Heitger, A., et al. (1995). Diabetes insipidus in Langerhans cell histiocytosis: results from the DAL-HX 83 study. *Med Pediatr Oncol*, **24**, 248–256.

Grois, N.G., Favara, B.E., Mostbeck, G.H., et al. (1998). Central nervous system disease in Langerhans cell histiocytosis. *Hematol Oncol Clin North Am*, **12**, 287–305.

Hadzic, N., Pritchard, J., Webb, D., et al. (2000). Recurrence of Langerhans cell histiocytosis in the graft after pediatric liver transplantation. *Transplantation*, **70**, 815–819.

Haupt, R., Fears, T.R., Heise, A., et al. (1997). Risk of secondary leukemia after treatment with etoposide (VP-16) for Langerhans' cell histiocytosis in Italian and Austrian – German populations. *Int J Cancer*, **71**, 9–13.

Haupt, R., Nanduri,V., Calevo, M.G., et al. (2004). Permanent consequences in Langerhans cell histiocytosis patients. A pilot study from the Histiocyte Society – late effects study group. *Pediatr Blood Cancer*, **42**, 438–444.

Hawkins, M.M., Kinnier-Wilson, L.M., Stovall, M.A., et al. (1992). Epipodophyllotoxins, alkylating agents and radiation and risk of secondary leukemia after childhood cancer. *Br Med J*, **304**, 951–958.

Hoeger, P.H., Nanduri, V.R., Harper, J.I., et al. (2000). Long term follow up of topical mustine treatment for cutaneous Langerhans cell histiocytosis. *Arch Dis Child*, **82**, 483–487.

Hoeger, P.H., Diaz, C., Malone, M., et al. (2001). Juvenile xanthogranuloma as a sequel to Langerhans cell histiocytosis: a report of three cases. *Clin Exp Dermatol*, **26**, 391–394.

Howarth, D.M., Gilchrist, G.S., Mullan, B.P., et al. (1999). Langerhans cell histiocytosis. Diagnosis, natural history, management, and outcome. *Cancer*, **85**, 2278–2290.

Kager, L., Heise, A., Minkov, M., et al. (1999). Occurrence of acute nonlymphoblastic leukemia in two girls after treatment of recurrent, disseminated Langerhans cell histiocytosis. *Pediatr Hematol Oncol*, **16**, 251–256.

Komp, D.M. (1981). Long-term sequelae of histiocytosis X. *Am J Pediatr Hematol/Oncol*, **3**, 165–168.

Komp, D.M., El Mahdi, A., Starling, K.A., et al. (1980). Quality of survival in histiocytosis X: a Southwest Oncology Group Study. *Med Pediatr Oncol*, **8**, 35–40.

Kusumakumary, P. (2000). Permanent disabilities in childhood survivors of Langerhans cell histiocytosis. *Ped Hematol Oncol*, **17**, 375–381.

Lopes, L.F. and de Camargo, B. (1999). Secondary acute promyelocytic leukemia after treatment with etoposide for Langerhans cell histiocytosis (LCH). *Med Pediatr Oncol*, **32**, 315.

Macedo Silva, M.L., Land, M.G., Maradei, S., et al. (2002). Translocation (11;11)(p13–p15;q23) in a child with therapy-related acute myeloid leukemia following chemotherapy with DNA-topoisomerase II inhibitors for Langerhans cell histiocytosis. *Cancer Genet Cytogenet*, **135**, 101–102.

Nanduri, V.R., Pritchard, J., Chong, W.K., et al. (1998). Labyrinthine involvement in Langerhans' cell histiocytosis. *Int J Ped Otorhinolaryngol*, **46**(1–2), 109–115.

Nanduri, V.R., Bareille, P., Pritchard, J., et al. (2000). Growth and endocrine disorders in Langerhans cell histiocytosis. *Clin Endocrinol*, **53**, 509–515.

Nanduri, V.R., Lillywhite, L., Chapman, C., et al. (2003). Cognitive outcome of long term survivors of multisystem Langerhans cell histiocytosis: a single-institution, cross-sectional study. *J Clin Oncol*, **21**, 2961–2967.

Nesbit, M.E., Keiffer, S., and D'Angio, G.J. (1969). Reconstitution of vertebral height in histiocytosis X: a long-term follow-up. *J Bone Joint Surg*, **51**, 1360–1368.

Ottaviano, F., and Finlay, J.L. (2003). Diabetes insipidus and Langerhans cell histiocytosis: a case report of reversibility with 2-chlorodeoxyadenosine. *J Pediatr Hematol Oncol*, **25**, 575–577.

Raj, A., Bendon, R., Moriarty, T., et al. (2001). Langerhans cell histiocytosis following childhood acute lymphoblastic leukemia. *Am J Hematol*, **68**, 284–286.

Rami, B., Schneider, U., Wandl-Vergesslich, K., *et al.* (1998). Primary hypothroidism, central diabetes insipidus and growth hormone deficiency in multisystem Langerhans cell histiocytosis: a case report. *Acta Paediatr*, **87**, 112–114.

Rosenzweig, K.E., Arceci, R.J. and Tarbell, N.J. (1997). Diabetes insipidus secondary to Langerhans' cell histiocytosis: is radiation therapy indicated? *Med Pediatr Oncol*, **29**, 36–40.

Sims, D.G. (1977). Histiocytosis X. Follow-up of 43 cases. *Arch Dis Child*, **52**, 433–440.

The French LCH Study group (1996). A multi-centre retrospective survey of Langerhans' cell histiocytosis: 348 cases observed between 1983 and 1993. *Arch Dis Child*, **75**, 17–24.

Titgemeyer, C., Grois, N., Minkov, M., *et al.* (2001). Pattern and course of single-system disease in Langerhans cell histiocytosis data from the DAL-HX 83- and 90- study. *Med Pediatr Oncol*, **37**, 108–114.

Whitsett, S.F., Kneppers, K., Coppes, M.J., *et al.* (1999). Neuropsychological deficits in children with Langerhans cell histiocytosis. *Med Pediatr Oncol*, **33**, 486–492.

Willis, B., Ablin, A., Weinberg, V., *et al.* (1996). Disease course and late sequelae of Langerhans' cell histiocytosis: 25-year experience at the University of California, San Francisco, *J Clin Oncol*, **14**, 2073–2082.

Wu, J.H., Lu, M.Y., Lin, K.H., *et al.* (1999). Development of acute lymphoblastic leukemia in a child after treatment of Langerhans cell histiocytosis: report of one case. *Acta Paediatr Taiwan*, **40**, 441–442.

15

Uncommon histiocytic disorder: the non-Langerhans cell histiocytoses

Sheila Weitzman and James Whitlock

The two major disorders of the monocyte/macrophage system are Langerhans cell histiocytoses (LCH) and hemophagocytic lymphohistiocytosis (HLH). All other non-malignant disorders are included in the group of conditions known as the non-Langerhans cell histiocytoses (non-LCH), and includes a long list of conditions that are diverse and confusing. Although overlap exists in some conditions, from a

Table 15.1 Classification of the non-LCH

(a) Non-LCH related predominantly to the DC line

  1 The JXG family

    Cutaneous
- JXG and adult XG
- Benign cephalic histiocytosis (early JXG)
- Generalized eruptive histiocytosis (GEH) (precursor of JXG, XD, PNH)
- Progressive nodular histiocytosis

    Cutaneous with a major systemic component
- Xanthoma disseminatum

    Systemic
- Systemic JXG
- Erdheim–Chester disease (ECD)

  2 Indeterminate cell histiocytoses

(b) Non-LCH related predominantly to the macrophage line

    Cutaneous
- Reticulohistiocytoma (may have features of both lines)
- CRD disease

    Cutaneous with a major systemic component
- Multicentric reticulohistiocytosis (MRH)

    Systemic
- Sinus histiocytosis with massive lymphadenopathy (SHML) (R-DD)

JXG: Juvenile Xanthogranuloma; CRO: Cutaneous Rosai–Dorfman disease. Reprinted from Weitzman, S., Uncommon Histiocytic Disorders (In Press) with permission from John Wiley & Sons.

practical viewpoint, most of the non-LCH can be considered as arising from either a dendritic cell (DC) or the macrophage/monocyte (Table 15.1). A recognizable DC, the dermal dendrocyte, has as a hallmark positive immunostaining for the blood clotting transglutaminase factor XIIIa (Chu, 2000), and is thought to be the precursor of many of the dendritic non-LCH. The term dermal dendrocyte may be a misnomer as this cell may be found in many tissues, and these cells may more correctly be termed interstitial dendrocytes (Banchereau *et al.*, 2003).

Clinically the non-LCH can be divided into three major groups: those that predominantly affect the skin, those that affect the skin but have a major systemic component, and those diseases that primarily involve extracutaneous sites, although skin involvement may be part of the disease (Table 15.1).

Non-LCH of dendritic lineage

The juvenile xanthogranuloma family

Studies have shown that most of the cutaneous non-LCH disorders namely juvenile xanthogranuloma (JXG), benign cephalic histiocytosis (BCH), GEH, xanthoma disseminatum (XD) progressive nodular hyperplasia (PNH) and their localized counterparts, as well as ECD, share the identical immunophenotype with expression of vimentin, CD14, CD68, CD163 and fascin. They are usually negative for CD1a, S100 and Birbeck granules. Factor XIIIa is consistently expressed on the constitutive cells, particularly at the early stages, suggesting derivation from the interstitial/dermal dendrocyte (Favara *et al.*, 1997; Chu, 2000). It is felt that these diseases, despite clinical differences, form a spectrum of the same disorder of which xanthogranuloma (XG) is the archetype (Zelger and Burgdorf, 2001).

Based on pathologic review of over 400 cases, Zelger *et al.* described five major morphologic types of histiocytes, schematically depicted in Figure 15.1, and grouped the non-LCH according to the constituent histiocyte (Zelger *et al.*, 1996). Chu took the concept forward by suggesting that the different morphologic types are the same cell at different stages of maturation, and that they form a continuum along a pathway of maturation, from the early scalloped cell through the vacuolated cells which then becomes xanthomatized and finally becomes mature spindle-shaped cells (Chu, 2000). Thus it appears that the JXG family form a spectrum of the same disease, with the various JXG family disorders arising from the dermal/interstitial dendrocyte at different stages of its maturation pathway (Figure 15.2), explaining why some disorders associated with the more immature dendrocyte, can evolve into disorders characteristically associated with a more mature stage of dendrocyte differentiation. Perhaps the strongest evidence for this concept, other than the identical immunohistochemistry, is the clinical picture of XG which changes from early reddish-brown lesions becoming increasingly xanthotomatous and eventually

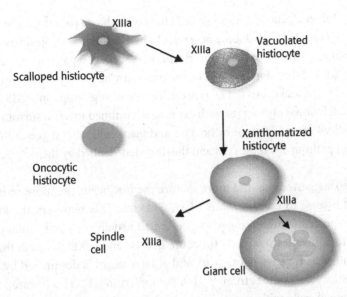

Figure 15.1   Maturation pathway of the constitutive histiocyte of the non-LCH (derived from Chu, 2000; Zelger *et al.*, 2001)

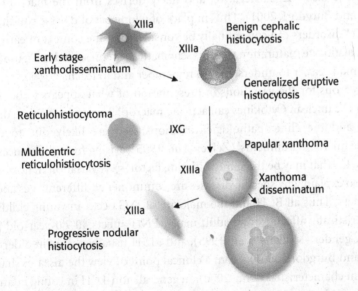

Figure 15.2   Schematic representation of JXG family by maturation stage of the histiocyte (Chu, 2000; Zelger *et al.*, 2001). Reprinted from Weitzman, S. (In Press) *Pediatr Blood Cancer*, with permission from John Wiley & Sons

heals often leaving a fibrous scar, mimicking the changes in histiocyte morphology. Numerous cases which show one type of lesion beside another (Mullans *et al.*, 1995; Chang, 1999), and cases following a time cycle with progression from immature histiocytes to the more mature cells, reinforce these concepts (Chu, 2000;

Gonzalez-Ruiz *et al.*, 2000). Lesions of BCH have been shown pathologically to mature to lesions typical of JXG, and some now refer to BCH as early JXG. Similarly, GEH has been shown to evolve from the monomorphous vacuolated pattern into XG, XD or MRH (Zelger and Burgdorf, 2001). The finding of strong MS-1 protein expression in all non-LCH cells tested, but not LCH, as well as the strong cytoplasmic MS-1 expression in small lesional histiocytes, with expression confined to a rim surrounding the xanthomatized center of large histiocytes and giant cells, also suggests a common maturation pathway for these cells and the disorders defined by them (Goerdt *et al.*, 1993).

Chu also suggested that the more mature the histiocyte, the more resistant the associated disease to therapy. Thus BCH, GEH and JXG represent the immature end of the spectrum, presenting with disease that usually resolves spontaneously or responds to adjuvant therapy. At the more mature end is XD in which the disease resolves, but usually after many years and at later stages is dominated by spindle-shaped histiocytes. At the extreme end of the spectrum is PNH, a disease of mature spindle-shaped cells with no tendency to spontaneous remission and which is resistant to treatment (Chu, 2000). The final cell, the oncocyte, the constitutive cell of MRH, is factor XIIIa negative, and likely derives from the macrophage line (Zelger and Burgdorf, 2001). Thus in place of a long list of diverse conditions, the non-LCH disorders can conceptually be considered in the context of early, middle and late histiocyte maturation stage, as schematically represented in Figure 15.2 and thus be made easier to understand, to remember and to teach.

The reasons for the variations in presentation of what appears to be the same disorder are unclear. Cytokines can activate macrophages and modulate their phenotype, and the clinicopathologic variations seen are likely due to differing 'cytokine microenvironments' (Zelger *et al.*, 1995), arising from differences in host response to what may be the same initiating factor(s). A variation in host response could also explain why specific diseases are commoner at different ages and different genders. Thus all BCH and the majority of JXG occur in young children, XD characteristically affects young adult males, PNH affects 40–60-year-old patients of either gender (Mullans *et al.*, 1995), and MRH usually occurs in older women (Zelger and Burgdorf, 2001). From a clinical point of view the diseases share some important characteristics (Chu, 2000). In general, non-LCH in young infants commonly are widespread, but tend to be benign and self-limited. Fatalities do occur in a minority of patients however. With increasing age, even in the young child, JXG is more likely to present as a solitary lesion, but most still involute spontaneously. In adults, non-LCH most commonly occur as single lesions which tend not to spontaneously involute. The majority are cured by excision. Generalized lesions in adults are less common, but when they occur they rarely regress spontaneously, and chemotherapy and radiation therapy often have no impact on the disease course (Chu, 2000). Finally, all the disorders may be associated with underlying infectious, autoimmune or malignant diseases, the likelihood of which increases with age (Zelger and Burgdorf, 2001).

Diagnosis of the non-LCH

While the conceptual framework proposed above is felt to be useful for putting the disorders into a form that will be better understood and remembered, many pathologists believe that the morphology alone is too variable to be used for diagnosis (as might be expected if the diseases are arising from cells at varying stages along a continuum).

From the pathologist's viewpoint therefore, the differential diagnosis of histiocytic lesions is based initially on the immunophenotype, by which they can be subdivided into LCH, JXG family and those that are neither LCH nor JXG. The non-LCH disorders are then divided based mainly on the clinical picture into the various JXG family members and non-JXG disorders (Tables 15.1 and 15.2).

JXG

JXG, the commonest of the non-LCH, is usually a benign proliferative disorder which resolves spontaneously. The prognosis depends on the extent of extracutaneous involvement. The pathogenesis is unknown, and the initiating stimuli may be one of many infectious or physical factors. It is not associated with lipid disorders. The factor(s) responsible for the spontaneous involution are unknown, but an immune response to the lesion may play a role. A report of a solitary JXG lesion maturing within 2 weeks of biopsy, suggests that maturation was accelerated by an inflammatory response to biopsy (Kubota et al., 2001). JXG has been associated with neurofibromatosis type 1 (NF1) and juvenile chronic myelogenous leukemia (JCML, today called juvenile myelomonocytic leukemia (JMML)). In these patients the JXG usually precedes or occurs concurrently with the JMML. Children with JXG and NF1 are estimated to have a 20–32-fold higher risk of JMML than patients with NF1 alone (Zvulunov et al., 1995).

Histopathology of JXG

The histopathology is described in Chapter 2. A characteristic feature, the Touton giant cell, seen in 85% of cases of JXG (Dehner, 2003), but not limited to JXG, is characterized by a wreath of nuclei around a homogenous eosinophilic center, while the periphery shows prominent xanthomatization (Figure 15.3). Although usually polymorphous, JXG can present with mainly vacuolated histiocytes, without foamy histiocytes or giant cells. This 'non-lipidized' or 'monomorphous' JXG occurs predominantly in infants less than 6 months of age (Escribano et al., 2002) and

Table 15.2 Clinical features important in the diagnosis of the non-LCH

Diagnosis	Age range	No. of lesions	Appearance	Sites of predilection	Natural history
DC lineage					
JXG	0–18 (median age 2 years)	Single:multiple 9:1	Reddish progressing to yellow brown	Head and neck, can be any site	Gradual involution
	<6 months, >M	Multiple-disseminated	Same	Same	Involution
Giant JXG	Young >F	Single	>2 cm	Upper extremity/back	Involution
Systemic JXG (4% of JXG)	Median age 0.3 years	Single to multiple	Almost 50% no skin	Subcutis, liver, spleen lung, CNS, ocular(iris)	May involute, CNS, ocular fatalities 4–10%
Adult XG	18–80 (median age 35 years)	Single	Same as JXG	Upper body (not legs)	No involution
BCH	Young child	Few to multiple	Reddish-tan papules	Head and neck	Involution or progression to XG
GEH	Young adult	Multiple-disseminated	Reddish-tan papules appears in crops	Face, trunk, arms spares flexures	Involution or progression to XG, XD, PNH
XD	Late teen–young adult usually <25 years, >M	Disseminated	Yellow/reddish brown grow forming plaques and nodules	Any skin, eyelids flexures, mucosa, viscera including CNS transient DI	Slow involution over years or progression rare fatalities
PNH	40–60 years M and F	Multiple-disseminated	1 Xanthomatous skin 2 Deeper subcut nodules	Any	Progression to disfigurement

ECD	7–84 (mean 53 years)	Mainly systemic	Xanthelasma xanthoma	Symmetrical long bone sclerosis, proptosis, lung, kidney retroperitoneal fibrosis, CNS including DI	High fatality rate – lung fibrosis resp/cardiac failure
Monocyte/macrophage cell lineage					
MRH	40+, >F 85% white	Multiple	Pink-reddish brown or yellow	Dorsum hands, 'coral bead' periungual vermicular around nostrils face, pinna, arms, legs symmetric erosive polyarthritis – usually precedes rash	Progression may involute after years Disabling arthritis in some patients
SHML	Mean 20.6 years wide range	Mainly systemic	Firm indurated papules	Cervical adenopathy 80% 'B' symptoms 43% extranodal – skin, soft tissue, upper respectively bone, eye, CNS (dural based), others	Exacerbations and remissions often self-limited (years) 5–11% fatalities

References: Szekeres (1988); Tahan et al. (1989); Foucar et al. (1990); Mullans et al. (1995); Freyer et al. (1996); Veyssier-Belot et al. (1996); Ferrando et al. (1998); Chang (1999); Gorman et al. (2000); Wee et al. (2000); Juskevicius and Finlay (2001); Luz et al. (2001); Shamburek et al. (2001); Zelger and Burgdorf (2001); Chang et al. (2002); Escribano et al. (2002); Outland et al. (2002); Dehner (2003); Rush et al. (2003). Reprinted from *Pediatr Blood Cancer* with permission from John Wiley & Sons.

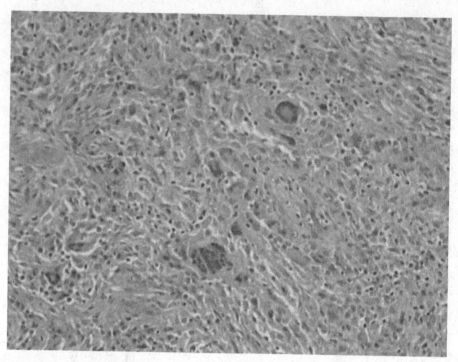

Figure 15.3   JXG with Touton giant cells

probably represent immature or evolving JXG. Serial biopsies of a patient showed increasing numbers of foamy histiocytes and giant cells over time (Tanz *et al.*, 1994), giving support to the concepts described above.

Clinical features of JXG

JXG is a disease of the young (median age 2 years), and may be present at birth. The M:F ratio is 1.5:1, however male preponderance was much higher (12:1) and median age lower (5 months) in children with multiple skin lesions (Dehner, 2003) (Figure 15.4). The incidence of JXG is unknown as solitary spontaneously regressing lesions may be missed.

Clinically JXG mainly involves the skin, but may be localized to a single extracutaneous site without skin involvement, or may have concurrent multiple organ and skin involvement (Dehner, 2003). The diagnosis is confirmed by biopsy, to exclude LCH and its self-healing variant, other benign histiocytoses, mastocytosis, dermatofibromas and dermatofibrosarcoma.

Cutaneous JXG

Cutaneous JXG presents as single to multiple papules or nodules, with a predilection for face, head and neck, followed by upper torso, upper extremities and lower extremities. It can present at any site, including the nails, on the penis, clitoris, eyelid, lips, palms and soles. The commonest presentation of JXG is as a single lesion (Figure 15.5).

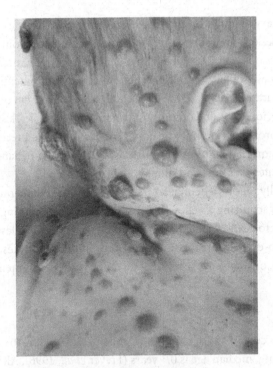

Figure 15.4   Multiple lesions of JXG in a neonate

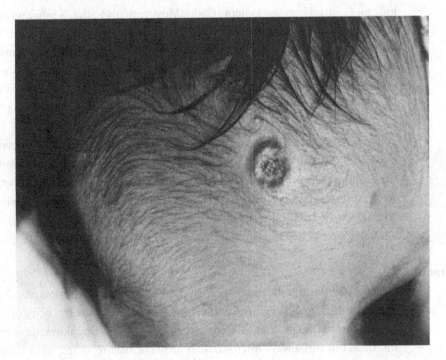

Figure 15.5   Solitary JXG-forehead of an infant

The overall ratio of solitary to multiple lesions is 9:1 in the first two decades (Dehner, 2003). In infancy, JXG lesions are more commonly multiple, ranging from a few to hundreds. Oral cavity lesions occur, usually at an older age (mean 9 years, less than 15% were infants), most are solitary. Oral JXG is not associated with systemic disease and excision is usually curative (Flaitz, 2002). Giant JXG is defined as 2 cm or more in diameter (Zelger and Cerio, 2001), and occur most commonly in females, less than 14 months of age, on the proximal extermity or upper back and may be preceded by a congenital precursor lesion leading to misdiagnosis as hemangioma (Chang, 1999). Giant JXG usually involutes over time and should not be overtreated.

Cutaneous JXG usually follows a benign course. With time the cutaneous lesions become xanthomatoid, acquiring a yellow-brown hue before undergoing gradual involution over months to years (Chang, 1999). In infants with multiple lesions, old and new lesions may co-exist and regression may occur at different rates. Lesions may resolve completely or may leave a residual atrophic or hyperpigmented scar (see also Chapter 8).

Systemic JXG

Systemic involvement occurs in 4% of children (Dehner, 2003) and 5–10% overall. It is a disease of the young, median age is 0.3 years (Freyer *et al.*, 1996). Almost half the patients have no skin lesions. The commonest site is a solitary mass in the sub-cutis and/or deeper soft tissues (deep JXG) (Dehner, 2003), followed by liver, spleen, lung and central nervous system (CNS). Most patients with CNS disease have multiple discrete intracranial/spinal cord lesions and/or leptomeningeal involvement. The majority exhibit a latent period of months to years between cutaneous and neurologic findings (Hernandez-Martin *et al.*, 1997). Lung JXG presents with multiple nodular opacities. Three of 174 children in Dehner's series presented with single bone lesions reminiscent of LCH, including one with vertebra plana (Dehner, 2003).

Systemic JXG may undergo spontaneous regression, however CNS involvement may result in significant problems with seizures, ataxia, increased intracranial pressure, subdural effusions, developmental delay, diabetes insipidus (DI) and other neurologic deficits (Freyer *et al.*, 1996). Fatalities have been reported. In one series two of 36 children died of progressive CNS disease (Freyer *et al.*, 1996) while in another, two neonates died of hepatic failure (Dehner, 2003).

Intraocular JXG

Ocular JXG occurs in the very young child, 90% of patients being less than 2 years old (Chang *et al.*, 1996). Skin involvement is seen in around 55%, but ocular JXG occurs in less than 1% of children with cutaneous JXG. Co-existing skin lesions are always multiple, but not always micronodular as previously reported. Skin lesions often develop after ocular, usually within 2 years of initial eye involvement (Chang *et al.*, 1996). Eye involvement is usually, but not always, unilateral. The commonest presentation is with an asymptomatic iris tumor, a red eye with uveitis, unilateral glaucoma, spontaneous hyphema, or heterochromia iridis (Hernandez-Martin *et al.*, 1997). Other areas of involvement include eyelid, epibulbar, cornea, orbit and rarely retina, optic nerve and choroid (Casteels *et al.*, 1993). Early diagnosis and treatment determine the final visual outcome. The diagnosis should not depend on finding typical skin lesions, and JXG should be part of the differential diagnosis of young children with unilateral hyphema, glaucoma or exophthalmos.

Therapy of JXG

JXG is usually a benign disorder with an excellent prognosis. For patients with isolated and accessible lesions, surgical excision appears to be curative, although most childhood lesions will disappear spontaneously.

Most children with multiple XG require no therapy, and an extensive work up in cutaneous JXG can be limited to patients in whom systemic disease is suspected clinically. Similarly, ophthalmologic consultation can be reserved for higher risk patients less than 2 years of age, who should undergo screening at diagnosis and every 3–6 months until age 2 (Hernandez-Martin *et al.*, 1997). The incidence of optic complications is low, but the consequences may be grave. Therapy includes topical, intralesional and subconjunctival corticosteroids, surgery may be required to treat complications such as hyphema and glaucoma, and systemic corticosteroids, chemotherapy or low-dose 'non-cataractogenic' radiation therapy (300–400 cGy in 50 cGy fractions) may be required (Casteels *et al.*, 1993; Chang *et al.*, 1996; Hernandez-Martin *et al.*, 1997).

Symptomatic patients with unresectable extracutaneous disease have been treated with systemic corticosteroids, LCH-like chemotherapy, radiation therapy and combinations of these. In general, patients with systemic JXG have fared well with some combination of steroids and vinca alkaloids (Dehner, 2003). The use of adjuvant therapy requires consideration of potential toxicity in these young infants, and a prudent approach may be to give emphasis to supportive care, with chemotherapy reserved for life threatening or progressive disease (Freyer *et al.*, 1996).

Adult XG

XG in adults commonly occurs as solitary skin lesions, mostly affecting 20–40-year olds. Typical lesions have been described up to 80 years of age (Tahan *et al.*, 1989). Adult XG affects either gender, and predominates in the head and neck region, with no reports of adult XG on the lower extremities (Chang, 1999). Affected adults are normolipemic. Pathologically there is no difference between juvenile and adult forms, but as a rule adult XG either does not resolve spontaneously (Zelger and Cerio, 2001) or regresses more slowly, and most lesions undergo surgical excision. Occasionally systemic XG involving lungs, long bones and peritoneum is seen in adults and must be differentiated from other histiocytic disorders (Chang, 1999). CNS and pericardial disease is associated with a poor prognosis.

Cutaneous disorders related to JXG

Benign cephalic histiocytosis (BCH)

BCH is a rare disorder which heals spontaneously and is not usually associated with systemic involvement. Pathologically the lesions vary over time and with age. BCH is considered to be an early form of JXG (Zelger and Cerio, 2001). Immunohisto-chemically BCH cells are identical to JXG. On electron microscopy they may show 'wormlike' cytoplasmic inclusions. Patients are typically young children with multiple tan papules on the cheeks, forehead and upper trunk (Figure 15.6). One patient with BCH and DI is described (Weston et al., 2000), but the condition is usually benign, self-limited and requires no therapy.

Generalized eruptive histiocytosis (GEH)

A rare benign histiocytic disorder characterized by asymptomatic, frequently symmetrical small red-brown papules on face, trunk, arms, usually sparing the flexures and sometimes involving mucosa. GEH mainly affects adults, but pediatric cases have

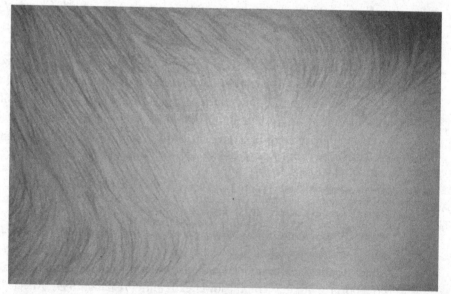

Figure 15.6 Benign cephalic histiocytosis

been described (Jang et al., 2000), ranging in age from 1 month (Jang et al., 1999) to 9 years (Wee et al., 2000). The distinguishing feature is the relatively rapid appearance of crops of lesions which disappear completely or resolve leaving a brown scar. New and old lesions may be present concurrently (Wee et al., 2000). Evolution of GEH to other non-LCH has been noted, and patients need to be rebiopsied if lesions become xanthomatoid, flexural or systemic symptoms develop (Wee et al., 2000). One pediatric case demonstrated healing in sun-exposed areas, suggesting the value of ultraviolet (UV) therapy, if therapy is necessary (Misery et al., 2001). It is important to distinguish GEH from the eruptive histiocytomas associated with hyperlipidemia.

Progressive nodular histiocytosis (PNH)

PNH consists of two types of lesions – superficial xanthomas showing foamy macrophages, and deeper subcutaneous nodules, mainly consisting of spindle-shaped histiocytes (Zelger and Cerio, 2001) with the same immunostaining as JXG. The disease is progressive with no tendency to spontaneous involution, and with time causes severe disfigurement. Chu suggests that the early stages of XD and PNH may be more sensitive to chemo- and radiation therapy and early aggressive treatment may help (Chu, 2000). This is unproven however. Large or painful lesions are usually excised.

The non-JXG cutaneous disorders

Indeterminate cell histiocytosis

This diagnosis includes histiocytic disorders in which the cells lack Birbeck granules and are CD1a-, Langerin- but otherwise have DC features similar to LCH. They may follow LCH or occur de novo, and appear to behave differently with a high incidence of local recurrence.

Indeterminate cell histiocytosis is sometimes seen years after LCH, with lesions occurring at the site of an earlier proven LCH lesion, but with a phenotype that suggests that the constitutive cells are more mature than the previous LCH cells, with loss of CD1a/Langerin, upregulation of surface HLA-DR, and increased fascin expression (Jaffe, personal communication).

Cutaneous non-LCH histiocytic disorders with a major systemic component

JXG family

Xanthoma disseminatum (XD)

XD is a variant of JXG, most often occurring in young adult males. It presents with widespread yellow/reddish-brown lesions which tend to first appear on the eyelids and in flexural areas (Szekeres, 1988). The lesions continue to grow forming distinctive plaques and nodules (Zelger and Burgdorf, 2001). The presence of mucosal and visceral involvement is characteristic of XD, almost any organ may be affected (Ferrando *et al.*, 1998). Ocular, CNS and meningeal involvement can cause significant morbidity (blindness, DI, exophthlmos, hydrocephalus, ataxia). DI occurs in 40% of cases but is usually transient from lesions compressing, but not destroying the hupothalamic-pituitary axis (Zelger and Burgdorf, 2001). XD also tends to involve the upper respiratory tract (trachea, larynx) rather than lower, and may produce respiratory obstruction. Caputo identified three clinical patterns, a rare self-healing form, a chronic often progressive form, and a progressive multi-organ form, fortunately the rarest, which may be fatal (Caputo and Grimalt, 1992).

Non-JXG family

Multicentric reticulohistiocytosis (MRH)

MRH is a rare multisystem disorder characterized by cutaneous involvement and a destructive arthropathy. Pathologically many giant cells with a ground glass eosinophilic cytoplasm, interspersed with mostly oncocytic histiocytes, is seen infil-trating dermis and synovium. Unlike the others, MRH histiocytes are XIIIa negative and an increase in lesional cytokines such as interleukin (IL)-12, tumor necrosis factor (TNF)-α, IL-1β, produced predominantly by activated macrophages, can be detected (Campbell and Edwaards, 1991). MRH is a disease of older adults, predom-inantly female, 85% of reported adults were white (Outland *et al.*, 2002). Rare cases in children have been described (Candell-Chalom *et al.*, 1998; Havill *et al.*, 1999; Outland *et al.*, 2002). The disease is associated with underlying malignancy in about 28% of cases, hyperlipidemia in 30–58% and autoimmune disease in 6–17% (Campbell and Edwaards, 1991; Gorman *et al.*, 2000).

Clinical features of MRH

Clinically two-thirds of patients present with symmetric polyarthritis, the skin lesions appearing an average of 3 years later. In 20% the skin nodules appear first, skin and joint lesions present simultaneously in the remainder (Outland *et al.*, 2002). See Chapter 8 for description of skin lesions. About one-third have mucosal lesions and 15% have characteristic vermicular lesions bordering the nostrils (Luz *et al.*, 2001). The arthritis is a polyarticular symmetric erosive arthritis, which may involve any joint. Although it often remits spontaneously, 15% (Candell-Chalom *et al.*, 1998) to 50% (Gorman *et al.*, 2000) progress to mutilating osteoarthropathy with disabling deformities. It has been postulated that release of urokinase from histiocytes plays a role in erosion of cartilage and bone (Luz *et al.*, 2001), and may explain the dis-parity between mildness of symptoms and extent of joint destruction. One-third of patients have symptoms of fever, weight loss and malaise. Differentiation of MRH from rheumatoid arthritis (RA) is important because of symmetric involvement frequently involving the interphalangeal joints of the hands, which may lead to a characteristic widening and shortening of the fingers known as the 'opera-glass' hand (Outland *et al.*, 2002).

Therapy of MRH

Exclusion of an underlying disease is important, although eradication does not usually influence disease course (Liang and Granston, 1996). Resolution of MRH was seen in a patient with renal-cell carcinoma following nephrectomy, however (Jansen and Kruithof, 2003). Disease activity may fluctuate spontaneously and effects of therapy are difficult to assess. Some patients, including most of the children, have self-limited disease with non-deforming arthritis. A 14-year-old girl treated with Naproxen alone, was left with residual deformities despite an apparent response (Outland *et al.*, 2002). Anti-inflammatory drugs (Havill *et al.*, 1999; Luz *et al.*, 2001) and corticosteroids (Liang and Granston, 1996) while palliative, have little effect on disease progression. Gold, tamoxifen and D-penicillamine failed in all cases (Luz *et al.*, 2001). Several reports suggest that methotrexate (MTX) alone or in combination may be effective (Liang and Granston, 1996; Cash *et al.*, 1997; Candell-Chalom *et al.*, 1998; Rentsch *et al.*, 1998; Havill *et al.*, 1999; Outland *et al.*, 2002). Cyclophosphamide alone produced a complete response (CR) in three cases (Liang and Granston, 1996) and prednisone and azathioprine resulted in a CR in one case (Hiramanek *et al.*, 2002). A recent review reported 11 of 16 cases having good results from combined therapy, usually including an alkylating agent (Luz *et al.*, 2001), and mentioned older studies in which psoralen with ultra-violet (PUVA) and topical nitrogen mustard improved skin lesions. A reasonable approach is to start therapy with a combination of corticosteroid and low-dose MTX, and to add or substitute cyclophosphamide for poor responders, as suggested by Liang. The finding of TNF-α positivity in the lesions suggests that anti-TNF agents or other 'anti-cytokine' therapy may be beneficial (Gorman *et al.*, 2000). A patient with systemic lupus erythematosus (SLE) and MRH (Saito *et al.*, 2001) and a 6-year-old girl with severe erosive arthritis responded to cyclosporine after failing standard therapy (Candell-Chalom *et al.*, 2000).

Solitary reticulohistiocytoma is morphologically the localized variant of MRH, treated by surgical excision. It occurs most commonly in young adult males, but may occur in the newborn where differentiation from LCH is important. Immunohistochemically it is S100 and CD1a negative (Jaffe, 1999).

Systemic non-LCH diseases

Systemic non-LCH diseases of the JXG family

Erdheim–Chester disease (ECD)

Morphologically and immunohistochemically ECD histiocytes are identical to those of JXG, with strong factor XIIIa positivity. CD1a and S100 are typically negative.

Some authorities consider ECD a variant of XG with mostly osseous and internal involvement (Zelger and Burgdorf, 2001) and differentiation is made on clinical and radiologic findings. As with JXG, LCH and ECD have been described simultaneously in patients at different sites (Kambouchner *et al.*, 1997) as has progression from LCH to ECD (Shamburek *et al.*, 2001). Factor XIIIa cells may normally be found in lung, in the areas where lung involvement by ECD occurs. They are known to stimulate fibroblast proliferation (Rush *et al.*, 2003), possibly accounting for the prominent fibrosis. A distinctive pattern of cytokine expression was described in one patient, consistent with histiocyte activation (Myra *et al.*, 2004).

Clinical features of ECD

ECD is predominantly a disease of adults (mean age 53 years, range 7–84) (Veyssier-Belot *et al.*, 1996).

Bilateral symmetrical long bone involvement is nearly always present and radiologic osteosclerosis and histology are the diagnostic features (Veyssier-Belot *et al.*, 1996). More than 50% of cases have extraskeletal involvement including kidney, retroperitoneum, skin, brain and lung, while retroorbital tissue, pituitary gland and heart are involved less frequently. The finding that lymph node, liver, spleen and axial skeleton disease is unusual, helps to distinguish ECD from LCH and other conditions with similar findings, including mucopolysaccharidoses, sarcoidosis, lymphoma and Pagets disease, as well as other histiocytic disorders such as sinus histiocytosis with massive lymphadenopathy (SHML).

The clinical picture ranges from asymptomatic infiltration to fulminant organ failure.

Bone pain in knees and ankles is the commonest presenting complaint and constitutional symptoms such as weakness, weight loss and fever are frequent (Veyssier-Belot *et al.*, 1996). Skin findings include pruritic rash, xanthelasma and periorbital xanthomata in the face of normal plasma lipids. Lung involvement may be asymptomatic, and presentation with cough and progressive dyspnea is associated with a poor prognosis (Veyssier-Belot *et al.*, 1996) as is the much less common pericardial infiltration (Gupta *et al.*, 2002). Other less common clinical manifestations include bilateral exophthalmos, sometimes with visual impairment, DI in 30% of cases, and CNS disease resulting in ataxia, behavioral disorders and even spastic paraplegia (Caparros-Lefebvre *et al.*, 1995). Dysuria, abdominal pain and bilateral nephromegaly from renal/ureteral obstruction by retroperitoneal fibrosis may occur.

On chest radiology, the localization of ECD is predominantly subpleural or septal (Egan *et al.*, 1999). Computed tomography (CT) chest shows smooth interlobular septal and visceral pleural thickening with patchy centrilobular opacities and an upper lung predominance (Devouassoux *et al.*, 1998; Gupta *et al.*, 2002). Radiographs of long bones show typical symmetric sclerosis at diaphyses and metaphyses, with

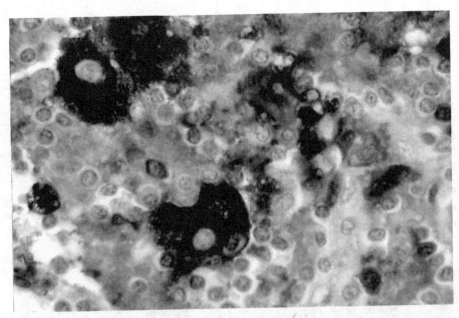

Fig. 15.10 SHML-sinus histiocytes staining positive with S100, showing emperipolesis

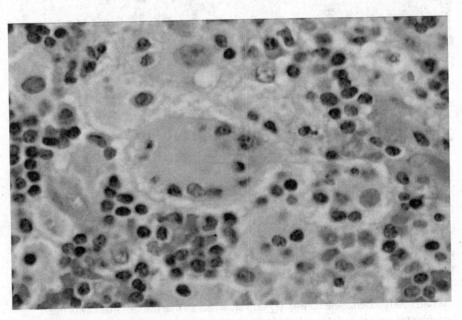

Fig. 15.11 SHML-sinus histiocytes with emperipolesis

Figures 15.10-16.9 in this section are available for download in colour from
www.cambridge.org/9780521184168

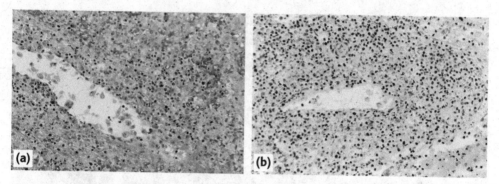

Fig. 16.1 Liver. (a) A lymphohistiocytic infiltrate is present. The presence of the large 'floating' macrophages within portal and central veins is characteristic but not invariable. (b) The infiltrate has no immunostaining for perforin in FHL-2 (perforin, diaminobenzidine (DAB))

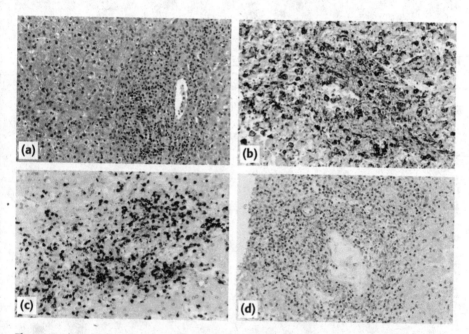

Fig. 16.3 Liver. (a) A mixed lymphohistiocytic infiltrate is concentrated on the portal areas. The large, pale, 'floating' macrophages are noted in a portal vein. (b) Immunostain for the macrophage marker CD163 reveals the extensive portal (and sinusoidal) macrophage infiltrate (diaminobenzidine (DAB)). (c) CD3 stain reveals that the vast majority of the lymphocytes are T-cells (DAB). (d) Perforin immunostain is negative in FHL-2 but not in the other variants or in cases of hepatitis in which many of the T-cells contain perforin

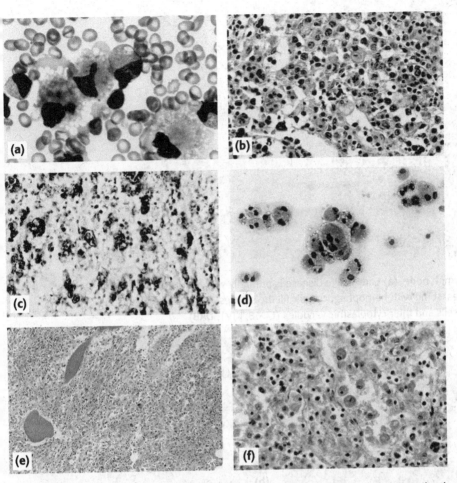

Fig. 16.2 Bone marrow. (a) The aspirate reveals large, cytoplasm-rich macrophages that have cytoplasmic pigment, vacuoles and cell remnants, most commonly erythroid. (b) The biopsy in early active disease contains scattered large and vacuolated macrophages that do not stand out. (c) These macrophages are best seen with anti-CD68 or CD163 staining (CD68, PGM-1, diaminobenzidine (DAB)). (d) Aspirate in late disease (autopsy) may show large numbers of macrophages in the absence of other hematopoietic elements. (e) Bone marrow at autopsy may show vast numbers of large macrophages and only sparse hematopoiesis in a damaged matrix. (f) Periodic acid and Schiff base (PAS) stain reveals the large macrophages, some in dilated vascular sinuses (PAS)

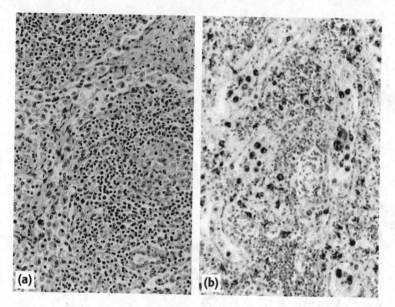

Fig. 16.4 Lymph node. (a) Early active disease is primarily sinus in distribution. Large macrophages, some with hemophagocytosis, fill the sinuses. (b) CD68 highlights the large phagocytic cells and their cytoplasmic vacuoles (CD68, KP-1, DAB)

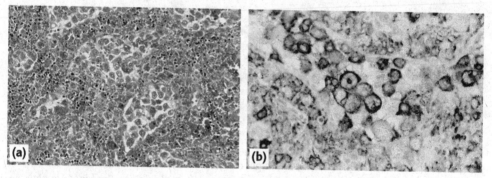

Fig. 16.5 Spleen. (a) The splenic sinuses are filled with large hemophagocytic (erythrophagocytic) macrophages. (b) CD163 immunostain highlights these cells and negative images of intracytoplasmic erythrocytes can be noted (DAB)

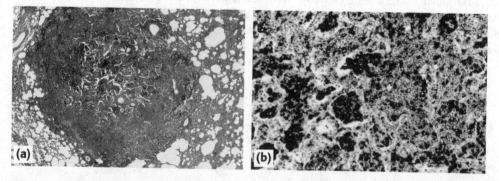

Fig. 16.6 Lung. (a) Nodular lesions with a peribronchial distribution are rarely seen in patients with HLH. These are not known to contain organisms after extensive search and culture. (b) Alveolar, but also interstitial, macrophages comprise the lesions (DAB, CD68)

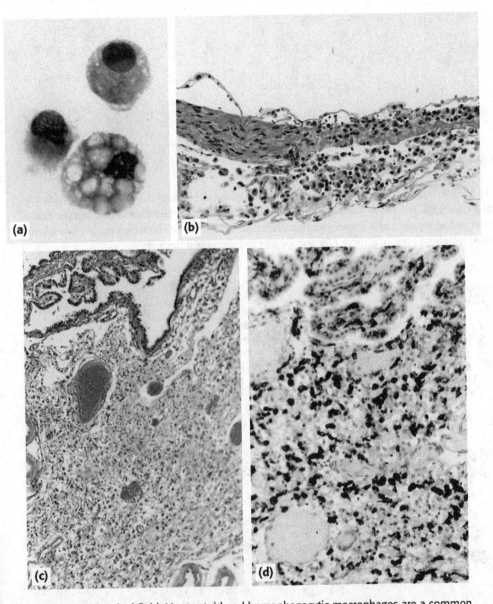

Fig. 16.7 CNS. (a) Spinal fluid. Monocytoid and hemophagocytic macrophages are a common finding in the CSF during active disease. (b) A spinal nerve root reveals the presence of macrophages within the leptomeninges. (c) Subchoroidal ventricular areas are a site for HLH infiltration. (d) Immunostaining for CD68 reveals the extensive macrophage presence in the area represented in (c) (DAB)

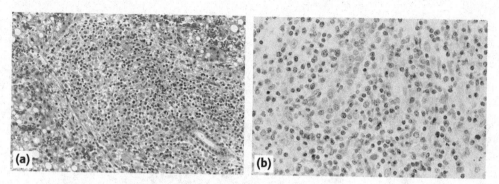

Fig. 16.8 EBV-related HLH, liver. (a) A mixed lymphohistiocytosis is seen that markedly expands the portal area. (b) EBER-1 probe highlights the intranuclear presence of EBV RNA in lymphocytic nuclei. This was not an instance of X-linked lymphoproliferative syndrome (XLPD) which usually has a more activated lymphoid presence, more EBV and greater hepatocellular necrosis

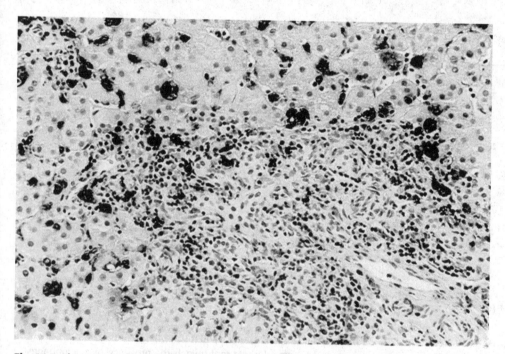

Fig. 16.9 Liver. Macrophage activation syndrome in a child with hepatitis shows the presence of phagocytic sinusoidal Kupffer cells, but lacks the presence of the portal macrophages typical of HLH (contrast with Figure 16.3(b)) (CD68, KP-1, DAB)

epiphyseal sparing, and sparing of the axial skeleton (Figure 15.7). A mixed osteolytic and sclerotic pattern is seen in about one-third of patients. Rarely lytic lesions involving the axial with sparing of the appendicular skeleton is seen (Klieger *et al.*, 2001) and distinction from LCH is made pathologically. Technetium99 scans show markedly increased uptake. Prolonged retention of gadolinium after magnetic resonance imaging (MRI) may be due to histiocyte uptake (Shamburek *et al.*, 2001). CT/MRI of orbits may show bilateral retroorbital involvement, while CNS findings are always located along the falx or dura.

Therapy of ECD

Many different therapeutic options have yielded varying degrees of success. These include surgical debulking, high-dose corticosteroid therapy, cyclosporine, interferon-α, chemotherapy and radiation therapy (Veyssier-Belot *et al.*, 1996; Devouassoux *et al.*, 1998). Surgical therapy of retroperitoneal disease is suboptimal because of the incidence of recurrence, and palliative percutaneous nephrostomies may be needed to preserve renal function (Fortman, 2001). The commonest chemotherapy drugs utilized have been vinca alkaloids, anthracyclines and

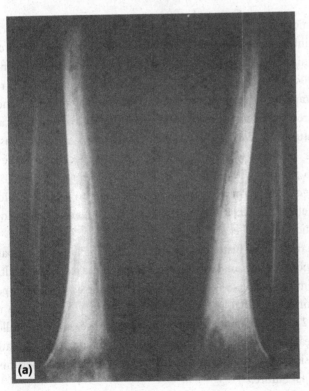

Figure 15.7   (a) Characteristic osteoseclerons of ECD. Symmetrical osteosclerosis diaphysis of long bones with epiphyseal sparing

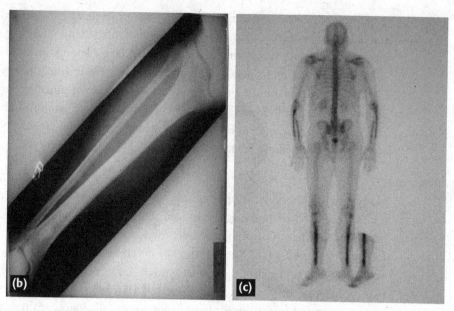

Figure 15.7   (b) X-ray and (c) Tc99 bone scan (courtesy of Dr E. Becker, Toronto)

cyclophosphamide (Gupta *et al.*, 2002). Responses to vincristine/prednisone (Gupta *et al.*, 2002), vinblastine/prednisone (Veyssier-Belot *et al.*, 1996) and cyclophosphamide/ prednisolone (Bourke *et al.*, 2003) and 2-chlorodeoxyadenosine (2-CdA) (Myra *et al.*, 2004) have been reported. Two patients were reported to respond to prolonged therapy with vinblastine and mycophenolate mofetil (Jendro *et al.*, 2004), another received clodronate and prednisone because of biochemical evidence of a high bone-turnover (Mossetti *et al.*, 2003). Interferon-α therapy has been recommended for patients who fail standard therapy because of the response reported in two patients with ECD and orbital involvement (Veyssier-Belot *et al.*, 1996; Esmaeli *et al.*, 2001). An 18-year-old boy refractory to corticosteroids, 2-CdA, interferon, and etoposide had a good partial remission after double autologous stem cell transplantation (Boissel *et al.*, 2001).

Variability in the natural history of the disease, the small number of patients and the lack of prospective trials, makes interpretation of these results difficult. Whether spontaneous remission occurs is unknown. The prognosis of ECD appears to be significantly worse than that reported in other histiocytoses. In the review by Veyssier-Belot, 22 of 37 patients died of progressive disease (mean follow-up 32 months), but death may occur after many years. The major cause of death appears to be lung fibrosis leading to respiratory or cardiac failure or retroperitoneal fibrosis leading to renal failure.

As with the other uncommon disorders, multi-institutional and multi-national trials may help to define the natural history and therapy of this disease.

Systemic non-LCH disorders not belonging to the JXG family

SHML (Rosai–Dorfman disease)

SHML is a non-neoplastic, polyclonal, usually self-limited disease, due to accumulation of S100+ histiocytes. The etiology of SHML is unknown. An increased incidence of autoimmune disorders including autoimmune hemolytic anemia and various rheumatologic disorders have been noted (Grabczynska *et al.*, 2001). Human herpesvirus 6 viral antigen gp106 has been demonstrated in SHML histiocytes (Levine *et al.*, 1992; Luppi *et al.*, 1998), but like the earlier demonstration of Epstein–Barr virus (EBV) genome, may be a spurious finding (Luppi *et al.*, 1998; Zelger and Cerio, 2001). Serologic evidence of EBV infection is present in over half the cases, but may represent an epiphenomenon of EBV reactivation due to the immune disturbance found commonly in SHML patients (Tsang *et al.*, 1994). Thirteen patients are reported with lymphoma and SHML, six had Hodgkins disease and two follicular non-Hodgkins lymphoma and SHML in the same lymph node (Lu *et al.*, 2000). Thus an infectious or malignant process may result in aberrant activation of the macrophage system with excessive cytokine-release by macrophages and T-cells.

Pathology of SHML

Involved lymph nodes show massive sinus infiltration of large histiocytes admixed with lymphocytes and plasma cells. Intact erythrocytes, lymphocytes and plasma cells may be engulfed by histiocytic cells (emperipolesis). Immunohistochemically SHML cells are S100+, CD68+, CD163+, HAM-56+, α_1-antichymotrypsin+ and α_1-antitrypsin+, but CD1a negative (Juskevicius and Finlay, 2001). SHML lesions show strong expression of IL-1, TNF-α and moderate expression of IL-6 (Foss *et al.*, 1996). IL-6 expression may be related to the polyclonal plasmacytosis and hypergammaglobulinemia observed. SHML must be distinguished from sinus hyperplasia (sinus histiocytosis) – a non-specific reaction to a wide variety of agents. In both conditions the histiocytes have strong macrophage antigen expression, but S100 positivity is limited to SHML (Eisen *et al.*, 1990) (Figure 15.8).

Although emperipolesis is not unique to SHML, its occurrence in histiocytes that express S100 in the appropriate clinico-pathologic setting, is considered diagnostic.

Clinical features of SHML

Most patients are young (mean age 20.6 years), but with a wide age distribution (Juskevicius and Finlay, 2001). Patients presenting with isolated intracranial disease appear to be older (mean age 37.5 years) (Deodhare *et al.*, 1998). The disease is slightly commoner in males (58%) and in blacks (Lauwers *et al.*, 2000). Around 80% of patients present with bilateral painless cervical adenopathy which may be associated

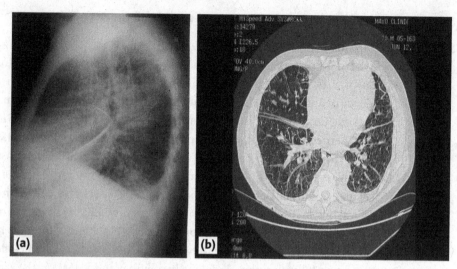

Figure 15.8   ECD: (a) lateral chest X-ray and (b) CT showing classical interlobular septal thickening and patchy centrilobular opacities (courtesy of Dr D Pearse, Toronto)

with fever, night sweats, malaise, weight loss, leukocytosis and hypergammaglobulinemia. Other nodal groups, including mediastinal and inguinal, may be involved. Involvement of extranodal tissue such as skin and soft tissue, upper respiratory tract, bone, eye and retroorbital tissue is found in 43%, with lymphadenopathy or as the sole initial manifestation of disease (Foucar *et al.*, 1990). Other reported sites include lung, urogenital tract, breast, gastrointestinal tract, liver and pancreas. Lung involvement usually comprises nodules associated with large airways, but interstitial disease may occur. Head and neck involvement occurs in approximately 22% of patients (Foucar *et al.*, 1990), the commonest site being nasal cavity, and the second commonest a major salivary gland such as parotid (Juskevicius and Finlay, 2001). Intracranial disease poses a significant diagnostic challenge, usually occurring without extracranial lymphadenopathy. Almost all reported intracranial lesions have been attached to dura, with only a few extending intraparenchymally. The disease clinically and radiologically resembles meningioma and histologically must be differentiated from LCH, infectious and lymphoproliferative disorders (Deodhare *et al.*, 1998).

Clinical course of SHML

The clinical course of SHML is unpredictable with episodes of exacerbation and remission which may extend over many years. The outcome is usually good and disease is often self-limiting, nonetheless about 5–11% of patients die from disease. A subset of patients with immunologic abnormalities at or prior to presentation, have a less favorable prognosis with more widespread nodal disease and a higher fatality rate (Foucar *et al.*, 1990; Goodnight *et al.*, 1996).

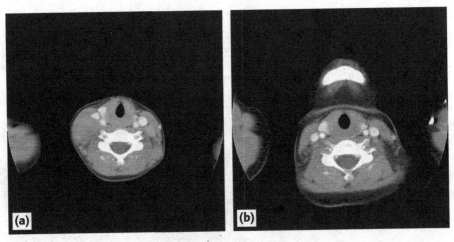

Figure 15.9 SHML: CT scan showing cervical lymphadenopathy: (a) at presentation and (b) post-steroid therapy

It has been suggested that SHML be divided into two categories. On the one hand, the disease may affect only lymph nodes which enlarge suddenly and which regress just as swiftly with no recurrences. Alternatively, it may involve several extranodal sites, usually with multinodal disease and with a protracted clinical course that lasts for years and is marked by intermittent remissions and relapses (Figure 15.9). The severity of disease is based on the number and type of extranodal sites (Lauwers *et al.*, 2000).

Cutaneous Rosai–Dorfman disease

While skin involvement occurs commonly, disease limited to skin is uncommon, and is called cutaneous Rosai–Dorfman (CRD) disease rather than SHML which implies nodal involvement. Skin lesions are mainly papules or nodules that are firm, indurated, ranging in size from 1 to 10 cm, but presentations with psoriasiform, pustular and acneiform lesions have been described (Cole and Finlay, 1999). CRD has a benign course with spontaneous resolution in most and therapy is indicated for cosmetic reasons only.

Therapy of SHML

Treatment is only necessary when nodal enlargement causes significant problems such as airway obstruction or for patients with extranodal disease with vital organ involvement (Pulsoni *et al.*, 2002). For intracranial dural-based lesions, surgical resection alone is successful in the majority (Deodhare *et al.*, 1998). A recent report recommended partial resection with adjuvant stereotactic radiosurgery, when complete resection carries the potential for excess morbidity (Hadjipanayis *et al.*, 2003). No standard approach has been delineated for other patients requiring treatment.

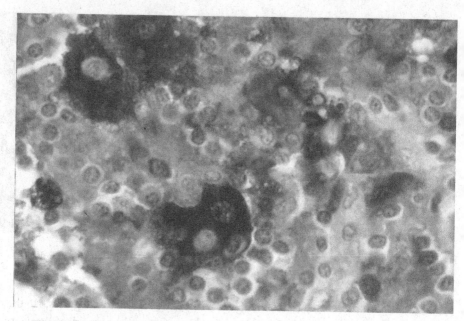

Figure 15.10 SHML: sinus histiocytes staining positive with S100, showing emperipolesis. See also color plates

Antibiotics are not useful. Surgical excision of resectable lesions achieved eight CR in nine patients (Pulsoni *et al.*, 2002). Systemic corticosteroids are useful in decreasing nodal size and symptoms, but regrowth often occurs within a short period of discontinuation (Scheel *et al.*, 1997). Different chemotherapeutic regimens have been tried with varying success (Figure 15.10). Pulsoni found that only 2 of 10 patients treated with chemotherapy achieved CR, both with combination low-dose MTX and 6-mercaptopurine (6MP). One, a 3-year old, had previously failed corticosteroids and etoposide (Horneff *et al.*, 1996). In other series a few patients achieved CR to different agents including vinblastine, MTX, 6MP and 6 thioguanine (Scheel *et al.*, 1997). It appears that anthracyclines and alkylating agent have little effect, and despite occasional reports of response, vinca alkaloids are of questionable value (Pulsoni *et al.*, 2002). There are two reports of success with prolonged interferon-α (Lohr *et al.*, 1995; Palomera *et al.*, 2001), but another patient failed interferon-α plus chemotherapy (Pulsoni *et al.*, 2002). There is a single report of CR from thalidomide (Viraben *et al.*, 1998) and one from acyclovir (Baildam *et al.*, 1992).

Recommendations for therapy

Lesions that do not involve vital organs should receive no active therapy. For patients with significant fever without a documented infection, or who have sudden enlargement of nodes, high-dose corticosteroids should be tried, with close observation for recurrence once therapy is discontinued. For those with vital organ compression

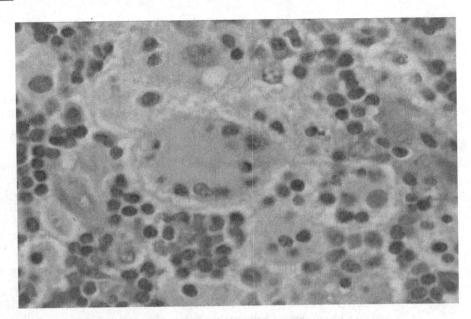

Figure 15.11 SHML: sinus histiocytes with emperipolesis. See also color plates

or other life-threatening involvement, surgery and high-dose corticosteroids can be tried, but emergency radiotherapy may be needed.

Radiotherapy alone has worked in some cases and should be tried if surgery is not possible (Pulsoni *et al.*, 2002).

The results of chemotherapy has not been encouraging, but when indicated, anti-metabolite therapy with combination 6MP and MTX may prove effective (Figure 15.11). It is possible that different patients with SHML will respond to different chemotherapy drugs. If anti-metabolites fail, different combinations can be tried.

Due to self-limited nature of the disease in most patients, however, chemotherapy should be restricted to patients with life-threatening disease, not responsive to other measures. Testing of combinations with lesser toxicity such as low-dose MTX and 6MP for patients without major complications, but with quality of life issues due to multiple reactivations or major cosmetic problems, would be justifiable within the context of a multinational trial.

In view of the single reports of success with immunomodulatory therapy, further trials of this mode of therapy would be of interest.

REFERENCES

Baildam, E.M., Ewing, C.I., D'Souza, S.W., *et al.* (1992). Sinus histiocytosis with massive lymphadenopathy (Rosai–Dorfman disease): response to acyclovir. *J Roy Soc Med*, **85**, 179–180.

Banchereau, J., Fay, J., Pascual, V., *et al.* (2003). Dendritic cells: controllers of the immune system and a new promise for immunotherapy. *Novartis Found Symp*, **252**, 226–235.

Boissel, N., Wechsler, B. and Leblond, V. (2001). Dendritic cells: controllers of the immune system and a new promise for immunotherapy. *Ann Int Med*, 844–845.

Bourke, S.C., Nicholson, A.G. and Gibson, G.J. (2003). Erdheim–Chester disease: pulmonary infiltration responding to cyclophosphamide and prednisolone. *Thorax*, **58**, 1004–1005.

Campbell, D.A. and Edwaards, N.L. (1991). Multicentric reticulohistiocytosis: a systemic macrophage disorder. *Baillieres Clin Rheumatol*, **5**, 301–319.

Candell-Chalom, E., Elenitsas, R., Rosenstein, E.D., *et al.* (1998). A case of multicentric reticulo-histiocytosis in a 6-year-old child. *J Rheumatol*, **25**, 794–797.

Candell-Chalom, E., Rosenstein, E.D. and Kramer, N. (2000). Cyclosporine as a treatment for multicentric reticulohistiocytosis. *J Rheumatol*, **27**, 556–556.

Caparros-Lefebvre, D., Pruvo, J.P., Remy, M., *et al.* (1995). Neuroradiologic aspects of Chester–Erdheim disease. *Am J Neuroradiol*, **16**, 735–740.

Caputo, R. and Grimalt, R. (1992). Solitary reticulohistiocytosis (reticulohistiocytoma) of the skin in children: report of two cases. *Arch Dermatol*, **128**, 689–699.

Cash, J.M., Tyree, J. and Recht, M. (1997). Severe multicentric reticulohisticytosis: disease stabilization achieved with methotrexate and hydroxychloroquine. *J Rheumatol*, **24**, 2250–2253.

Casteels, I., Olver, J., Malone, M., *et al.* (1993). Early treatment of juvenile xanthogranuloma of the iris with subconjunctival steroids. *Br J Ophthalmol*, **77**, 57–60.

Chang, M.W. (1999). Update on juvenile xanthogranuloma: unusual cutaneous and systemic variants. *Semin Cutan Med Surg*, **18**, 195–205.

Chang, M.W., Frieden, I.J. and Good, W. (1996). The risk of intraocular juvenile xanthogranuloma: survey of current practices and assessment of risk. *J Am Acad Dermatol*, **34**, 445–449.

Chang, S.E., Koh, G.J., Choi, J.H., *et al.* (2002). Widespread skin-limited adult Langerhans cell histiocytosis: long term follow up with good response to interferon alpha. *Clin Expt Dermatol*, **27**, 135–137.

Chu, A.C. (2000). The confusing state of the histiocytoses. *Br J Dermatol*, **143**, 475–476.

Cole, S. and Finlay, J. (1999). 2-Chlorodeoxyadenosine for adults with multi-system Langerhans cell histiocytosis. *Med Pediatr Oncol*, **33**, 512.

Dehner, L.P. (2003). Juvenile xanthogranulomas in the first two decades of life: a clinicopathologic study of 174 cases with cutaneous and extracutaneous manifestations. *Am J Surg Pathol*, **27**, 579–593.

Deodhare, S.S., Ang, L.C. and Bilbao, J.M. (1998). Isolated intracranial involvement in Rosai–Dorfman disease: a report of two cases and review of the literature. *Arch Pathol Lab Med*, **122**, 161–165.

Devouassoux, G., Lantejoul, S., Chatelain, P., *et al.* (1998). Erdheim–Chester disease: a primary macrophage cell disorder. *Am J Resp Crit Care Med*, **157**, 650–653.

Egan, A.J., Boardman, L.A., Tazelaar, H.D., *et al.* (1999). Erdheim–Chester disease: clinical, radiologic and histopathologic findings in five patients with interstitial lung disease. *Am J Surg Pathol*, **23**, 17–26.

Eisen, R.N., Buckley, P.J. and Rosai, J. (1990). Immunophenotypic characterization of sinus histiocytes with massive lymphadenopathy (Rosai–Dorfman disease). *Semin Diagn Pathol*, **7**, 74–82.

Escribano, L., Pérez de Oteyza, J., Núñez, R., et al. (2002). Cladribine induces immunopheno-typical changes in bone marrow mast cells from mastocytosis. Report of a case of mastocyto-sis associated with a lymphoplasmacytic lymphoma. *Leuk Res*, **26**, 1043–1046.

Esmaeli, R., Ahmadi, A., Tang, R., et al. (2001). Interferon theory for orbital infiltration second-ary to Erdheim–Chester disease. *Am J Ophthalmol*, **132**, 945–947.

Favara, B.E., Feller, A.C., Pauli, M., et al. (1997). Contemporary classification of histiocytic disorders. Reclassification Working Group of the Histiocyte Society. *Med Pediatr Oncol*, **29**, 157–166.

Ferrando, J., Campo-Voegeli, A., Soler-Carrillo, J., et al. (1998). Systemic xanthohistiocytoma: a variant of xanthoma disseminatum? *Br J Dermatol*, **138**, 155–160.

Flaitz, C. (2002). Juvenile xanthogranuloma of the oral cavity in children: a clinicopathologic study. *Oral Surg Oral Med Oral Pathol Oral Radiol Endod*, **94**, 345–352.

Fortman, B.J. (2001). Erdheim Chester disease of the retroperitoneum: a rare cause of ureteral obstruction. *Am J Roentg*, **176**, 1330–1331.

Foss, H.D., Herbst, H., Araujo, I., et al. (1996). Monokine expression in Langerhans' cell histiocytosis and sinus histiocytosis with massive lymphadenopathy (Rosai–Dorfman disease). *J Pathol*, **179**, 60–65.

Foucar, E., Rosai, J. and Dorfman, R. (1990). Sinus histiocytosis with massive lymphadenopathy (Rosai–Dorfman disease): review of the entity. *Semin Diagn Pathol*, **7**, 19–73.

Freyer, D.R., Kennedy, R., Bostrom, B.C., et al. (1996). Juvenile xanthogranuloma: forms of sys-temic disease and their clinical implications. *J Pediatr*, **129**, 227–237.

Goerdt, S., Kolde, G., Bonsmann, G., et al. (1993). Immunohistochemical comparison of cuta-neous histiocytoses and related skin disorders: diagnostic and histogenetic relevance of MS-1 high molecular weight protein expression. *J Pathol*, **170**, 421–427.

Gonzalez-Ruiz, A., Bernal Ruiz, A.I., Aragoneses Fraile, H., et al. (2000). Progressive nodular his-tiocytosis accompanied by systemic disorders. *Br J Dermatol*, **143**, 628–631.

Goodnight, J.W., Wang, M.B., Sercarz, J.A., et al. (1996). Extranodal Rosai–Dorfman disease of the head and neck. *Laryngoscope*, **106**, t-6.

Gorman, J.D., Danning, C., Schumacher, H.R., et al. (2000). Multicentric reticulohistiocytosis: case report with immunohistochemical analysis and literature review. *Arthritis Rheum*, **43**, 930–938.

Grabczynska, S.A., Toh, C.T., Francis, N., et al. (2001). Rosai–Dorfman disease complicated by autoimmune haemolytic anaemia: case report and review of a multisystem disease with cuta-neous infiltrates. *Br J Dermatol*, **145**, 323–326.

Gupta, A., Kelly, B. and McGuigan, J.E. (2002). Erdheim–Chester disease with prominent peri-cardial involvement. Clinical, radiologic, and histologic findings. *Am J Med Sci*, **324**, 96–100.

Hadjipanayis, C.G., Bejjani, G., Wiley, C., et al. (2003). Intracranial Rosai–Dorfman disease treated with microsurgical resection and stereotactic radiosurgery. Case report. *J Neurosurg*, **98**, 165–168.

Havill, S., Duffill, M. and Rademaker, M. (1999). Multicentric reticulohistiocytosis in a child. *Australas J Dermatol*, **40**, 44–46.

Hernandez-Martin, A., Baselga, E., Drolet, B.A., et al. (1997). Juvenile xanthogranuloma. *J Am Acad Dermatol*, **36**, t-67.

Hiramanek, N., Kossard, S. and Barnetson, R.St.C. (2002). Multicentric reticulohistiocytosis pre-senting with a rash and arthralgia. *Austral J Dermatol*, **43**, 136–139.

Horneff, G., Jurgens, H., Hort, W., *et al.* (1996). Sinus histiocytosis with massive lymphadenopathy (Rosai–Dorfman disease): response to methotrexate and mercaptopurine. *Med Pediatr Oncol*, **27**, 187–192.

Jaffe, R. (1999). The histiocytoses. *Clin Lab Med*, **19**, 135–155.

Jang, K.A., Lee, H.J., Choi, J.H., *et al.* (1999). Generalized eruptive histiocytoma of childhood. *Br J Dermatol*, **140**, 174–176.

Jang, K.A., Ahn, S.J., Choi, J.H., *et al.* (2000). Histiocytic disorders with spontaneous regression in infancy. *Pediatr Dermatol*, **17**, 364–368.

Jansen, T.L. and Kruithof, I.G. (2003). Diagnostic image (141). Nodules in a patient with rheumatoid arthritis. Multicentric reticulohistiocytosis as a paraneoplastic manifestation [Dutch]. *Ned Tijdschr voor Geneeskd*, **147**, 1067.

Jendro, M.C., Zeidler, H. and Rosenthal, H., *et al.* (2004). Improvement of Erdheim–Chester disease in two patients with sequential treatment with vinblastine and mycophenolate mofetil. *Clin Rheumatol*, **23**, 52–56.

Juskevicius, R. and Finlay, J.L. (2001). Rosai–Dorfman disease of the parotid gland, cytologic and histopathologic findings with immunohistochemical correlation. *Arch Pathol Lab Med*, **125**, 1348–1350.

Kambouchner, M., Colby, T.V., Domenge, C., *et al.* (1997). Erdheim–Chester disease with prominent pulmonary involvement associated with eosinophilic granuloma of mandibular bone. *Histopathology*, **30**, 353–358.

Klieger, M.R., Elkowitz, D.E., Arlen, M., *et al.* (2001). Erdheim–Chester disease: a unique presentation with multiple osteolytic lesions of the spine and pelvis that spared the appendicular skeleton. *Am J Roentg*, **178**, 429–432.

Kubota, Y., Kiryu, H., Takayama, J., *et al.* (2001). Histopathologic maturation of juvenile xanthogranuloma in a short period. *Pediatr Dermatol*, **18**, 127–130.

Lauwers, G.Y., Perez-Atayde, A., Dorfman, R.F., *et al.* (2000). The digestive system manifestations of Rosai–Dorfman disease (sinus histiocytosis with massive lymphadenopathy): review of 11 cases. *Hum Pathol*, **31**, 380–385.

Levine, P.H., Jahan, N., M.i.P., *et al.* (1992). Detection of human Herpesvirus 6 in tissues involved by sinus histiocytosis with massive lymphadenopathy (Rosai–Dorfman disease). *J Infect Dis*, **166**, 291–295.

Liang, G.C. and Granston, A.S. (1996). Complete remission of multicentric reticulohistiocytosis with combination therapy of steroid, cyclophosphamide, and low-dose pulse methotrexate. Case report, review of the literature, and proposal for treatment. *Arthritis Rheum*, **39**, 171–174.

Lohr, H.F., Godderz, W., Wolfe, T., *et al.* (1995). Long-term survival in a patient with Rosai–Dorfman disease treated with interferon-alpha. *Eur J Cancer*, **31A**, 2427–2428.

Lu, D., Estalilla, O.C., Manning, J.T.J., *et al.* (2000). Sinus histiocytosis with massive lymphadenopathy and malignant lymphoma involving the same lymph node: a report of four cases and review of the literature. *Mod Pathol*, **13**, 414–419.

Luppi, M., Barozzi, P., Garber, R., *et al.* (1998). Expression of human herpesvirus-6 antigens in benign and malignant lymphoproliferative diseases. *Am J Pathol*, **153**, 815–823.

Luz, F.B., Gaspar, A.P., Kalil-Gaspar, N., *et al.* (2001). Multicentric reticulohistiocytosis. *J Eur Acad Dermatol Venereol*, **15**, 524–531.

Misery, J., Kanitakis, J., Hermier, C., *et al.* (2001). Generalized eruptive histiocytoma in an infant with healing in summer: long term follow-up. *Br J Dermatol*, **144**, 435–437.

Mossetti, G., Rendina, D., Numis, F.G., *et al.* (2003). Biochemical markers of bone turnover, serum levels of interleukin-6/interleukin-6 soluble receptor and bisphosphonate treatment in Erdheim–Chester disease. *Clin Exp Rheumatol*, **21**, 232–236.

Mullans, E.A., Helm, T.N., Taylor, J.S., *et al.* (1995). Generalized non-Langerhans cell histiocytosis: four cases illustrate a spectrum of disease. *Int J Dermatol*, **34**, 106–112.

Myra, C., Sloper, L., Tighe, P.J., *et al.* (2004). Treatment of Erdheim–Chester disease with cladribine: a rational approach. *Br J Ophthalmol*, **88**, 844–846.

Outland, J.D., Keiran, S.J., Schikler, K.N., *et al.* (2002). Multicentric reticulohistiocytosis in a 14-year-old girl. *Pediatr Dermatol*, **19**, 527–531.

Palomera, L., Domingo, M., Soria, J., *et al.* (2001). Long term survival in a patient with aggressive Rosai–Dorfman disease treated with interferon alpha [Spanish]. *Med Clin (Barc)*, **116**, 797–798.

Pulsoni, A., Anghel, G., Falcucci, P., *et al.* (2002). Treatment of sinus histiocytosis with massive lymphadenopathy (Rosai–Dorfman disease): report of a case and literature review. *Am J Hematol*, **69**, 67–71.

Rentsch, J.L., Martin, E.M., Harrison, L.C., *et al.* (1998). Prolonged response of multicentric reticulohistiocytosis to low dose methotrexate. *J Rheumatol*, **25**, 1012–1015.

Rush, W.L., Andriko, J.A.W., Galateau-Salle, F., *et al.* (2003). Pulmonary pathology of Erdheim–Chester disease. *Mod Pathol*, **13**, 747–754.

Saito, K., Fujii, K., Awazu, Y., *et al.* (2001). A case of systemic lupus erythematosus complicated with multicentric reticulohistiocytosis (MRH): successful treatment of MRH and lupus nephritis with cyclosporine A. *Lupus*, **10**, 129–132.

Scheel, M.M., Rady, P.L., Tyring, S.K., *et al.* (1997). Sinus histiocytosis with massive lymphadenopathy: presentation as giant granuloma annulare and detection of human herpesvirus 6. *J Am Acad Dermatol*, **37**, 643–646.

Shamburek, R.D., Brewer, H.B.J. and Gochuico, B.R. (2001). Erdheim–Chester disease: a rare multisystem histiocytic disorder associated with interstitial lung disease. *Am J Med Sci*, **321**, 66–75.

Szekeres, E. (1988). Xanthoma disseminatum: a rare condition with non-X, non-lipid cutaneous histiocytopathy. *Dermatol Surg Oncol*, **14**, 1021–1024.

Tahan, S.R., Pastel-Levy, C., Bhan, A.K., *et al.* (1989). Juvenile xanthogranuloma. Clinical and pathologic characterization. *Arch Pathol Lab Med*, **113**, 1057–1061.

Tanz, W.S., Schwartz, R.A. and Janniger, C.K. (1994). Juvenile xanthogranuloma. *Cutis*, **54**, 241–245.

Tsang, W.Y., Yip, T.T. and Chan, J.K. (1994). The Rosai–Dorfman disease histiocytes are not infected by Epstein–Barr virus. *Histopathology*, **25**, 88–90.

Veyssier-Belot, C., Cacoub, P., Caparros-Lefebvre, D., *et al.* (1996). Erdheim–Chester disease, clinical and radiologic characteristics of 59 cases. *Medicine (Baltimore)*, **75**, 157–169.

Viraben, R., Dupre, A. and Gorguet, B. (1998). Pure cutaneous histiocytosis resembling sinus histiocytosis. *Clin Exp Dermatol*, **13**, 197–199.

Wee, S.H., Kim, H.S., Chang, S.N., *et al.* (2000). Generalized eruptive histiocytoma: a pediatric case. *Pediatr Dermatol*, **17**, 453–455.

Weston, W.L., Travers, S.H., Mierau, G.W., *et al.* (2000). Benign cephalic histiocytosis with diabetes insipidus. *Pediatr Dermatol*, **17**, 296–298.

Zelger, B.W.H. and Burgdorf, W.H. (2001). The cutaneous 'histiocytoses'. *Adv Dermatol*, **17**, 77–114.

Zelger, B.W.H. and Cerio, R. (2001). Xanthogranuloma is the archetype of non-Langerhans cell histiocytosis. *Br J Dermatol*, **45**, 369–370.

Zelger, B.G., Zelger, B., Steiner, H., *et al.* (1995). Solitary giant xanthogranuloma and benign cephalic histiocytosis – variants of juvenile xanthogranuloma. *Br J Dermatol*, **133**, 598–604.

Zelger, B.W., Sidoroff, A., Orchard, G., *et al.* (1996). Non-Langerhans cell histiocytoses. A new unifying concept. *Am J Dermatopathol*, **18**, 490–504.

Zvulunov, A., Barak, Y. and Metzker, A. (1995). Juvenile xanthogranuloma, neurofibromatosis, and juvenile chronic myelogenous leukemia. World statistical analysis. *Arch Dermatol*, **131**, 904–908.

16

The histopathology of hemophagocytic lymphohistiocytosis

Ronald Jaffe

Introduction

Although the earliest report of the inherited condition, now known as familial hemo-phagocytic lymphohistiocytosis (FHL) (OMIM 603552, 603553, 602782, 170280), is traditionally attributed to Farquhar and Claireaux (1952), it was not until 1995 that a logical framework for the understanding of these conditions was provided (Henter and Elinder, 1995; Henter, 2002). According to this schema, hemophagocytic lym-phohistiocytosis (HLH) with an underlying genetic defect is regarded as 'primary HLH'. All other forms are reactive, examples of the macrophage activation syndrome, and hence, 'secondary HLH'. The 'contemporary classification of histiocytic disorders' (Favara et al., 1997) lists primary HLH as including a clearly familial form as well as a sporadic form without a clear family history, nonetheless thought to be genetic, and secondary hemophagocytic syndromes that are infection or malignancy associated. Curiously, it is not the histiocyte (monocyte-macrophage) that is abnormal in either form. In primary HLH there is a defect in the control of the inflammatory process, such as perforin mutations, that leads to the activation and accumulation of macrophages. In secondary HLH, the macrophage activation appears to be driven by cytokines following a trigger. It is however, becoming apparent that even in second-ary, reactive macrophage activation type HLH, there may be an inherited predisposi-tion in the form of reactive versus non-reactive polymorphisms for certain receptors and response molecules such as IL-10, IL-12 and IL-18 (Lammas et al., 2002; Fujihara et al., 2003; Goldstein et al., 2003). It is also now clear that FHL can be triggered by an infectious or inflammatory stimulus (Henter et al., 1991; Henter et al., 1993).

The histopathology will be described for familial HLH; that is the pathology of children who are known to have a family history or one of the causative molecular genetic defects (Janka, 1983; Goldberg and Nezelof, 1986; Favara, 1992). The histo-pathology of secondary hemophagocytic syndromes will be described separately. It is important to note that hemophagocytosis (the presence of various blood-derived cells in macrophages) and especially, erythrophagocytosis (the presence of erythrocytes in macrophages) is neither sensitive nor specific for HLH, but an epiphenomenon.

Hemophagocytosis is not found in all children with HLH (Aricò et al., 1996; Ost et al., 1998), particularly at presentation, and may be episodic in any individual. Erythrophagocytosis is seen in regional nodes most commonly following minor blood transfusion reactions and after surgery, even in the absence of other features of sepsis or macrophage activation (Listinsky, 1988; Suster et al., 1988). Patients with HLH commonly have had blood transfusions, so it is not always clear whose cells are being phagocytosed.

Erythrocyte sequestration and erythrophagocytosis can also follow intravenous immunoglobulin administration (Kessary-Shoham et al., 1999).

Primary HLH

The inherited hemophagocytic lymphohistiocytic syndromes are listed in Table 16.1, along with other inherited syndromes that confer a susceptibility to macrophage activation (Feldmann et al., 2003).

Familial hemophagocytic lymphohistiocytosis (FHL-1–FHL-3)

The diagnosis of HLH is not primarily a tissue diagnosis and is made by compiling a number of clinical and laboratory features that raise the possibility of HLH. The histopathologic features may (or may not) be contributory (Henter et al., 1991). The major features include a family history, if one exists, fever, splenomegaly, varying cytopenias, hypertriglyceridemia, hypofibrinogenemia and high serum ferritin levels (see Chapter 18). Although hemophagocytosis is most commonly found in the spleen and lymph nodes, and not as frequently in the bone marrow, it can be focal or even

Table 16.1 Inherited hemophagocytic lymphohistiocytic syndromes and macrophage activation susceptibility

OMIM	Locus	Defect
Inherited HLH syndromes		
FHL-1 (HPLH1) 603552	9q21.3–22	Unknown
FHL-2 (HPLH2) 603553	10q21–22	Perforin mutations
FHL-3	17q25	Hmunc 13-4 mutations
Faisalabad (HJACD) 602782	11q25	Unknown
With macrophage activation susceptibility		
Chediak–Higashi (CHS1) 214500	1q42.1–42.2	Lysosomal trafficking regulator
Griscelli (GS1) 214450	15q21	Myosin or Ras-associated protein
X-linked lymphoproliferative syndrome (XLPD) 308240	Xq25	SH2 D1A mutations
Omenn 603554 (RAG1/RAG2)	11p13	Recombination activating genes

absent, especially early in the condition and when there has been some therapy. It is thus no longer considered an essential finding in the revised diagnostic guidelines (Chapter 18).

Phenotypic and molecular genetic diagnosis is now available for a number of genes known to underlie the HLH phenotype. Stepp *et al.* (1999) linked the FHL locus at 10q21–22 (FHL-2) to defects in the perforin gene and the absence of stainable perforin in lymphocyte granules. Most of the mutations identified to date are associated with complete absence or marked reduction in the content of perforin (Feldmann *et al.*, 2002). In patients who have the perforin gene mutation, absence or reduction of perforin can be demonstrated in all cytotoxic cells by flow cytometry (Kogawa *et al.*, 2002) by quantitative fluorescence (Maher *et al.*, 2002) or by rapid polymerase chain reaction (PCR) (zur Stadt *et al.*, 2003). Immunostaining of tissues for perforin expression is also markedly reduced or absent (Figure 16.1) but the absence of perforin staining is not specific for FHL-2, since it is also seen in some instances of human immunodeficiency virus (HIV) in children (Haridas *et al.*, 2003). Perforin mutation has also been noted in an instance of HLH associated with chronic active Epstein–Barr virus (EBV) infection, blurring the line between primary and secondary HLH (Katano *et al.*, 2003). The absence of perforin pertains only to FHL-2, and not to patients with FHL-1 and FHL-3 (see Chapter 17). Now that there is a 'gold-standard' diagnosis, at least for a subset of HLH, the relative importance of morphologic features, especially hemophagocytosis, can be reassessed.

Bone marrow

According to the original diagnostic guidelines (Henter *et al.*, 1991) it was described as follows: 'In the bone marrow, histiocytes are initially unevenly distributed but later become more diffuse. In early stages, the bone marrow may only show slight

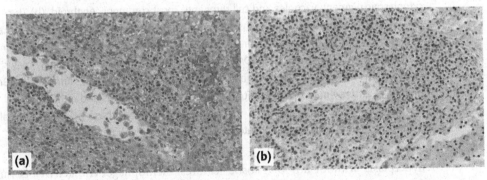

Figure 16.1 Liver. (a) A lymphohistiocytic infiltrate is present. The presence of the large 'floating' macrophages within portal and central veins is characteristic but not invariable. (b) The infiltrate has no immunostaining for perforin in FHL-2 (perforin, diaminobenzidine (DAB)). See also color plates

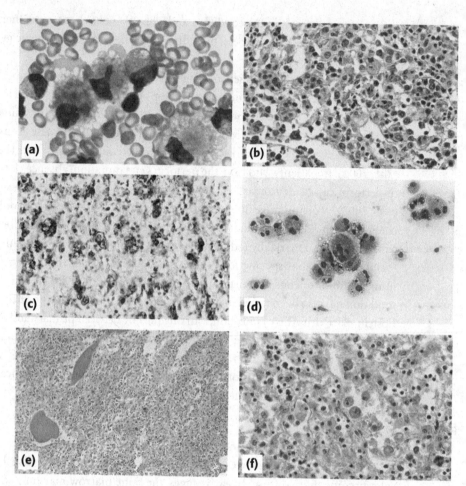

Figure 16.2 Bone marrow. (a) The aspirate reveals large, cytoplasm-rich macrophages that have cytoplasmic pigment, vacuoles and cell remnants, most commonly erythroid. (b) The biopsy in early active disease contains scattered large and vacuolated macrophages that do not stand out. (c) These macrophages are best seen with anti-CD68 or CD163 staining (CD68, PGM-1, diaminobenzidine (DAB)). (d) Aspirate in late disease (autopsy) may show large numbers of macrophages in the absence of other hematopoietic elements. (e) Bone marrow at autopsy may show vast numbers of large macrophages and only sparse hematopoiesis in a damaged matrix. (f) Periodic acid and Schiff base (PAS) stain reveals the large macrophages, some in dilated vascular sinuses (PAS). See also color plates

hyperplasia without any diagnostic features. Hemophagocytic activity is rarely found at this stage'. Features that mimic myelodysplasia, dyserythropoiesis and abnormal granulocytes with Pelger–Huet change have been described early in the disease (Imashuku *et al.*, 2000). The activated and enlarged macrophages are more easily seen on marrow aspirates in early disease (Figure 16.2) but if the marrow biopsy is immunostained to reveal the macrophages, the increased number and large size of regularly spaced macrophages are evident. CD163 and CD68 are useful markers for macrophages. CD68–PGM-1 antibody is preferable because, unlike the KP-1 antibody, early myeloid precursors are not stained. With progression of disease, the macrophages become more prominent as the marrow is progressively depleted of hematopoietic elements. As in other sites, the macrophages are accompanied by an infiltrate of small lymphocytes (Chang *et al.*, 2003) but without plasma cells; and hemophagocytosis can be prominent. Fibrin deposits are said to be characteristic of HLH (Goldberg and Nezelof, 1986). Importantly, the macrophages are always cytologically bland (Henter *et al.*, 1998). Histiocytes may come to dominate the marrow due to disease progression or, in part, to cytotoxic therapy. Bone marrow involvement was only found in about 40% of children at autopsy, although the marrow was severely hypoplastic in some (Ost *et al.*, 1998).

Liver

Liver involvement is common in all forms of childhood HLH (Favara, 1996; Ost, 1998; deKerguenec *et al.*, 2001; Jaffe, 2004). Hepatosplenomegaly is one of the defining clinical findings (Henter *et al.*, 1991), and is accompanied by elevated hepatocellular enzyme levels, hyperbilirubinemia, hypofibrinogenemia, hypertriglyceridemia and hyperferritinemia. FHL can present as fulminant hepatic failure in the infant and the high ferritin levels mimic neonatal hemochromatosis (Parizhskaya *et al.*, 1999; Natsheh *et al.*, 2001). Recurrence of primary HLH in the liver, after liver transplantation is described (Parizhskaya *et al.*, 1999). All reports accentuate the fact that liver involvement in FHL is primarily portal, with a dominant lymphocytic element that simulates chronic hepatitis. The pattern of chronic hepatitis on liver biopsy in an infant is said to be distinctive enough to raise suspicion of FHL (Favara, 1996). The portal infiltrate is mostly T-lymphocytes with admixed histiocytes that have little, if any, hemophagocytosis (Ost *et al.*, 1998). FHL-2 infants will generally have a T-cell infiltrate that lacks perforin staining, a feature not seen in other forms of HLH (Figure 16.3). Staining of the portal macrophages (CD163+, CD68+) reveals coarse granular cytoplasmic staining of large numbers of cells in contrast to the more vacuolar and hemophagocytic appearance displayed by the Kupffer cells although this pattern is not always present (Ost *et al.*, 1998). Central venulitis and the presence of large, vacuolated 'floating' intravascular cells are well demonstrated with the macrophage stains (Favara, 1996). Bile duct damage is not a feature, ductular proliferation is not seen and cholestasis, if present, is canalicular.

Lymph node

Lymph nodes are conspicuously enlarged in less than one-third of HLH patients (Favara, 1992). Definitive involvement of nodes has, however, been found in about 75% of children at autopsy (Ost *et al.*, 1998). The natural history suggests that nodal enlargement is an early phenomenon, with progressive infiltration of sinuses and the interfollicular paracortex with macrophages (Figure 16.4). Hemophagocytosis

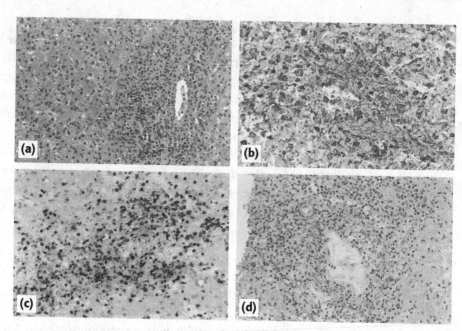

Figure 16.3   Liver. (a) A mixed lymphohistiocytic infiltrate is concentrated on the portal areas. The large, pale, 'floating' macrophages are noted in a portal vein. (b) Immunostain for the macrophage marker CD163 reveals the extensive portal (and sinusoidal) macrophage infiltrate (diamino-benzidine (DAB)). (c) CD3 stain reveals that the vast majority of the lymphocytes are T-cells (DAB). (d) Perforin immunostain is negative in FHL-2 but not in the other variants or in cases of hepatitis in which many of the T-cells contain perforin. See also color plates

is more prominent in the sinuses than the paracortex. Immunostaining for CD163 or CD68 will highlight the bland macrophages but also accentuates the negative unstained contours of the phagocytosed cells within their vacuolar cytoplasm.

As the disease progresses, even without treatment, there is depletion of lymphocytes, with preservation of the general architecture (Janka, 1983; Henter and Elinder, 1991; Favara, 1992; Ost et al., 1998). The paracortex is depleted, follicles become small and inconspicuous, and follicular germinal centers disappear (Ost et al., 1998) or become epithelioid. The sinuses dilate as the lymphoid depletion becomes more extreme and hemophagocytosis may become more evident.

Fine-needle aspirations (FNA) of lymph nodes may increase the chances of documenting hemophagocytosis when the bone marrow is not diagnostic, and can assist in establishing the diagnosis (Arico et al., 1996).

Spleen

Splenic enlargement is an early finding in 84–98% of HLH cases (Janka, 1983; Henter and Elinder, 1991). Splenomegaly ≥3 cm below the costal margin is one of the diagnostic criteria for HLH, and the splenomegaly can reach massive proportions.

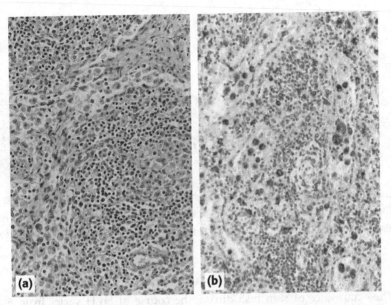

Figure 16.4 Lymph node. (a) Early active disease is primarily sinus in distribution. Large macrophages, some with hemophagocytosis, fill the sinuses. (b) CD68 highlights the large phagocytic cells and their cytoplasmic vacuoles (CD68, KP-1, DAB). See also color plates

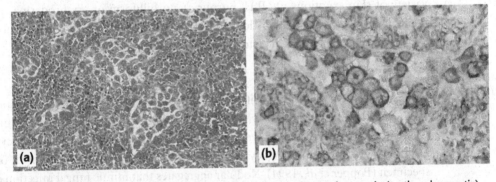

Figure 16.5 Spleen. (a) The splenic sinuses are filled with large hemophagocytic (erythrophagocytic) macrophages. (b) CD163 immunostain highlights these cells and negative images of intracytoplasmic erythrocytes can be noted (DAB). See also color plates

Splenic involvement was found in 71% of cases at autopsy (Ost *et al.*, 1998), although diagnostic features may be masked by extensive hemosiderin deposition. The disease involves the red pulp that is markedly expanded, in part by accumulation of hemophagocytic macrophages in the splenic sinuses (Figure 16.5). The white pulp, like lymphoid tissue elsewhere, undergoes progressive depletion with time. Splenic puncture to increase the chance of finding hemophagocytosis (Henter and Elinder, 1991; Arico *et al.*, 1996) may be dangerous in view of the coexisting coagulopathy.

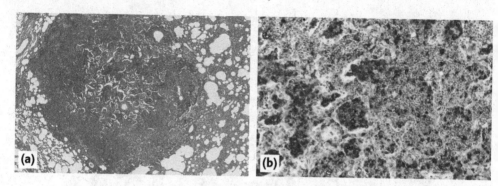

Figure 16.6   Lung. (a) Nodular lesions with a peribronchial distribution are rarely seen in patients with HLH. These are not known to contain organisms after extensive search and culture. (b) Alveolar, but also interstitial, macrophages comprise the lesions (DAB, CD68). See also color plates

Skin

The occurrence of skin rash during the course of HLH varies from 6% (Janka, 1983) to 65% (Morrell *et al.*, 2002), and is usually described as 'non-specific and maculopapular'. Favara (1992) reported a lymphohistiocytic infiltrate without hemophagocytosis in the reticular dermis. Morell *et al.* (2002) catalogs a wider variety of skin eruptions in HLH, purpuric, morbilliform or erythroderma, and their biopsies had non-diagnostic features with perivascular lymphohistiocytosis and no detectable hemophagocytosis.

Lung

Lung 'involvement' without specific details is mentioned in various reviews (Janka 1983; Henter *et al.*, 1998; Ost *et al.*, 1998). Symptomatic lung involvement in three children, with biopsy in two, showed peribronchial and interstitial lymphohistiocytic infiltrates without hemophagocytosis, with a granulomatous component in one specimen (Popper *et al.*, 1994). Nodular aggregates that mimic fungal infection do occur, and should be recognizable with CD163 or CD68 immunostaining of the infiltrate (Figure 16.6).

Central nervous system and spinal fluid

Pleocytosis of the spinal fluid is common in HLH, though frank hemophagocytosis is not. A count of $<50 \times 10^6$ cell/l of mainly mononuclear cells is regarded as supporting diagnostic evidence. Central nervous system (CNS) involvement can occur in the absence of cerebrospinal fluid (CSF) pleocytosis, the pleocytosis is thought to represent meningeal infiltration (Favara, 1992). CNS involvement can be present in about 20% of patients at presentation and in half or more during the disease course (Haddad *et al.*, 1997; Henter *et al.*, 1998). In a small number of children the cerebromeningeal involvement may precede systemic disease which may even be

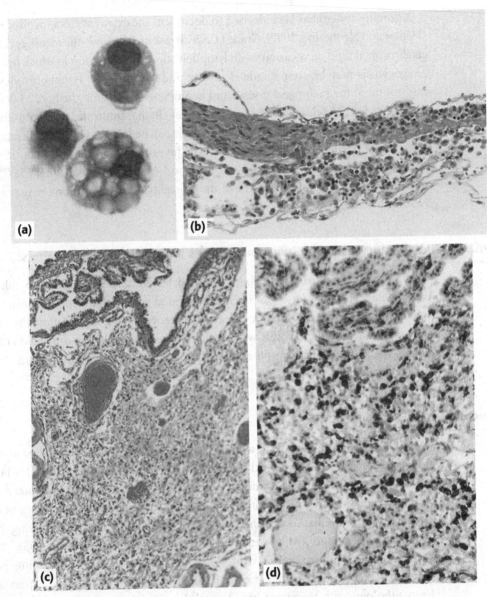

Figure 16.7   CNS. (a) Spinal fluid. Monocytoid and hemophagocytic macrophages are a common finding in the CSF during active disease. (b) A spinal nerve root reveals the presence of macrophages within the leptomeninges. (c) Subchoroidal ventricular areas are a site for HLH infiltration. (d) Immunostaining for CD68 reveals the extensive macrophage presence in the area represented in (c) (DAB). See also color plates

restricted to the CNS (Henter and Elinder, 1992). Combined with the fact that cerebromeningeal disease can be accompanied by ocular features that include retinal infiltrates or hemorrhage, this has led to suspicion of child abuse in some instances (Rooms *et al.*, 2003) (Figure 16.7).

A grading system has been devised to document the extent of CNS involvement (Henter and Nennesmo, 1997). Grade I CNS disease involves only the meninges (and cerebrospinal fluid on occasion) with lymphohistiocytic infiltration in which hemophagocytosis may be seen. Grade II disease adds perivascular lymphohistiocytic infiltration to the meningeal disease and hemophagocytosis may be hard to document. Grade III disease adds diffuse intraparenchymal infiltrates with multifocal necrosis and reactive astrogliosis. Leukomalacia can be followed by mineralization. The sites of particular vulnerability include the posterior pituitary (Janka, 1983) and the pineal (Favara, 1992) sites where the blood–brain barrier is lacking. The CNS involvement is responsible for some of the mortality in this condition (Henter and Nennesmo, 1997).

Primary HLH, histiocytosis with joint contractures and sensorineural deafness

A Pakistani kindred from Faisalabad had the defect localized to 11q25 (Moynihan *et al.*, 1998). The disorder began in early childhood with eyelid involvement in the index child, followed by systemic disease with generalized lymphadenopathy and hypergammaglobulinemia, but without hepatosplenomegaly. An unrelated child with similar features had lymph node pathology that simulated Rosai–Dorfman's histiocytosis.

Secondary HLH

Macrophage activation may occur secondary to a number of disorders including infection- and malignancies-associated hemophagocytic syndrome (IAHS and MAHS, respectively) and rheumatic disorders (Grom, 2003). The macrophage activation and resulting hypercytokinemia accounts for the secondary hemophagocytic syndromes (secondary HLH) (Chapters 18 and 19). There has been progress in identifying the different T-cell subsets involved in the macrophage activation (Mosser, 2003).

Most authors emphasize that clinical and cytokine profiles do not distinguish between primary and secondary hemophagocytic syndromes. The same is true for histopathology, with the single broad generalization, that secondary HLH often has less of a lymphocytic presence than primary HLH; although this is not true for EBV-associated disease.

In documenting the secondary HLH that can accompany systemic Langerhans cell histiocytosis (LCH), five categories of involvement were described (Favara *et al.*, 2002). Category I included cases with fully defined hemophagocytic syndrome that meets the diagnostic guidelines. These patients had hemophagocytosis as well as fever, hepatosplenomegaly, cytopenias, hypofibrinogenemia and hypertriglyceridemia. Category II consisted of cases with hemophagocytosis and at least two, but not all of the features in Category I. Category III included cases with hemophago-cytosis in any tissue and signs of macrophage activation in the liver, enlarged Kupffer cells that have light S100+ staining. Category IV cases had only hemophagocytosis in marrow, lymph node or liver but no other signs of macrophage activation. Category V documented instances of macrophage activation limited to the liver, but without hemophagocytosis.

Histopathology of secondary HLH

Since secondary HLH may be triggered by infectious or neoplastic stimuli, the presence of the responsible agent or malignancy may be an important finding. In this category, EBV is probably the most important (Janka *et al.*, 1998) and some of these patients may have mutations in the SH2 D1A gene leading to the molecular defect characteristic of the X-linked lymphoproliferative syndrome. It is important to stain for EBV by doing an EBER-1 probe in all instances of HLH to exclude or document the presence of viral RNA (Figure 16.8). The association with malignancy is complex; in most instances the macrophage activation occurs before or during treatment for a known malignancy. Occasionally HLH is the herald of a masked and undiagnosed malignancy. Of these, the NK/T-cell leukemia/lymphomas which are linked to EBV are probably the most common in childhood (Janka *et al.*, 1998).

Bone marrow

The histologic features can be progressive with time but also cyclical, so that a wide spectrum of findings is noted in secondary HLH as it is in primary HLH. Enlarged macrophages with abundant cytoplasm are widely scattered in the early stages and the degree of hemophagocytosis can vary (Chang *et al.*, 2003). Stromal damage

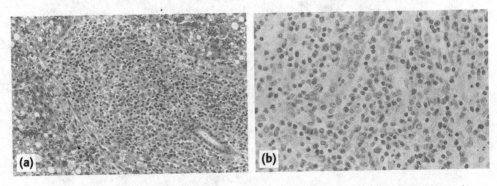

Figure 16.8 EBV-related HLH, liver. (a) A mixed lymphohistiocytosis is seen that markedly expands the portal area. (b) EBER-1 probe highlights the intranuclear presence of EBV RNA in lymphocytic nuclei. This was not an instance of X-linked lymphoproliferative syndrome (XLPD) which usually has a more activated lymphoid presence, more EBV and greater hepatocellular necrosis. See also color plates

with edema and 'pink fat' can be an early feature. As the marrow becomes more depleted, the numbers of large phagocytic macrophages become increased and even confluent. CD163 and CD68 are useful markers. Dilated vascular sinuses may contain large floating phagocytic macrophages.

Liver

Macrophage activation causes functional and histopathologic changes in the liver. Hepatic features were described in 30 patients with secondary HLH (deKerguenec et al., 2001). Hepatomegaly was noted in half, and raised hepatocellular enzyme levels and ferritin were noted in all. The triad of high levels of bilirubin and alkaline phosphatase associated with low levels of factor V was associated with a poor outcome. Increased numbers of enlarged Kupffer cells with prominent hemophagocytic activity were accompanied by sinusoidal dilation.

These large activated Kupffer cells are S100+, and are well seen with CD68 (KP-1) or CD163 staining (Favara, 1996). 'Floating' phagocytic macrophages are seen in central and portal veins. There are no studies to date that clearly separate the histopathology of the liver in the primary from those of secondary HLH. Review of familial cases, including those with perforin defect, demonstrate that most instances of primary

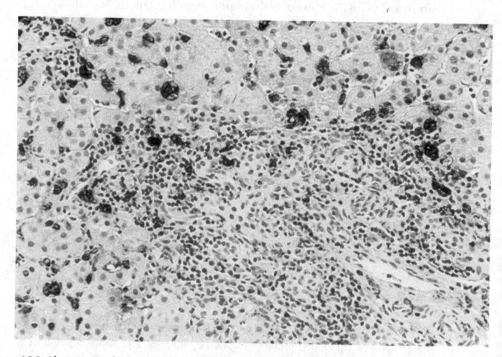

Figure 16.9 Liver. Macrophage activation syndrome in a child with hepatitis shows the presence of phagocytic sinusoidal Kupffer cells, but lacks the presence of the portal macrophages typical of HLH (contrast with Figure 16.3(b)) (CD68, KP-1, DAB). See also color plates

HLH have a prominent portal lymphoid infiltrate whereas, secondary HLH has Kupffer cell hyperplasia without the portal component (Figure 16.9) (Jaffe, 2004). This is less true for EBV-related disorders or those associated with leukemic infiltrates.

Canalicular and intracellular cholestasis can be been in the absence of biliary obstructive changes (Tsui *et al.*, 1992; deKerguenec *et al.*, 2001). Occasionally, there are hepatocellular necroses that can reach massive proportions, especially in the x-linked lymphoproliferative syndrome (Markin, 1994).

Apart from the instances of massive hepatic necrosis, all features of the hemophagocytic syndromes in the liver appear to be reversible without consequence.

Skin

Smith *et al.* (1992) described 10 patients with skin involvement as part of secondary HLH associated with viral infections or lymphoma. A variety of changes was seen, some of diagnostic value. Hemorrhage with or without associated hemophagocytosis and microthrombi may be present. In some, edema and hemorrhage extend from the dermis into the subcutaneous fat and hemophagocytosis can be prominent at this site – the so-called 'cytophagic histiocytic panniculitis'. The bland histiocytes are usually accompanied by a sparse to moderate T-cell infiltrate. EBER-1 probe for EBV is positive in the lymphocytes in some instances, and malignant cells are usually present in those cases of macrophage activation associated with leukemia.

Summary

In general, the histopathology of the primary and secondary hemophagocytic syndromes is only contributory to the diagnosis. Not only are their manifestations largely similar in all sites, but hemophagocytosis is not specific to the HLH. The macrophages themselves are cytologically bland and are not the cells that harbor the defect in most instances.

REFERENCES

Arico, M., Janka, H., Fischer, A., *et al.* (1996). Hemophagocytic lymphohistiocytosis: diagnosis, treatment and prognostic factors. Report of 122 children from the international registry. *Leukemia*, **10**, 197–203.

Chang, K.L., Gaal, K.K., Huang, Q., *et al.* (2003). Histiocytic lesions involving the bone marrow. *Semin Diagn Pathol*, **20**, 226–236.

deKerguenec, C., Hillaire, S., Molinié, V., *et al.* (2001). Hepatic manifestations of hemophagocytic syndrome. A study of 30 cases. *Am J Gastroenterol*, **3**, 852–857.

Farquhar, J.W. and Claireaux, A.E. (1952). Familial haemophagocytic reticulosis. *Arch Dis Child*, **27**, 519–525.

Favara, B.E. (1992). Hemophagocytic lymphohistiocytosis: a hemophagocytic syndrome. *Semin Diagn Pathol*, **9**, 63–74.

Favara, B.E. (1996). Histopathology of the liver in histiocytosis syndromes. *Pediatr Pathol Lab Med*, **16**, 413–433.

Favara, B.E., Feller, A.C., Pauli, M., *et al.* (1997). Contemporary classification of histiocytic disorders. *Med Pediatr Oncol*, **29**, 157–166.

Favara, B.E., Jaffe, R. and Egeler, R.M. (2002). Macrophage activation and hemophagocytic syndrome in Langerhans cell histocytosis: report of 30 cases. *Pediatr Dev Pathol*, **5**, 130–140.

Feldmann, J., Le Diest, F., Ouchee-Chardin, M., *et al.* (2002). Functional consequences of perforin gene mutations in 22 patients with familial haemophagocytic lymphohistiocytosis. *Br J Haematol*, **117**, 965–972.

Feldmann, J., Callebaut, I., Raposo, G., *et al.* (2003). Munc 13-4 is essential for cytolytic granules fusion and is mutated in a form of familial hemophagocytic lymphohistiocytosis (FHL3). *Cell*, **115**, 461–473.

Fujihara, M., Muroi, M., Tanamoto, K., *et al.* (2003). Molecular mechanisms of macrophage activation and deactivation by lipopolysaccharide: roles of the receptor complex. *Pharmacol Ther*, **100**, 171–194.

Goldberg, J. and Nezelof, C. (1986). Lymphohistiocytosis: a multi-factorial syndrome of macrophagic activation. Clinico-pathological study of 38 cases. *Hematol Oncol*, **4**, 275–289.

Goldstein, J.I., Goldstein, K.A., Wardwell, K., *et al.* (2003). Increase in plasma and surface CD163 levels in patients undergoing coronary artery bypass graft surgery. *Atherosclerosis*, **170**, 325–332.

Grom, A.A. (2003). Macrophage activation syndrome and reactive hemophagocytic lymphohistiocytosis: the same entities? *Curr Opin Rheumatol*, **15**, 587–590.

Haddad, E., Sulis, M.L., Jabado, N., *et al.* (1997). Frequency and severity of central nervous system lesions in hemophagocytic lymphohistiocytosis. *Blood*, **89**, 794–800.

Haridas, V., McCloskey, T.W., Pahwa, R., *et al.* (2003). Discordant expression of perforin and granzyme A in total and HIV-specific CD8 T lymphocytes of HIV infected children and adolescents. *AIDS*, **17**, 2313–2322.

Henter, J.I. (2002). Biology and treatment of familial hemophagocytic lymphohistiocytosis: importance of perforin in lymphocyte-mediated cytotoxicity and triggering of apoptosis. *Med Pediatr Oncol*, **38**, 305–309.

Henter, J.I. and Elinder, G. (1991). Familial hemophagocytic lymphohistiocytosis. Clinical review based on the findings in seven children. *Acta Paediatr Scand*, **80**, 269–277.

Henter, J.I. and Elinder, G. (1992). Cerebromeningeal hemophagocytic lymphohistiocytosis. *Lancet*, **339**, 104–107.

Henter, J.I. and Elinder, G. (1995). Haemophagocytic lymphohistiocytosis: an inherited primary form and a reactive secondary form. *Br J Haematol*, **91**, 774–775.

Henter, J.I. and Nennesmo, I. (1997). Neuropathologic findings and neurologic symptoms in twenty-three children with hemophagocytic lymphohistiocytosis. *J Pediatr*, **130**, 358–365.

Henter, J.I., Elinder, G., Ost, A., and the FHL Study Group of the Histiocyte Society. (1991). Diagnostic guidelines for hemophagocytic lymphohistiocytosis. *Semin Oncol*, **18**, 29–33.

Henter, J.I., Ehrnst, A., Andersson, J., *et al.* (1993). Familial hemophagocytic lymphohistiocytosis and viral infections. *Acta Paediatr*, **82**, 369–372.

Henter, J.I., Arico, M., Elinder, G., *et al.* (1998). Familial hemophagocytic lymphohistiocytosis. Primary hemophagocytic lymphohistiocytosis. *Hematol Oncol Clin North Am*, **12**, 417–433.

Imashuku, S., Kitazawa, K., Ishii, M., *et al.* (2000). Bone marrow changes mimicking myelodysplasia in patients with hemophagocytic lymphohistiocytosis. *Int J Hematol*, **72**, 353–357.

Jaffe, R. (2004). Liver involvement in the histiocytic disorders of childhood. *Pediatr Dev Pathol.* **7**, 214–225.

Janka, G. (1983). Familial hemophagocytic lymphohistiocytosis. *Eur J Pediatr*, **140**, 221–230.

Janka, G., Imashuku, S., Elinder, G., *et al.* (1998). Infection- and malignancy-associated hemophagocytic syndromes. Secondary hemophagocytic lymphohistiocytosis. *Hematol Oncol Clin North Am*, **12**, 435–444.

Katano, H., Ali, M.A., Patera, A.C., *et al.* (2004). Chronic active Epstein–Barr virus infection associated with mutations in perforin that impair its maturation. *Blood*, **103**, 1244–1252.

Kessary-Shoham, H., Levy, Y., Shoenfeld, Y., *et al.* (1999). *In vivo* administration of intravenous immunoglobulin (IVIg) can lead to enhanced erythrocyte sequestration. *J Autoimmun*, **13**, 129–135.

Kogawa, K., Lee, S.M., Villanueva, J., *et al.* (2002). Perforin expression in cytotoxic lymphocytes from patients with hemophagocytic lymphohistiocytosis and their family members. *Blood*, **99**, 61–66.

Lammas, D.A, DeHeer, E., Edgar, J.D., *et al.* (2002). Heterogeneity in the granulomatous response to mycobacterial infection in patients with defined genetic mutations in the interleukin 12-depende interferon-gamma production pathway. *Int J Exp Pathol*, **83**, 1–20.

Listinsky, C.M. (1988). Common reactive erythrophagocytosis in axillary lymph nodes. *Am J Clin Pathol*, **90**, 189–192.

Maher, K.J., Klimas, N.G., Hurwitz, B., *et al.* (2002). Quantitative fluorescence measures for determination of intracellular perforin content. *Clin Diagn Lab Immunol*, **9**, 1248–1252.

Markin, R.S. (1994). Manifestations of Ebstein–Barr virus-associated disorders of liver. *Liver*, **14**, 1–13.

Morrell, D.S., Pepping, M.A., Scott, J.P., *et al.* (2002). Cutaneous manifestations of hemophagocytic lymphohistiocytosis. *Arch Dermatol*, **138**, 1208–1212.

Mosser, D.M. (2003). The many faces of macrophage activation. *J Leukoc Biol*, **73**, 209–212.

Moynihan, L.M., Bundey, S.E., Heath, D., *et al.* (1998). Autozygosity mapping, to chromosome 11q25, of a rare autosomal recessive syndrome causing histiocytosis, joint contractures, and sensorineural deafness. *Am J Hum Genet*, **62**, 1123–1128.

Natsheh, S.E., Roberts, E.A., Ngan, B., *et al.* (2001). Liver failure with marked hyperferritinemia; 'ironing out' the diagnosis. *Can J Gastroenterol*, **15**, 537–540.

Ost, A., Nilsson-Ardnor, S. and Henter, J.I. (1998). Autopsy findings in 27 children with haemophagocytic lymphohistiocytosis. *Histopathology*, **32**, 310–316.

Parizhskaya, M., Reyes, J. and Jaffe, R. (1999). Hemophagocytic syndrome presenting as acute hepatic failure in two infants: clinical overlap with neonatal hemochromatosis. *Pediatr Dev Pathol*, **2**, 360–366.

Popper, H.H., Zenz, W., Mache, C., *et al.* (1994). Familial haemophagocytic lymphohistiocytosis. A report of three cases with unusual lung involvement. *Histopathology*, **25**, 439–445.

Rooms, L., Fitzgerald, N. and McClain, K.L. (2003). Hemophagocytic lymphohistiocytosis masquerading as child abuse: presentation of three cases and review of central nervous system findings of hemophagocytic lymphohistiocytosis. *Pediatrics*, **111**, 636–640.

Smith, K.J., Skelton, H.G., Yeager, J., *et al.* (1992). Cutaneous histopathologic, immunohistochemical, and clinical manifestations in patients with hemophagocytic syndrome. *Arch Dermatol*, **128**, 193–200.

Stepp, S.E., Dufourcq-Lagelouse, R., Le Diest, F., *et al.* (1999). Perforin gene defects in familial hemophagocytic lymphohistiocytosis. *Science*, **286**, 1957–1959.

Suster, S., Hilsenbeck, S. and Rywlin, A.M. (1988). Reactive histiocytic hyperplasia with hemophagocytosis in hematopoietic organs: a reevaluation of the benign hemophagocytic proliferations. *Hum Pathol*, **19**, 705–712.

Tsui, W.M., Wong, K.F. and Tse, C.C. (1992). Liver changes in reactive haemophagocytic syndrome. *Liver*, **12**, 363–367.

zur Stadt, U., Kabisch, H., Janka, G., *et al.* (2003). Rapid LightCycler assay for identification of the perforin codon 375 Trp → stop mutation in patients and families with hemophagocytic lymphohistiocytosis (HLH). *Med Pediatr Oncol*, 41, 26–29.

17

Genetics and pathogenesis of hemophagocytic lymphohistiocytosis

Kim Ericson, Bengt Fadeel and Jan-Inge Henter

Introduction

Farquhar and Claireaux published a report in 1952 of a disease characterized by progressive erythropaenia, neutropaenia and thrombocytopaenia, despite a reactive bone marrow, and named it familial hemophagocytic reticulosis (Farquhar and Claireaux, 1952). In the 50 years since their seminal report, the knowledge and understanding of this condition, now termed hemophagocytic lymphohistiocytosis (HLH), has increased rapidly. It is now well established that familial HLH (FHL) is a primary immunodeficiency, characterized by hypercytokinemia (elevated serum levels of inflammatory cytokines) and a concomitant defect in natural killer (NK) cell cytotoxicity (Perez et al., 1984; Arico et al., 1988; Eife et al., 1989; Henter et al., 1998; Sullivan et al., 1998; Kogawa et al., 2002). Recent genetic studies have revealed underlying molecular defects in FHL patients, greatly improving our understanding of the basic pathogenesis of this disease. Deciphering the underlying molecular mechanism of immunodeficiency in FHL patients may also teach us more about the role of cellular cytotoxicity in immune homoeostasis under normal conditions.

Pathogenesis of HLH

Cytotoxic T lymphocytes- and NK cell-mediated apoptosis

Lymphocyte-mediated cytotoxicity is the main pathway for tumour surveillance and for eradicating virus-infected cells and intracellular pathogens. The effector lymphocytes are the cytotoxic T lymphocytes (CTLs) and NK cells, which act by killing their cellular targets through induction of apoptosis. CTLs and NK cells utilize either of two mechanisms for killing, both of which require direct contact between effector and target cells. The first pathway is non-secretory, and depends on the engagement and aggregation of target cell death receptors, such as Fas, and its cognate ligand, Fas ligand (FasL), on the killer cell membrane. The cytoplasmic tail of

Fas contains a motif called the 'death domain', able to mediate a death signal upon oligomerization with subsequent activation of the caspase cascade, resulting in classical caspase-dependent apoptosis (as reviewed in Russell and Ley, 2002). The main function of the Fas–FasL pathway is to eliminate self-reactive lymphoid cells. The second pathway involves a cytoplasmic granule toxin, perforin, and a family of structurally related serine proteases (granzymes). Adhesion of the CTLs to the target cell, via interaction of the T-cell receptor (TCR) and the antigen–MHC (major histocompatability complex) complex, triggers a Ca^{2+}-dependent degranulation. Perforin and granzymes are then secreted and together induce apoptosis of the target cell in a caspase-dependent or -independent manner (as reviewed in Lieberman, 2003). This pathway operates mainly in viral defence and immune surveillance against cancer, but recent studies in mice and humans indicate that perforin may also play a role in the maintenance of immune homoeostasis (Smyth *et al.*, 2001).

The immune system has a remarkable capacity to maintain a state of dynamic equilibrium despite recurrent exposure to a diverse array of organisms and constant exposure to self-antigens. In HLH, the state of dynamic equilibrium has been disrupted, causing an unbalanced expansion and activation of CTLs and macrophages, resulting in hemophagocytosis. Importantly, recent molecular characterizations reveal that some of the inherited forms of HLH can be explained by defects in the perforin–granzyme cell death pathway.

Lymphocyte cytotoxicity dysfunction: a basic defect

The pathophysiology of HLH is characterized by markedly decreased or absent CTL and NK cell activity (Perez *et al.*, 1984; Arico *et al.*, 1988; Eife *et al.*, 1989; Henter *et al.*, 1998; Sullivan *et al.*, 1998; Kogawa *et al.*, 2002). The defect in CTL and NK cell cytotoxicity is restored by bone marrow transplantation. The recent discovery of mutations in the genes-encoding perforin and MUNC13-4 (discussed below) offers a plausible explanation for the defect in cytotoxicity, at least in some cases of HLH. Perforin is an apoptosis-triggering agent required for granzyme B to induce apoptosis in target cells and MUNC13-4 has been shown to be important for the exocytosis of the perforin-containing granules from effector lymphocytes. Lack of perforin expression or absence of perforin release will ultimately have the same outcome: a defect in CTL and NK cell-dependent induction of apoptosis in target cells.

A recent study described four distinct defects in cellular cytotoxicity in HLH patients. These authors defined groups 1, 2 and 4 as a reduced or absent cytolytic function against K562 target cells that could be reconstituted by mitogen, interleukin (IL)-2 or prolonged effector-to-target incubation time, respectively. The majority of the patients, however, belonged to so-called group 3, in which the cytotoxic activity could not be reconstituted. Perforin mutations were found in some patients in the latter group, while the genetic defect in the remaining patients was unknown (Schneider *et al.*, 2003). Nevertheless, one may speculate that the heterogeneity of defects in cellular cytotoxicity in HLH patients may be associated with distinct molecular defects.

Hypercytokinemia: a consequence of immune dysregulation

Hypercytokinemia is a central part of HLH pathophysiology (Henter *et al.*, 1991). NK-cells and CTLs belong to different lymphocyte lineages, but share a common mechanism to exert their cytotoxic function. NK cell triggering results in cytotoxicity and in the production of cytokines that exert a regulatory role in immune and inflammatory responses. CTLs are important mediators of adaptive immunity. During the initial encounter with an intracellular microbe, CTLs bearing TCRs specific for pathogen-derived antigens are selected to undergo clonal expansion. As a result, pathogen-specific CTLs rapidly increase under cytokine influence. These expanded populations of effector CTLs contribute to the clearance of the pathogen and then decline in numbers to a memory level, through a process of activation-induced cell death (apoptosis). In HLH, the expansion of CTLs under the influence of elevated Th1 cytokines is sustained and the decline fails to occur. It is reasonable to assume that the cytokine alterations in HLH are linked to the defect in cytotoxicity and apoptosis triggering in these individuals (Fadeel *et al.*, 2001).

The NK-cell stimulatory cytokine, IL-12, is elevated in HLH patients. It has a broad array of activities, acting on both T- and NK cells to induce production of interferon (IFN)-γ, leading to further enhancement of IL-12 production. The elevated levels of IL-12 and IFN-γ in HLH skew the immune response towards a Th1-type response (Osugi *et al.*, 1997). Several other inflammatory cytokines are elevated, including IL-1 receptor antagonist, soluble IL-2 receptor, IL-6 and tumour necrosis factor (TNF)-α (Henter *et al.*, 1998). The Th2 cytokines, IL-4 and IL-10, are not elevated in HLH. In a proposed hypothesis of a cytokine network in HLH, Th1 cells, initially stimulated with pathogens, secrete IL-2 and IFN-γ. IFN-γ stimulates macrophages to induce rapid production of IL-12, IL-1 and TNF-α (Osugi *et al.*, 1997). Emminger *et al.* have described an expansion of monocytes producing the inflammatory cytokines TNF-α, IL-1β and IL-6 in HLH, but almost no anti-inflammatory IL-10. IL-1, in turn, is known to activate T-cells and to induce the production of IL-2 (Emminger *et al.*, 2001).

Molecular genetics of HLH

Linkage analyses in HLH patients

Primary or familial HLH is an autosomal recessive disease. In 1999, two different disease loci were identified by homozygosity mapping. Ohadi *et al.* showed linkage to 9q21.3–22 (FHL1) in four of five families with a maximum LOD score of 6.05.

So far, only a few FHL patients have been reported showing linkage to FHL1 and the responsible gene is still unknown (Ohadi *et al.*, 1999; Goransdotter Ericson *et al.*, 2001). A French group described linkage to 10q21–22 (FHL2) in 10 of 17 families with a maximum multipoint LOD score of 11.22 at the marker D10S1650 (Dufourcq-Lagelouse *et al.*, 1999). At this locus the gene-encoding perforin, a protein known to be important for lymphocyte cytotoxicity, was subsequently found to be mutated in FHL2 patients (Stepp *et al.*, 1999). Several groups have reported further evidence of genetic heterogeneity in HLH, with at least three possible loci (Graham *et al.*, 2000; Goransdotter Ericson *et al.*, 2001). Sequencing of the perforin gene and genetic linkage in a cohort of 34 patients with FHL and their parents have shown that only 10% of patients map to chromosome 9q21.3–22 and approximately 20–40% to chromosome 10 (Goransdotter Ericson *et al.*, 2001). Recently, mutations in the gene MUNC13-4 at chromosome 17q25 were identified (Feldmann *et al.*, 2003) (see below). The proportion of HLH patients carrying this mutation remains to be determined.

The role of perforin for granule-mediated killing

Perforin is one of the major cytolytic proteins in lytic granules in NK cells and CTLs. Recent studies indicate some expression also in CD4+ T lymphocytes and neutrophils (Wagner *et al.*, 2004). Perforin is synthesized as a 70 kDa precursor that is cleaved at the carboxyl terminus to yield the active 60 kDa form (Uellner *et al.*, 1997). The protein shows partial homology in structure to complement component C9 and other components of the complement system (Podack, 1992; Liu *et al.*, 1995) (Figure 17.1). Therefore, in the original paradigm, perforin was thought to directly induce target cell death by damaging the target cell membrane, causing cell lysis similar to that induced by complement or by acting as a pore-forming protein allowing granzymes to enter the target cell. However, recent studies have shown that granzyme B can enter target cells without perforin (Motyka *et al.*, 2000; Metkar *et al.*, 2002; Pinkoski and Green, 2002). The revised hypothesis holds that granzyme B can enter target cells without perforin; however, perforin is required for the release of granzymes from the endolysosomal compartment into the cytosol of the target cell. Granzyme B is then apparently rapidly trafficked to the nucleus (Trapani *et al.*, 1996), where it induces target cell DNA fragmentation and apoptosis, both in cells that contain caspases and those that do not. Caspases, however, appear to amplify the granzyme B signal (Talanian *et al.*, 1997; Trapani *et al.*, 1998).

Functional consequences of perforin deficiency

Mice lacking the perforin gene have been used to evaluate the role of perforin for granule-mediated cytotoxicity. These mice are healthy; however, the cytotoxic activity of CTLs and of NK cells is impaired. Perforin-deficient mice infected with

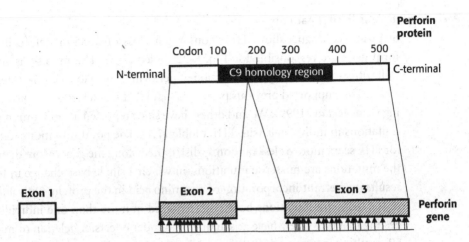

Figure 17.1   Schematic representation of the genomic organization of the perforin gene and the corresponding perforin protein. The gene has three exons, but only exons 2 and 3 are transcribed. The position of the C9 homology region in the protein is indicated by the filled box in the protein and positioned schematically by the codon numbering. The sites of identified disease-causing mutations in HLH patients are indicated by arrows

lymphocytic choriomeningitis virus (LMCV) exhibit an HLH-like phenotype driven by IFN-γ and TNF-α with an uncontrolled expansion of activated CTLs (Kagi *et al.*, 1999; Matloubian *et al.*, 1999). Studies in these mice indicate that perforin is involved in downregulating T-cell responses during chronic LMCV infection; however, the expansion of antigen-specific T lymphocytes might also be a result of reduced clearance and increased antigen load (Badovinac and Harty, 2000, 2002). Similarly, it has been suggested that viral infections may precipitate HLH in genetically predisposed individuals (Henter *et al.*, 1993). A recent study showed that perforin-deficient mice cleared infections with *Listeria monocytogenes* as effectively as wild-type mice. Importantly, the expansion of CTLs in perforin-deficient mice was 3- to 4-fold higher than in wild-type mice, while the downregulation of CTLs after clearance of infection was indistinguishable in the two groups (Badovinac *et al.*, 2002). Thus, a regulatory role for perforin in the process of antigen-specific T lymphocyte regulation is proposed from several studies, but the influence of other factors such as pathogen virulence, cytokine modulation and genetic factors remains to be elucidated. Interestingly, recent studies of mice deficient for myeloid Elf-1-like factor (MEF), a member of the erythroblast transformation-specific domain (ETS) family of transcription factors, have revealed a critical role for MEF in NK and NK–T-cell development as well as for perforin expression in NK cells. Despite a normal perforin gene status, perforin expression is severely impaired in NK cells from these mice, likely accounting for the lack of NK-mediated killing of tumour cells (Lacorazza *et al.*, 2002).

Perforin mutations in HLH patients

Stepp and colleagues showed that homozygous loss-of-function defects in the perforin gene are responsible for 10q21–22-linked HLH. The mutations correlated well with reduced or absent expression of perforin from cytotoxic cells (Stepp *et al.*, 1999). This supported previous proposals that HLH is a defect in apoptosis triggering (Fadeel *et al.*, 1999). We and others have since reported a spectrum of perforin mutations in individuals with FHL (Table 17.1). The point mutations responsible for FHL seem more or less randomly distributed along the gene. More than 70% of the mutations are missense mutations, in which a single base change in the DNA results in aberrant incorporation of an amino acid in the protein. Only a minority of the missense mutations have been reported in more than one individual, suggesting that only a few have arisen due to founder effects. A deletion of nucleotide 50, resulting in a frameshift at codon 17 and a truncated protein (Stepp *et al.*, 1999; Clementi *et al.*, 2001; Feldmann *et al.*, 2002; Kogawa *et al.*, 2002; Molleran Lee *et al.*, 2004), and a nonsense mutation, resulting in a premature stop codon and a truncated protein at codon 374 (Stepp *et al.*, 1999; Clementi *et al.*, 2001; Goransdotter Ericson *et al.*, 2001; Feldmann *et al.*, 2002; Suga *et al.*, 2002), are so far the most commonly reported mutations. The Leu17Fshft mutation has been reported in five different studies in a total of 14 patients of African origin. The Trp374Stop mutation has been identified in 13 patients of Turkish origin and one Japanese patient. The fact that these mutations were identified in patients of mainly African and Turkish origin, respectively, speaks in favour of a founder effect, although this remains to be proven. In the Japanese population, a 1090–1091delCT mutation has been observed in five FHL patients, of which at least four had ancestors originating from the same geographic area in south-western Japan (Suga *et al.*, 2002; Ueda *et al.*, 2003). The Ala91Val and the Asp252Ser mutations have been reported as potential disease-causing mutations (Stepp *et al.*, 1999; Clementi *et al.*, 2001; Feldmann *et al.*, 2002; Busiello *et al.*, 2004) as well as polymorphisms (Feldmann *et al.*, 2002; Molleran Lee *et al.*, 2004). The identification of mutations in the perforin gene has thus, for the first time, given rise to the possibility of a molecular diagnosis in FHL patients and prenatal diagnostics in affected families.

Genotype–phenotype correlation studies

In autosomal recessive disorders, which show a diverse array of mutations, clinical heterogeneity is not uncommon. Interestingly, a recent study aiming to characterize the genotype–phenotype correlation in 14 unrelated families with perforin deficiency concluded that clinical and biological analyses did not differentiate between patients with missense and nonsense mutations. The only manifestation that differed was age at diagnosis, which showed a higher variability in the missense group. In all patients the perforin gene mutations lead to absence of intracellular perforin

Table 17.1 Perforin mutations reported as disease-causing in the literature

	Nucleotide change	Mutation	Missense/nonsense/frameshift
1	1A > G	Met1Val	Missense
2	3G > A	Met1Leu	Missense
3	50delT	Leu17Fsht > Stop	Frameshift
4	116C > A	Pro39His	Missense
5	133G > A	Gly45Arg	Missense
6	134G > A	Gly45Glu	Missense
7	148G > A	Val50Met	Missense
8	160C > T	Arg54Ser	Missense
9	190C > T	Gln64Stop	Nonsense
10	207delC	Pro69Fshft > Stop	Frameshift
11	208G > T	Asp70Tyr	Missense
12	217T > C	Cys73Arg	Missense
13	265C > A	Pro89Thr	Missense
14♠	272C > T	Ala91Val	Missense
15	283T > C	Trp94Arg	Missense
16	445G > A	Gly149Ser	Missense
17	449C > A	Ser150Stop	Nonsense
18	469T > G	Phe157Val	Missense
19	548T > G	Val183Gly	Missense
20	657C > A	Tyr219Stop	Nonsense
21	658G > A	Gly220Ser	Missense
22	662C > T	Thr221Ile	Missense
23	665A > G	His222Arg	Missense
24	666C > A	His222Gln	Missense
25	671T > A	Ile224Asp	Missense
26	673C > T	Arg255Trp	Missense
27	694C > T	Arg232Cys	Missense
28	695G > A	Arg232His	Missense
29♠	755A > G	Asp252Ser	Missense
30	781G > A	Glu261Lys	Missense
31	836G > A	Cys279Tyr	Missense
32	853–855delAAG	ΔLys285	Frameshift
33	895C > T	Arg299Cys	Missense
34	938A > T	Asp313Val	Missense
35	949G > A	Gly317Arg	Missense
36	1034G > T	Pro345Thr	Missense
37	1081A > T	Arg361Trp	Missense
38	1083delG	Arg361Fshft > Stop	Frameshift

(*continued*)

Table 17.1 (*continued*)

	Nucleotide change	Mutation	Missense/nonsense/frameshift
39	1090–1091delCT	Leu364Fshft > Stop	Frameshift
40	1122G > A	Trp374Stop	Nonsense
41	1182insT	Glu394Fsht > Stop	Frameshift
42	1246C > T	Glu416Stop	Nonsense
43	1286G > A	Gly429Glu	Missense
44	1442A > C	Gln481Pro	Missense
45	1491T > A	Cys497Stop	Nonsense
46	1628insT	Leu543Fsht	Frameshift
47	1636delC	Gln546Fsht	Frameshift

♠ These mutations have been reported as disease-causing mutations as well as polymorphisms.

expression in cytotoxic cells, and in most individuals this correlated to an absence of cytotoxic activity. In a few patients, correlating to certain missense mutations, cytotoxic activity was still detectable, albeit significantly reduced (Feldmann *et al.*, 2002). This might be one explanation for the delayed onset of the disease for some of the patients carrying missense mutations. Other explanations might be the influence of environmental factor(s) such as infectious-triggering agents that might cause different phenotypes and differences in the severity of manifestations of the disease. In support of this, a patient diagnosed at birth by genetic analysis did not show features of an HLH phenotype (Feldmann *et al.*, 2002) and it is well known that siblings may develop quite different clinical pictures (Henter and Elinder, 1992).

Molecular biology of MUNC13-4 deficiency

The MUNC13-4 gene

MUNC13-4 is a mammalian homologue of the *Caenorhabditis elegans* gene-encoding UNC-13; mutations in the *unc-13* gene cause severely uncoordinated movements in the worm, hence the name. The human gene is mapped to chromosome 17q25 and encodes a protein likely to be important for the vesicle–plasma membrane fusion during exocytosis of cytotoxic granules from CTLs and NK cells. The mRNA encodes a 1088 amino acid protein (Figure 17.2). MUNC13-4 is expressed in various tissues, both haematopoietic and non-haematopoietic. In haematopoietic tissue, expression was seen in spleen, thymus and peripheral leucocytes with high levels of expression in CD19+ B lymphocytes, CD4+ lymphocytes, CD8+ lymphocytes and mononuclear cells (Feldmann *et al.*, 2003). MUNC13-1, -2 and -3 are

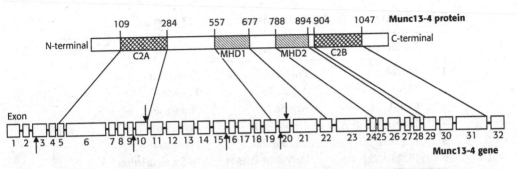

Figure 17.2   Schematic representation of the genomic organization of the Munc13-4 gene and the corresponding Munc13-4 protein. The position of the C2 domains (C2A and C2B) and the Munc homology domain (MHD1 and MHD2) in the Munc13-4 protein are represented by the filled boxes and positioned in relationship to the amino acid numbering. The sites of identified disease-causing mutations in HLH patients are indicated by arrows

other members of the MUNC13-like family (Li and Chin, 2003). These proteins are located in the cytosol. Subcellular localization studies of MUNC13-4 show that it differs from MUNC13-1, -2 and -3 insofar as MUNC13-4 partially co-localizes with perforin and cytotoxic granules in lymphocytes (Feldmann *et al.*, 2003).

The role of MUNC13-4 in cytotoxic granule exocytosis

The exact mechanism leading to synaptic vesicle exocytosis is not fully understood, but an essential step is the priming event. In neurosecretory cells the priming event requires MUNC13-1, -2 and -3. MUNC13-1 interacts with the SNARE (soluble N-ethylmaleimide-sensitive factor attachment protein receptor) complex, suggesting that the MUNC13 family of proteins might be of importance for priming of synaptic vesicles for fusion. The SNARE complex is known to play a central role in membrane fusion events. There are 36 different SNAREs in the human genome encoding proteins found in distinct compartments of the secretory and endocytic trafficking pathways, contributing to intracellular membrane fusion processes. In the SNARE model, t-SNAREs and v-SNAREs (present on target and vesicle membranes, respectively) assisted by several different proteins, are thought to recognize each other specifically and to form a core complex that brings the two membranes together, ultimately leading to fusion (Li and Chin, 2003). In addition, another protein, Rab27a, has been shown to be crucial for the exocytosis events, acting in the late stages. Mutations in the RAB27A gene in humans cause Griscelli disease, an inherited condition with similarities to HLH (Menasche *et al.*, 2000; Stinchcombe *et al.*, 2001). In a related condition, known as Chediak–Higashi syndrome (CHS), mutations in the LYST (lysosomal trafficking regulator)/CHS gene lead to enlarged and functionally abnormal lytic granules in CTLs and NK cells (Certain *et al.*, 2000; de Saint Basile and Fischer, 2003). Both conditions are associated with defective cellular cytotoxicity; RAB27A- and

Table 17.2 Disease-causing mutations in the Munc 13-4 gene

	Nucleotide change	Mutation	Missense/nonsense/frameshift
1	214delC	Pro72Fshft > Stop	Frameshift
2	753 + 1(G > T)	Asp252Fshft	Frameshift
3	C766T	Arg256X	Nonsense
4	1389 + 1(G > A)	Thr464Fshft	Frameshift
5	1755insT	His586Fshft	Frameshift
6	1822del12bp	DelVal608–Ala611	In-frame deletion

LYST/CHS-dependent defects in intracellular melanosome transport also occur, accounting for the partial albinism seen in these patients.

In MUNC13-4-deficient CTLs, the lytic granules polarize towards the point of contact with the target cell, as frequently as do granules from control cells. Thus, MUNC13-4 is not required for the microtubule-mediated movement of lytic granules to the site of contact with the target cell membrane. This suggests that MUNC13-4 is involved in the last steps of the secretory process (i.e. vesicle docking, priming or membrane fusion). The Golgi complex was found to be polarized close to the site of membrane contact and the granules were closely associated with the plasma membrane both in control and in MUNC13-4-deficient CTLs (Feldmann *et al.*, 2003). However, exocytic fusion of lytic granules and the release of granule contents into the cellular cleft were observed only in control conjugates. MUNC13-4 is thus likely important for the priming event, occurring between the Rab cycle and the SNARE complex.

MUNC13-4 mutations in HLH patients

Feldmann *et al.* (2003) sequenced the coding region of MUNC13-4 in 10 HLH patients, previously linked to the 17q25 locus (FHL3). MUNC13-4 mutations were identified in all 10 patients. A total of six different mutations have been described in MUNC13-4-deficient HLH patients (Table 17.2). A homozygous 12 bp deletion in exon 20 has been observed in four patients from three unrelated families of Moroccan origin. This in-frame deletion preserved the open reading frame and is predicted to encode a protein lacking V608 to A611. In two families nucleotide changes in the canonical splice-donor sequence have been identified, which results in an out-of-frame splicing of exons 8 to 10 and an out-of-frame splicing of exons 14 to 16, respectively. In addition, a nonsense mutation, a single nucleotide deletion and a single nucleotide insertion were identified (Feldmann *et al.*, 2003).

Feldmann and colleagues showed that the mutations in MUNC13-4 are directly related to the defect in cytotoxicity specific for HLH patients. Cells from three of the patients were transfected with cDNA encoding the wild-type MUNC13-4, which fully restored cytotoxic activity. Cytotoxic granules are regulated secretory-storage

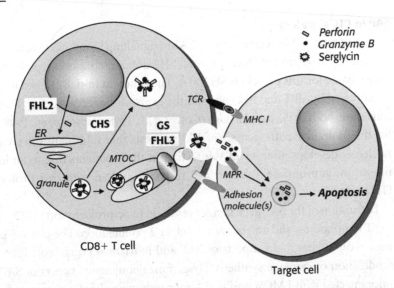

Figure 17.3   Schematic representation of the secretory pathway of CTLs affected in inherited hemophagocytic syndromes (consult text for details). ER, endoplasmic reticulum; GS, Griscelli disease; MPR, mannose 6-phosphate receptor; MTOC, microtubule organizing center; CHS, Chediak-Higashi Syndrome; FHL, familial hemophagocytic lymphohistiocytosis; MHC, major histocompatibility complex

organelles that release their content upon TCR activation. This process is defective in HLH patients with MUNC13-4 mutations. The release of granzyme A, a protease that co-localizes with perforin in lytic granules, was also investigated. Granzyme A was undetectable in the supernatant of activated CTLs from HLH patients carrying MUNC13-4 mutations, suggesting that exocytosis is impaired (Feldmann *et al.*, 2003) (Figure 17.3).

Molecular biology of X-linked lymphoproliferative disease

Epstein–Barr virus-triggered hemophagocytosis

X-linked lymphoproliferative disease (XLP) is an inherited primary immunodeficiency, in which patients have an increased susceptibility to Epstein–Barr virus (EBV). There are three main phenotypes: a fulminant fatal infectious mononucleosis, malignant B-cell lymphoma and dysgammaglobulinemia. Other associated symptoms are aplastic anaemia, vasculitis and pulmonary lymphomatoid granulomatosis. Patients can display more than one phenotype, particularly after exposure to EBV. XLP patients who develop fulminant fatal infectious mononucleosis have a pronounced polyclonal proliferation of T- and B-cells, resulting in liver necrosis and bone marrow failure and leading to a virus-associated hemophagocytosis syndrome with a close resemblance to HLH (Engel *et al.*, 2003; Sharifi *et al.*, 2004).

The role of SAP in CTL signalling

The gene mutated in XLP encodes SLAM (signalling lymphocyte activation molecule)-associated protein (SAP), a small SH2 domain-containing protein. An alternative name for this protein is SH2D1A. The gene was initially linked to Xq25. SAP is expressed by all T and NK cells and the expression increases after T and NK cell activation, both *in vitro* and *in vivo* (Coffey *et al.*, 1998; Nichols *et al.*, 1998). A model for the molecular pathogenesis of XLP suggests that fulminant infectious mononucleosis develops after an EBV infection in these patients due to an inability to mount an appropriate T helper cell response and an extended proliferation of CTLs (Engel *et al.*, 2003).

Disruption of the SAP gene in mice results in hyperproliferation of IFN-γ-producing T lymphocytes and an aberrant T helper 2 proliferation. The phenotype of these mice recapitulates many aspects of XLP and indicates a crucial role for SAP in the modulation of cytokine synthesis. Dysgammaglobulinemia occurs in SAP-deficient mice infected with LMCV, and is also seen in humans harbouring mutations in the SAP gene, although not always in association with EBV infection (Engel *et al.*, 2003).

SAP gene mutations in XLP and HLH patients

Most of the 50 mutations in SAP that have been reported in patients with XLP consist of large or small deletions resulting in complete loss of the gene, or nonsense, splice site or missense mutations that lead to premature arrest of protein synthesis or to a non-functional SAP. Analyses of missense mutations provided information about the functionally important amino acid residues in SAP, but have indicated that there is no correlation between genotype and phenotype. In fact, identical mutations result in different phenotypes in the same family. Therefore, environmental factors determine disease expression and these factors are not limited to infection with EBV, as the XLP phenotype can develop in its absence (Engel *et al.*, 2003).

Among 25 male patients fulfilling the diagnostic criteria for HLH, four patients (16%) were found to harbour mutations in SAP (Arico *et al.*, 2001). No clinical or laboratory signs at presentation distinguished the patients carrying SAP mutations from the remaining cohort of patients. Only two of the patients with SAP mutation were known to have a history of EBV infection. Therefore, XLP is an important differential diagnosis in male patients with a family history of previously affected males, but also in families lacking family history.

Concluding remarks

Studies in recent years have served to unravel the underlying genetic defect in some forms of FHL. Thus, the disease is due, in a proportion of cases, to mutations in the gene-encoding perforin, a lytic granule constituent, while in other patients, mutations in MUNC13-4, encoding a protein that is important for lytic granule exocytosis, have been identified. These findings have provided an explanation for the defective cytotoxic cell function in HLH. Moreover, this provides an opportunity for a molecular diagnosis, including prenatal diagnosis, in affected families. Understanding the underlying molecular defect may also facilitate the development of alternative therapeutic strategies, including gene therapy of HLH. Future studies should aim to characterize genetic defect(s) in HLH patients that do not display perforin or MUNC13-4 mutations, with particular emphasis on the role of other molecules involved in cytotoxic cell function. Also it will be important to investigate whether impaired CTL and NK cell activity *per se* may serve as a surrogate marker of HLH, in cases where the underlying molecular defect remains unknown.

Frequently asked questions

How should FHL patients that do not harbour mutations in perforin or MUNC13-4 be diagnosed if there is no family history?

The identification of mutations in the perforin and MUNC13-4 genes offers a possibility of a molecular diagnosis. However, not all FHL patients harbour perforin mutations: the incidence is likely to be about 30%, although there may be differences among ethnic groups. Moreover, the relative number of FHL patients carrying MUNC13-4 mutations is not yet known. Patients in whom neither perforin mutations nor MUNC13-4 mutations are identified should be diagnosed based upon the diagnostic criteria established by the Histiocyte Society, and NK-cell function, as determined by conventional *in vitro* testing of patient cells.

Is a prenatal diagnosis of FHL possible?

Yes, for families in whom perforin or MUNC13-4 mutations have been identified, a prenatal diagnosis is a possibility. If the mutation(s) in the previously affected child or in the heterozygous parents are known the result will be available within a few days. The analysis requires a chorion villous biopsy that is usually taken during the first trimester. For consanguineous families that do not harbour perforin or MUNC13-4 mutations there is a (theoretical) possibility to establish a prenatal diagnosis based on linkage analysis. This type of analysis usually requires DNA from both affected and healthy siblings.

REFERENCES

Arico, M., Lanfranchi, A., Molinari, E., *et al.* (1988). Cell-mediated cytotoxicity in children during and after therapy for acute lymphoblastic leukemia. *Pediatr Hematol Oncol*, **5**, 279–286.

Arico, M., Imashuku, S., Clementi, R., *et al.* (2001). Hemophagocytic lymphohistiocytosis due to germline mutations in SH2D1A, the X-linked lymphoproliferative disease gene. *Blood*, **97**, 1131–1133.

Badovinac, V.P. and Harty, J.T. (2000). Intracellular staining for TNF and IFN-gamma detects different frequencies of antigen-specific CD8(+) T cells. *J Immunol Method*, **238**, 107–117.

Badovinac, V.P. and Harty, J.T. (2002). CD8(+) T-cell homeostasis after infection: setting the 'curve'. *Microbes Infect*, **4**, 441–447.

Badovinac, V.P., Porter B.B. and Harty, J.T. (2002). Programmed contraction of CD8(+) T cells after infection. *Nat Immunol*, **3**, 619–626.

Busiello, R., Adriani, M., Locatelli, F., *et al.* (2004). Atypical features of familial hemophagocytic lymphohistiocytosis. *Blood*, **103**, 4610–4612.

Certain, S., Barrat, F., Pastural, E., *et al.* (2000). Protein truncation test of LYST reveals heterogenous mutations in patients with Chediak–Higashi syndrome. *Blood*, **95**, 979–983.

Clementi, R., zur Stadt, U., Savoldi, G., *et al.* (2001). Six novel mutations in the PRF1 gene in children with haemophagocytic lymphohistiocytosis. *J Med Genet*, **38**, 643–646.

Coffey, A.J., Brooksbank, R.A., Brandau, O., *et al.* (1998). Host response to EBV infection in X-linked lymphoproliferative disease results from mutations in an SH2-domain encoding gene. *Nat Genet*, **20**, 129–135.

de Saint Basile, G. and Fischer, A. (2003). Defective cytotoxic granule-mediated cell death pathway impairs T lymphocyte homeostasis. *Curr Opin Rheumatol*, **15**, 436–445.

Dufourcq-Lagelouse, R., Jabado, N., Le Deist, F., *et al.* (1999). Linkage of familial hemophagocytic lymphohistiocytosis to 10q21–22 and evidence for heterogeneity. *Am J Hum Genet*, **64**, 172–179.

Eife, R., Janka, G.E., Belohradsky, B.H., *et al.* (1989). Natural killer cell function and interferon production in familial hemophagocytic lymphohistiocytosis. *Pediatr Hematol Oncol*, **6**, 265–272.

Emminger, W., Zlabinger, G.J., Fritsch, G., *et al.* (2001). CD14(dim)/CD16(bright) monocytes in hemophagocytic lymphohistiocytosis. *Eur J Immunol*, **31**, 1716–1719.

Engel, P., Eck, M.J. and Terhorst, C. (2003). The SAP and SLAM families in immune responses and X-linked lymphoproliferative disease. *Nat Rev Immunol*, **3**, 813–821.

Fadeel, B., Orrenius, S. and Henter, J.I. (1999). Induction of apoptosis and caspase activation in cells obtained from familial haemophagocytic lymphohistiocytosis patients. *Br J Haematol*, **106**, 406–415.

Fadeel, B., Orrenius, S. and Henter, J.I. (2001). Familial hemophagocytic lymphohistiocytosis: too little cell death can seriously damage your health. *Leuk Lymphoma*, **42**, 13–20.

Farquhar, J.W. and Claireaux, A.E. (1952). Familial haemophagocytic reticulosis. *Arch Dis Child*, **27**, 519–525.

Feldmann, J., Le Deist, F., Ouachee-Chardin, M., *et al.* (2002). Functional consequences of perforin gene mutations in 22 patients with familial haemophagocytic lymphohistiocytosis. *Br J Haematol*, **117**, 965–972.

Feldmann, J., Callebaut, I., Raposo, G., *et al.* (2003). Munc13-4 is essential for cytolytic granules fusion and is mutated in a form of familial hemophagocytic lymphohistiocytosis (FHL3). *Cell*, **115**, 461–473.

Goransdotter Ericson, K., Fadeel, B., Nilsson-Ardnor, S., *et al.* (2001). Spectrum of perforin gene mutations in familial hemophagocytic lymphohistiocytosis. *Am J Hum Genet*, **68**, 590–597.

Graham, G.E., Graham, L.M., Bridge, P.J., *et al.* (2000). Further evidence for genetic heterogeneity in familial hemophagocytic lymphohistiocytosis (FHLH). *Pediatr Res*, **48**, 227–232.

Henter, J.I. and Elinder, G. (1992). Cerebromeningeal haemophagocytic lymphohistiocytosis. *Lancet*, **339**, 104–107.

Henter, J.I., Elinder, G., Soder, O., *et al.* (1991). Hypercytokinemia in familial hemophagocytic lymphohistiocytosis. *Blood*, **78**, 2918–2922.

Henter, J.I., Ehrnst, A., Andersson, J., *et al.* (1993). Familial hemophagocytic lymphohistiocytosis and viral infections. *Acta Paediatr*, **82**, 369–372.

Henter, J.I., Arico, M., Elinder, G., *et al.* (1998). Familial hemophagocytic lymphohistiocytosis. Primary hemophagocytic lymphohistiocytosis. *Hematol Oncol Clin North Am*, **12**, 417–433.

Kagi, D., Odermatt, B. and Mak, T.W. (1999). Homeostatic regulation of CD8+ T cells by perforin. *Eur J Immunol*, **29**, 3262–3272.

Kogawa, K., Lee, S.M., Villanueva, J., *et al.* (2002). Perforin expression in cytotoxic lymphocytes from patients with hemophagocytic lymphohistiocytosis and their family members. *Blood*, **99**, 61–66.

Lacorazza, H.D., Miyazaki, Y., Di Cristofano, A., *et al.* (2002). The ETS protein MEF plays a critical role in perforin gene expression and the development of natural killer and NK-T cells. *Immunity*, **17**, 437–449.

Li, L. and Chin, L.S. (2003). The molecular machinery of synaptic vesicle exocytosis. *Cell Mol Life Sci*, **60**, 942–960.

Lieberman, J. (2003). The ABCs of granule-mediated cytotoxicity: new weapons in the arsenal. *Nat Rev Immunol*, **3**, 361–370.

Liu, C.C., Walsh, C.M. and Young, J.D. (1995). Perforin: structure and function. *Immunol Today*, **16**, 194–201.

Matloubian, M., Suresh, M., Glass, A., *et al.* (1999). A role for perforin in downregulating T-cell responses during chronic viral infection. *J Virol*, **73**, 2527–2536.

Menasche, G., Pastural, E., Feldmann, J., *et al.* (2000). Mutations in RAB27A cause Griscelli syndrome associated with haemophagocytic syndrome. *Nat Genet*, **25**, 173–176.

Metkar, S.S., Wang, B., Aguilar-Santelises, M., *et al.* (2002). Cytotoxic cell granule-mediated apoptosis: perforin delivers granzyme B-serglycin complexes into target cells without plasma membrane pore formation. *Immunity*, **16**, 417–428.

Molleran Lee, S., Villanueva, J., Sumegi, J., *et al.* (2004). Characterisation of diverse PRF1 mutations leading to decreased natural killer cell activity in North American families with haemophagocytic lymphohistiocytosis. *J Med Genet*, **41**, 137–144.

Motyka, B., Korbutt, G., Pinkoski, M.J., *et al.* (2000). Mannose 6-phosphate/insulin-like growth factor II receptor is a death receptor for granzyme B during cytotoxic T cell-induced apoptosis. *Cell*, **103**, 491–500.

Nichols, K.E., Harkin, D.P., Levitz, S., *et al.* (1998). Inactivating mutations in an SH2 domain-encoding gene in X-linked lymphoproliferative syndrome. *Proc Natl Acad Sci USA*, **95**, 765–770.

Ohadi, M., Lalloz, M.R., Sham, P., *et al.* (1999). Localization of a gene for familial hemophago-cytic lymphohistiocytosis at chromosome 9q21.3–22 by homozygosity mapping. *Am J Hum Genet*, **64**, 165–171.

Osugi, Y., Hara, J., Tagawa, S., *et al.* (1997). Cytokine production regulating Th1 and Th2 cytokines in hemophagocytic lymphohistiocytosis. *Blood*, **89**, 4100–4103.

Perez, N., Virelizier, J.L., Arenzana-Seisdedos, F., *et al.* (1984). Impaired natural killer activity in lymphohistiocytosis syndrome. *J Pediatr*, **104**, 569–573.

Pinkoski, M.J. and Green, D.R. (2002). Lymphocyte apoptosis: refining the paths to perdition. *Curr Opin Hematol*, **9**, 43–49.

Podack, E.R. (1992). Perforin: structure, function, and regulation. *Curr Top Microbiol Immunol*, **178**, 175–184.

Russell, J.H. and Ley, T.J. (2002). Lymphocyte-mediated cytotoxicity. *Annu Rev Immunol*, **20**, 323–370.

Schneider, E.M., Lorenz, I., Walther, P., *et al.* (2003). Natural killer deficiency: a minor or major factor in the manifestation of hemophagocytic lymphohistiocytosis? *J Pediatr Hematol Oncol*, **25**, 680–683.

Sharifi, R., Sinclair, J.C., Gilmour, K.C., *et al.* (2004). SAP mediates specific cytotoxic T cell func-tions in X-linked lymphoproliferative disease. *Blood*, **103**, 3821–3827.

Smyth, M.J., Kelly, J.M., Sutton, V.R., *et al.* (2001). Unlocking the secrets of cytotoxic granule proteins. *J Leukoc Biol*, **70**, 18–29.

Stepp, S.E., Dufourcq-Lagelouse, R., Le Deist, F., *et al.* (1999). Perforin gene defects in familial hemophagocytic lymphohistiocytosis. *Science*, **286**, 1957–1959.

Stinchcombe, J.C., Barral, D.C., Mules, E.H., *et al.* (2001). Rab27a is required for regulated secre-tion in cytotoxic T lymphocytes. *J Cell Biol*, **152**, 825–834.

Suga, N., Takada, H., Nomura, A., *et al.* (2002). Perforin defects of primary haemophagocytic lymphohistiocytosis in Japan. *Br J Haematol*, **116**, 346–349.

Sullivan, K.E., Delaat, C.A., Douglas, S.D., *et al.* (1998). Defective natural killer cell function in patients with hemophagocytic lymphohistiocytosis and in first degree relatives. *Pediatr Res*, **44**, 465–468.

Talanian, R.V., Yang, X., Turbov, J., *et al.* (1997). Granule-mediated killing: pathways for granzyme B-initiated apoptosis. *J Exp Med*, **186**, 1323–1331.

Trapani, J.A., Browne, K.A., Smyth, M.J., *et al.* (1996). Localization of granzyme B in the nucleus. A putative role in the mechanism of cytotoxic lymphocyte-mediated apoptosis. *J Biol Chem*, **271**, 4127–4133.

Trapani, J.A., Jans, D.A., Jans, P.J., *et al.* (1998). Efficient nuclear targeting of granzyme B and the nuclear consequences of apoptosis induced by granzyme B and perforin are caspase-dependent, but cell death is caspase-independent. *J Biol Chem*, **273**, 934–938.

Ueda, I., Morimoto, A., Inaba, T., *et al.* (2003). Characteristic perforin gene mutations of haemophagocytic lymphohistiocytosis patients in Japan. *Br J Haematol*, **121**, 503–510.

Uellner, R., Zvelebil, M.J., Hopkins, J., *et al.* (1997). Perforin is activated by a proteolytic cleavage during biosynthesis which reveals a phospholipid-binding C2 domain. *Embo J*, **16**, 7287–7296.

Wagner, C., Iking-Konert, C., Denefleh, B., *et al.* (2004). Granzyme B and perforin: constitutive expression in human polymorphonuclear neutrophils. *Blood*, **103**, 1099–1104.

18

Clinical aspects and therapy of hemophagocytic lymphohistiocytosis

Gritta Janka, Jan-Inge Henter and Shinsaku Imashuku

Hemophagocytic lymphohistiocytosis (HLH) is a hyperinflammatory condition resulting from an uncontrolled ineffective immune response. The underlying immune deficiency can be inherited or acquired, but whatever the defect, the result is an unbalanced expansion, and activation of cytotoxic lymphocytes and macrophages, resulting in hypercytokinemia and hemophagocytosis, and the classic clinical syndrome of HLH (Figure 18.1). Initial symptoms are non-specific often leading to a delay in diagnosis.

Incidence and epidemiology

In a retrospective study the incidence of primary, familial HLH (FHLH) was estimated as 0.12/100,000 children per year (Henter *et al.*, 1991a). It can be assumed

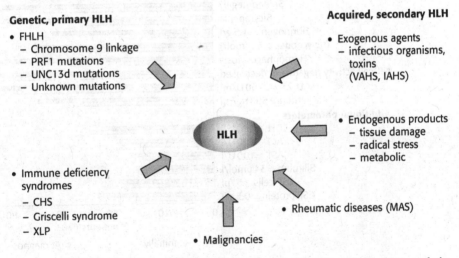

Genetic, primary HLH

- FHLH
  - Chromosome 9 linkage
  - PRF1 mutations
  - UNC13d mutations
  - Unknown mutations

- Immune deficiency syndromes
  - CHS
  - Griscelli syndrome
  - XLP

HLH

- Malignancies

Acquired, secondary HLH

- Exogenous agents
  - infectious organisms, toxins (VAHS, IAHS)

- Endogenous products
  - tissue damage
  - radical stress
  - metabolic

- Rheumatic diseases (MAS)

Figure 18.1 HLH: classification and underlying conditions (Janka and Schneider, 2004). *PFR1*: perforin gene; *UNC13d*: Munc13-4 gene; CHS: Chediak Higashi syndrome; XLP: x-linked lymphoproliferative syndrome; VAHS: virus-associated hemophagocytic syndrome; IAHS: infection-associated hemophagocytic syndrome; MAS: macrophage-activation syndrome. Reprinted with permission from Blackwell Publishing, Oxford

that this is a minimal figure as there are still patients who are undiagnosed. There is a slight male preponderance (Janka, 1983; Henter *et al.*, 2002). FHLH has been reported from many different countries. As an autosomal recessive disease, it is found especially in ethnic groups where consanguineous marriages are common.

The incidence of secondary HLH is unknown, but in the authors' experience an increasing number of older children, previously healthy or with underlying conditions such as auto-immune diseases or malignancies, are being diagnosed.

Age at onset, clinical symptoms and natural course of disease

Most patients with FHLH develop the disease very early; 70–80% are below 1 year of age (Janka, 1983; Aricò *et al.*, 1996). Characteristically there is a symptom-free interval after birth, in <10% HLH manifests itself in the first week of life. However, late-onset cases have been reported (Allen *et al.*, 2001). Secondary HLH has been described at all ages including many adults.

The cardinal symptoms are prolonged high fever, hepatosplenomegaly and cytopenias (Figure 18.2). In more than one-third of the patients the fever subsides spontaneously but recurs within days to weeks (Müeller-Rosenberger, 2004). On

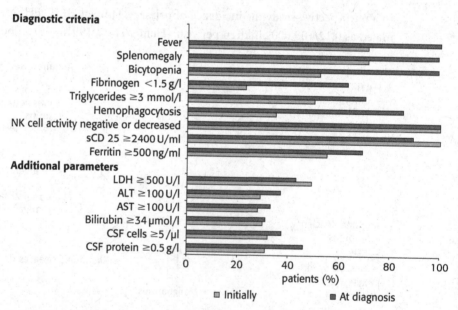

Figure 18.2 Symptoms and laboratory values in HLH. Symptoms at first presentation and at time of diagnosis. The bars denote the percentage of patients in whom the symptoms are present. ALT: alanine aminotransferase; AST: aspartate aminotransferase; CSF: cerebrospinal fluid; LDH: lactate dehydrogenase. Janke G.E. (In Press). Reprinted with permission from Springer-Verlag ©

first presentation there is usually only moderate organomegaly. Lymphadenopathy, a non-specific rash, icterus, edema, or neurologic symptoms such as irritability, cranial nerve palsies or seizures may be present. Many patients develop neurologic symptoms later in the course. In some children, hepatic failure (Parizhskaya et al., 1999) or neurologic abnormalities (Henter and Elinder, 1992; Kieslich et al., 2001) may be the leading symptoms at presentation or remain the sole manifestation of HLH (Henter and Elinder, 1992; Rostasy et al., 2004).

Whereas the clinical condition of the patient is often not severely impaired initially, and respiratory or gastrointestinal symptoms suggest a harmless viral infection, the progression of clinical symptoms and conspicuous laboratory values should alert the physician to the possibility of HLH. Initially patients may improve with non-specific therapies such as transfusions or antibiotics, but responses are usually short-lived. Some children may even enjoy prolonged intervals without need for treatment between exacerbations of the disease (Janka-Schaub et al., 1999).

In children with a presumed or proven genetic defect, HLH is usually rapidly fatal. The terminal events are bacterial or fungal infections, pneumonia and bleeding as well as cerebral dysfunction (Janka, 1983). Presumed secondary forms may also have a high-mortality rate without treatment (Janka et al., 1998).

Laboratory values

Anemia or thrombocytopenia is usually present initially. In spite of markedly increased erythropoiesis, often with maturation defects, there is an inadequate reticulocyte response documenting ineffective erythropoiesis. A positive Coombs test and platelet antibodies are found in some patients. Up to 28% have leukocytosis with either neutrophilia or lymphocytosis. Neutropenia ($<1 \times 10^9$/l), present initially in about 30% of patients, afflicts most children eventually and is responsible for fatalities due to infections. Pancytopenia is progressive in untreated children (Janka, 1983; Müeller-Rosenberger, 2004).

An isolated low fibrinogen, not expected with uncomplicated infections, develops in more than 60% of patients (Janka, 1983; Müller-Rosenberger, 2004). In addition some patients exhibit a global coagulation disorder, which may be life-threatening (Hadchouel et al., 1985; Chen et al., 1998; Janka et al., 1998). Hypertriglyceridemia is present in most children (Janka, 1983; Henter et al., 1991b; Müeller-Rosenberger, 2004) and may reach levels >10 mmol/l. In children with febrile illnesses, triglycerides do not normally exceed 3 mmol/l (Garbagnati, 1993). Hyperferritinemia >500 ng/ml, probably upregulated by oxidative stress (Tsuji et al., 2000), is found in more than half the patients. Less frequent are elevated lactate dehydrogenase (LDH), serum transaminases, bilirubin, low total protein and hyponatremia.

A bone marrow examination is mandatory but only a minority shows hemophagocytosis at presentation (Janka, 1983; Müeller-Rosenberger, 2004). A lumbar puncture should also be performed as more than 50% of the patients will have pathologic findings (Janka, 1983; Aricò *et al.*, 1996; Haddad *et al.*, 1997) many in the absence of neurologic symptoms (Müeller-Rosenberger, 2004).

Elevated levels of the alpha chain of the soluble interleukin-2 receptor (sCD25) and of the soluble FAS (CD178) ligand reflect stimulation of histiocytes and T-cells (Komp *et al.*, 1989; Imashuku *et al.*, 1998; Schneider *et al.*, 2002). Impaired natural killer (NK)-cell function is found in all cases in our experience and that of others (Eife *et al.*, 1989; Aricò *et al.*, 1996; Sullivan *et al.*, 1998; Schneider *et al.*, 2002) whereas not all patients reported from Japan or the USA had decreased NK-cell activity (Imashuku *et al.*, 1998; Molleran Lee *et al.*, 2004). Residual cellular toxicity can be shown to be present in some patients after prolonged effector/target incubation or with the addition of mitogen or interleukin-2 (Schneider *et al.*, 2002). The defect is permanent in primary FHLH (Eife *et al.*, 1989; Schneider *et al.*, 2002) and usually resolves in secondary HLH. However, even in some of these patients, long-lasting defects have been described (Janka *et al.*, 2000).

Underlying conditions and classification

HLH is not a single disease but can be encountered secondary to a variety of underlying conditions leading to the same hyperinflammatory phenotype.

FHLH, first described in 1952 (Farquhar and Claireaux, 1952) is an autosomal recessive disease for which several gene defects have been described (see Chapter 17). In addition, well-characterized immune deficiencies such as Griscelli syndrome, Chediak-Higashi syndrome (CHS), and X-linked lymphoproliferative (XLP) syndrome may present initially as HLH (Dufourcq-Lagelouse *et al.*, 1999). In a substantial number of patients, thought to have genetic disease based on a positive family history or a relapsing course, the gene defect is as yet unknown.

A clinical picture with symptoms of HLH has also been described in several inborn metabolic diseases (Mandel *et al.*, 1990; Ikeda *et al.*, 1998; Duval *et al.*, 1999). The clinical picture of HLH can be induced by a variety of infectious organisms, mostly viruses, but also bacteria, protozoa and fungi (Reiner and Spivac, 1988; Janka *et al.*, 1998; Fisman, 2000), thus the term virus-associated hemophagocytic syndrome (VAHS) (Risdall *et al.*, 1979) was replaced by infection-associated hemophagocytic syndrome (IAHS). Like FHLH, IAHS has proven to be a dangerous disease with a fatality rate of more than 50% in children (Janka *et al.*, 1998). In the first report by Risdall *et al.*, the majority of patients with IAHS had an acquired iatrogenic immune-deficiency, however in subsequent reports most patients had no underlying genetic or acquired immune defect. Epstein-Barr virus (EBV)-associated HLH is by far the most frequent and dangerous form of IAHS (see later).

Originally the presence of an infection was thought to differentiate familial and acquired HLH. However, it is now clear that even in the genetic form, most episodes of HLH are triggered by an infectious agent (Henter *et al.*, 1993; Aricò *et al.*, 1996). As clinical symptoms and laboratory findings do not allow discrimination between familial and secondary disease, the diagnosis of IAHS should be made with caution.

Patients with systemic inflammatory rheumatic disorders may develop a life-threatening HLH syndrome (Hadchouel *et al.*, 1985; Mouy *et al.*, 1996; Stephan *et al.*, 2001) for which the term macrophage-activation syndrome (MAS) has been commonly used. It has recently been suggested that this condition be included as a separate entity in the category of secondary HLH (Ramanan and Baildam, 2002) (see Chapter 19).

Secondary HLH may also be associated with malignancies, mostly hematopoietic. Lymphoma-associated HLH is the commonest form of secondary HLH in adults (see later in this chapter).

Diagnostic management

In non-familial cases, a thorough history and diagnostic work-up is necessary to rule out an underlying disease predisposing to HLH. CHS or Griscelli syndrome should be suspected in patients with albinism. In males, EBV-associated HLH suggests the possibility of XLP; mental retardation, developmental delay or aminoaciduria suggests a metabolic disease, and a history of rheumatic or other auto-immune diseases, an associated MAS. As discussed later, lymphoma-associated HLH may present a difficult diagnostic problem.

Although identification of an infection does not help to distinguish primary from secondary HLH, a rigorous search for an infectious agent, including polymerase chain reaction (PCR) for viruses, is encouraged, as the elimination of a triggering agent may be an important part of therapy. In HLH associated with leishmaniasis, specific drug therapy without additional anti-inflammatory therapy is usually curative. Whether HLH-oriented immunosuppressive therapy should be added, however, ultimately depends on the severity of the clinical symptoms.

Diagnostic criteria

In 1991, the FHL Study Group of the Histiocyte Society proposed diagnostic guidelines for HLH (Henter *et al.*, 1991c). Although it was emphasized that the lack of hemophagocytosis should not exclude ill patients from treatment, the requirement of hemophagocytosis for a definite diagnosis of HLH often delayed treatment. The criteria have been revised for the open HLH-2004 protocol (Table 18.1) and ferritin, sCD25 and NK-cell activity have been added. A value >2400 U/ml for sCD25 proved to have high sensitivity (93%) and specificity (1.00) for HLH compared to sepsis or other infections (Janka and Schneider, 2004). Although NK-cell activity is measured by specialized laboratories and is usually not available in time for

Table 18.1 Diagnostic criteria for HLH[1]

Familial disease/known genetic defect
Clinical and laboratory criteria (five of eight criteria)
- Fever
- Splenomegaly
- Cytopenia ≥2 cell lines
    Hemoglobin <90 g/l (below 4 weeks <120 g/l)
    Platelets <100 × 10^9/l
    Neutrophils <1 × 10^9/l
- Hypertriglyceridemia and/or hypofibrinogenemia
    Fasting triglycerides ≥3 mmol/l
    Fibrinogen <1.5 g/l
- Ferritin ≥500 μg/l
- sCD25[2] ≥2400 U/ml
- Decreased or absent NK-cell activity
- Hemophagocytosis in bone marrow
    CSF or lymphnodes

[1]Janka and Schneider, (2004). [2]For method see Schneider *et al.*, (2002). Supportive evidence are cerebral symptoms with moderate pleocytosis and/or elevated protein, elevated transaminases and bilirubin, LDH > 1000 U/l. Reprinted with permission from Blackwell Publishing, Oxford

treatment decisions, it should be included as an important marker. Pretreatment blood samples should be obtained to confirm the diagnosis by NK-cell activity or sCD25, retrospectively. In parents of supposedly genetic cases, restricted NK-cell function is a frequent finding and helps to confirm familial disease (Sullivan *et al.*, 1998; Schneider *et al.*, 2002).

In the absence of familial disease or a verified genetic mutation, five of eight criteria are required for a diagnosis of HLH. Supportive evidence includes cerebral symptoms with moderate cerebrospinal fluid (CSF) pleocytosis and/or elevated protein, elevated transaminases, bilirubin and LDH. Consanguinity is often found in Turkish patients with or without known familial disease. Age below 1 year was associated with either familial or persisting/relapsing disease in 90% of the patients in the German registry.

Perforin expression in NK-cells and cytotoxic lymphocytes, measured by flow-cytometry, is helpful in identifying patients with perforin gene mutations (Aricò *et al.*, 2002; Kogawa *et al.*, 2002). However, decreased perforin expression and NK-cell impairment was recently reported in patients with systemic juvenile arthritis (Grom *et al.*, 2003; Wulffraat *et al.*, 2003), although no genetic defects were found.

Mutation analysis of the genes currently identified in HLH is available at specialized laboratories.

Whereas the diagnosis is not difficult when the full-blown syndrome is present, an incomplete picture is frequent at initial presentation (Figure 18.2). In particular, hemophagocytosis is lacking in many patients, and splenomegaly and bicytopenia may be absent. Transient improvement with non-specific therapies such as transfusion may contribute further to the diagnostic uncertainty. Moreover the identification of an infectious organism may distract from the possible diagnosis of HLH.

Therapy of HLH

Therapeutic background

FHLH is usually a rapidly fatal disease, if untreated. In the early 1980s, the median survival of all patients reported in the literature was <2 months, irrespective of whether treatment was administered (Janka, 1983). Various treatments including cytotoxic agents were tried with limited effect, and it was not until the epipodophyllotoxin-derivative etoposide in combination with corticosteroids, was introduced into HLH therapy (Ambruso et al., 1980) that major improvements in survival were achieved.

A treatment protocol that included etoposide, corticosteroids, intrathecal methotrexate (IT MTX) and cranial irradiation was shown to be successful in prolonging survival (Fischer, 1985). Subsequently other therapeutic regimens using similar drugs but without cranial irradiation (Janka, 1989; Henter and Elinder, 1991) were effective in prolonging survival for more than 5 years after onset in some patients, but no child with familial disease was cured with chemotherapy alone. It was therefore a major advance when allogeneic hematopoietic stem cell transplantation (SCT) was shown to induce not only prolonged resolution but also cure (Fischer et al., 1986).

Therapeutic problems

As emphasized earlier, the diagnosis of HLH may be very difficult, particularly when there is no family history and no evidence of a molecular defect. As a result children with HLH may die without treatment, because of late diagnosis or lack of correct diagnosis (Janka, 1983; Henter et al., 1991a). Moreover, the attempts to differentiate FHLH from secondary forms, particularly IAHS, often results in further significant therapeutic delays. The development of the Histiocyte Society diagnostic guidelines for HLH (Henter et al., 1991c) which did not separate FHL and IAHS, was thus an important advance. As the presentation may be atypical in some patients, such as patients with mainly central nervous system (CNS) symptoms, it is possible that even the new revised criteria may not be fulfilled. This may also be the case very early in the course of HLH in the second affected child in a family. *Treatment therefore, must sometimes be commenced on a strong clinical suspicion even when the diagnostic criteria are not completely fulfilled.*

Therapy

Study HLH-94

In 1994, the Histiocyte Society opened treatment protocol HLH-94 (Figure 18.3) (Henter *et al.*, 1997). The basic strategy underlying the therapy included prompt control of the hypercytokinemic disorder, treatment of any underlying disease and full supportive care. In brief, it included an initial phase with etoposide and

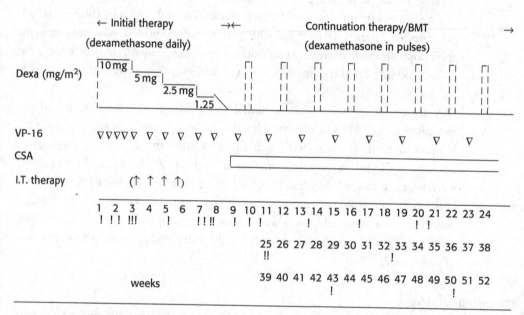

Figure 18.3 Overview of the treatment protocol HLH-94. Day of death for 23 patients who died the first year of therapy, except those who underwent BMT, is marked with an '!'. BMT: Go to BMT during continuation therapy as soon as an acceptable donor is available, preferably when the disease is non-active; Dexa: dexamethasone daily (pulses are 10 mg/m² for 3 days); VP-16: etoposide 150 mg/m² iv; I.T. therapy: IT MTX (if progressive neurologic symptoms or if an abnormal CSF has not improved). This research was originally published by Henter *et al.* (2002) © the American Society of Hematology

corticosteroids, followed by a continuation phase. Cyclosporin A (CSA) was added after the initial therapy, since CSA had earlier been shown to be effective in FHL (Stephan *et al.*, 1993; Loechelt *et al.*, 1994). An important advance in this protocol was that, as per the published guidelines, and in contrast to previous recommendations, FHL and IAHS no longer had to be differentiated before therapy was started. Instead, therapy to improve the patients condition was started immediately and the final diagnosis could safely be delayed. All children with HLH were thus started on chemotherapy regardless of the presence of an associated infection. After 8 weeks of initial treatment, patients with positive familial history and/or verified molecular-based FHLH, and those with *persistent or relapsing* non-familial disease proceeded to continuation therapy and allogeneic SCT. Children with a *resolved* non-familial, non-genetically verified disease after 8 weeks of therapy, discontinued therapy and restarted only in case of a reactivation. In this way the clinical course decided the need for SCT in non-familial patients and patients without verified genetic mutations. An important role for continuation therapy was to keep the patient stable while a bone marrow donor was sought. Since survival in FHLH depends on a SCT, a family haploidentical donor was deemed acceptable, if no other donor was available. Intensive supportive care was an important part of therapy.

CNS disease

Cerebral involvement may cause severe and irreversible damage (Henter and Elinder, 1992; Haddad *et al.*, 1997; Henter and Nennesmo, 1997) and IT therapy has been used although its therapeutic effect is questionable. In children with HLH, CNS disease at diagnosis often resolves with systemic therapy, while IT therapy appears to be less effective. Systemic therapy including dexamethasone, which penetrates the blood–brain barrier well, was therefore the suggested first line therapy in HLH-94, even in cases with CNS involvement. IT MTX, for a maximum of four doses, was recommended only if there were progressive neurologic symptoms, or if an abnormal CSF had not improved after 2 weeks of dexamethasone. This approach has been continued in the current open protocol.

Results of study HLH-94

The outcome of children treated for HLH during the first 4 years of the HLH-94 protocol was recently published (Henter *et al.*, 2002). At a median follow-up of 3.1 years, the estimated 3-year probability of survival for all 113 eligible patients recruited during the period July 1994–June 1998 was 55% ($\pm$9%) (Figure 18.4). In children with an affected sibling, that is verified familial disease, the 3-year

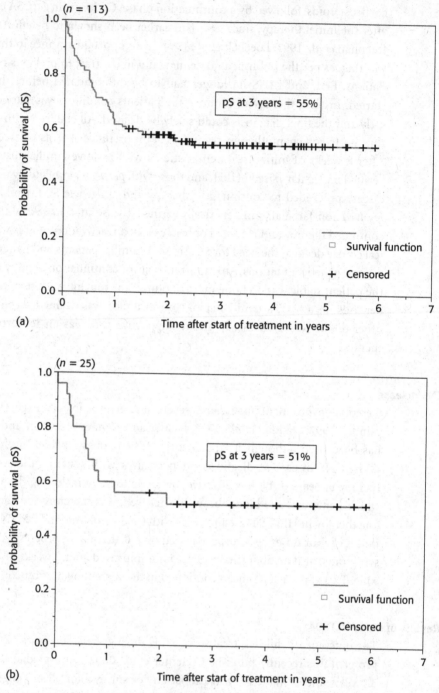

Figure 18.4 Kaplan–Meier survival curve for (a) all eligible study patients treated with HLH-94 (*n* = 113), and (b) patients with an affected sibling (*n* = 25). This research was originally published by Henter *et al.* (2002) © the American Society of Hematology

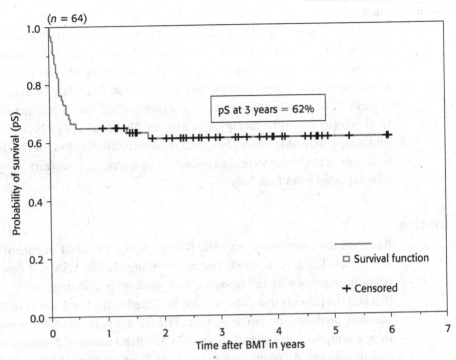

Figure 18.5 Kaplan–Meier survival curve for patients who underwent SCT, starting at the time of SCT (missing date of SCT in one of the 65 patients, leaving 64 patients for analysis). This research was originally published by Henter *et al.* (2002) © the American Society of Hematology

probability of survival was 51% (±9%). Twenty-five patients (22%) died prior to SCT. The 3-year probability of survival after SCT was 62% (±12%) (*n* = 65) (Figure 18.5).

The median time from therapy start to SCT was 187 days (range 65–995). There was no difference in survival when SCT was performed early (*n* = 32, 62 ± 17% estimated 3-year survival) versus late (*n* = 32, 61 ± 18%) after onset of therapy. Ten of 15 (67%) with matched related donors were alive as compared to 17 of 25 (68%) with matched unrelated donors, and 6 of 14 (43%) with family haploidentical donors. All surviving SCT patients were free of disease. In the 25 deceased SCT patients, death occurred prior to day +100 in 20 patients, mostly caused by SCT complications (*n* = 17).

The results of HLH-94 thus confirmed that allogeneic SCT can cure children with FHLH (Fischer *et al.*, 1986; Blanche *et al.*, 1991; Baker *et al.*, 1997; Jabado *et al.*, 1997; Duerken *et al.*, 1999; Henter *et al.*, 2002).

Patients without SCT

In the first 4 years of HLH-94 there were 23 children, all without a positive family history, that were alive without a SCT, 20 of whom were off therapy and without evidence of disease for more than 12 months, and three who were on therapy for more than 1 year. These children most probably had secondary HLH but were sufficiently ill to require HLH-specific treatment; 10 of the 20 patients off therapy, received only the initial therapy over 8 weeks. Almost all (19 of 20) of the patients off therapy were older than 12 months at onset (including four of the six children in the entire study that were aged 6 years or more), and the majority ($n = 12, 60\%$) were reported from East Asia.

HLH-2004

Based on the experiences with HLH-94, a slightly modified treatment protocol, HLH-2004, has been opened. The major change is that CSA will now be given up-front together with the etoposide and corticosteroid therapy, based on the fact that half the patients that did not reach SCT, died in the first 8 weeks of therapy. In addition, prednisolone will be added to IT MTX for patients with progressive neurologic symptoms or residual abnormal CSF after 2 weeks of dexamethasone. The patient flow and decisions with regard to SCT are unchanged but the SCT conditioning regimen has been slightly modified. As in HLH-94, a family haploidentical donor is acceptable if no other donor is available. The experience with a non-myeloablative approach is limited, and cannot be generally recommended at this point, but may be a future alternative.

Reactivation therapy

Genetic forms of HLH are characterized by frequent reactivations prior to SCT, or more or less continuous disease activity. Reactivation may occur following immune response triggering, as may occur from infections. In particular, reactivation of the disease is common as the therapeutic intensity is reduced, and should not be regarded as an ominous treatment failure, but rather as a sign indicating that the present treatment intensity is insufficient. A reactivation will commonly respond to an intensification of the usual therapy. One possible way to intensify therapy is to restart the induction therapy but with a therapy duration of <8 weeks. In the case of a CNS reactivation, urgent treatment, including corticosteroids, is needed to avoid CNS sequelae. One method is to administer dexamethasone daily or every second day between the dexamethasone pulses. Although the value of IT therapy has not been clearly established, responses in patients with CNS relapse have been observed and IT MTX plus prednisolone are therefore being recommended for CNS disease progression.

Other therapeutic regimens and salvage therapy

A regimen that includes corticosteroids, CSA and anti-thymocyte globulin (ATG), has been successful in inducing remission in experienced hands (Stephan *et al.*, 1993; Jabado *et al.*, 1997). A small fraction of patients do not respond to the HLH-94 protocol induction, but it seems unfortunately, that many of these also do not respond to ATG. Experience has shown that some patients, who failed induction on HLH-94, responded to increased doses of the same drugs, such as higher dose dexamethasone.

Frequently asked questions about HLH

Question: How do we know if a patient with HLH will need a SCT?

SCT is necessary for children with affected siblings, patients with bi-allelic mutations in the perforin gene, the hMunc 13-4 gene or other genes causing the disease. All patients with HLH who have familial disease should receive SCT. Recent preliminary data also suggests that HLH patients with a non-reversible defect in NK- and T-cell activity, defined as NK-cell activity deficiency type 3 (Schneider *et al.*, 2002), will also need a SCT (Zheng *et al.*, 2004). In addition, SCT is also recommended for a patient with HLH and a diagnosis of XLP syndrome, CHS or Griscelli syndrome. In addition, patients without any evidence of (a) mutation defects, (b) family history and (c) NK-cell activity deficiency type 3, are also candidates for SCT if their HLH is persistent or recurrent, and there is no known underlying condition such as rheumatic or metabolic disease.

Question: How to treat a mild form of HLH?

Certain patients, such as older children or adolescents/adults with mild symptoms and a non-familial disease, could be started on treatment with corticosteroids alone or in combination with intravenous immunoglobulin (IVIG). If they fail to respond or progress, other immunosuppressive drugs such as CSA or etoposide can be added. (See Chapter 19 for discussion of HLH associated with rheumatic diseases.) It has to be kept in mind that in patients with EBV-associated HLH the probability of long-term survival was significantly higher when etoposide treatment was begun <4 weeks from diagnosis. Thus this aforementioned form of reduced therapy should be undertaken with caution.

Question: How do we treat a patient with an HLH reactivation?

Reactivations indicate that the present treatment intensity is insufficient. Therapy should be reintensified with etoposide once or twice weekly and dexamethasone daily, but initial therapy may now be shorter than 8 weeks. In patients with CNS relapse on continuation therapy, IT therapy is recommended and dexamethasone, given daily or every second day between the dexa-pulses, should be considered.

Prolonged corticosteroid therapy may lead to severe side-effects. In patients with HLH reactivation, SCT should be performed as soon as possible. If there is inadequate response to therapy intensification, other induction protocols could be considered, as discussed above.

EBV-associated HLH

Among the various infection-associated HLH, EBV-HLH is the most common and problematic in children and young adults. Although an immunocompromised status is suspected in the development of EBV-HLH, precise mechanisms of host's vulnerability to EBV is largely unknown and the majority of EBV-HLH occurs in apparently immunocompetent and previously healthy children (Imashuku, 2002). Exceptionally, it develops in association with hereditary XLP.

Clinical features

EBV plays the central role in the development of HLH through augmentation of hypercytokinemia, however, EBV-related HLH is distinct from other VAHS because of its clonal characteristics. VAHS, including EBV-HLH, was initially described as a non-neoplastic disorder associated with systemic viral infection (Risdall *et al.*, 1979). However, the concept has changed markedly in patients with EBV-HLH. Over the last decade it has become clear that EBV can infect not only B-cells but also T-and NK-cells. Such EBV-infected T/NK-cells appear to play a major role in the development of EBV-HLH as well as hemophagocytic syndrome associated with malignant lymphoma (Quintanilla-Martinez *et al.*, 2000; Mitarnun *et al.*, 2002; Kawa, 2003). The EBV-infected T/NK-cells proliferate mono- or oligoclonally (Kawaguchi *et al.*, 1993; Dolezal *et al.*, 1995), and both EBV-HLH and T/NK-lymphoma-associated HLH show similar pathogenesis and clinical features.

Compared to non-EBV-HLH, clinical symptoms and signs are generally more severe in EBV-HLH patients. Some EBV-HLH patients have a rapidly fatal primary EBV infection distinct from classical infectious mononucleosis (IM). Many reports on fatal cases of EBV-HLH are available in the literature (Mroczek *et al.*, 1987; Kikuta *et al.*, 1993; Su *et al.*, 1994). However, the majority of EBV-HLH cases have a prolonged atypical IM-like, rather slowly progressing disease course. EBV-HLH associated with XLP (Sumazaki *et al.*, 2001), or with chronic active EBV infection (CAEBV) (Ishihara *et al.*, 1995; Kanegane *et al.*, 2002) is generally severe and fatal.

It is important that any HLH patient suspected to have an EBV-association should be examined for clonality by cytogenetic analysis, for T-cell receptor (TCR) gene rearrangements and for the fused termini of the EBV genome by Southern analysis. Clonality was determined in 27 of our 32 patients with EBV-HLH, 23 were proven to have clonal disease (21 monoclonal and 2 biclonal). TCR rearrangements were positive in 15 of the 25 cases studied (TCR beta in 11, TCR gamma in 3 and TCR delta in 1) (Imashuku *et al.*, 2000b). No specific molecular abnormalities were identified in the majority of EBV-HLH or CAEBV cases. Exceptionally SAP mutation was noted in XLP-associated EBV-HLH (Sumegi *et al.*, 2000; Sumazaki *et al.*, 2001) and perforin mutation was identified in one case of CAEBV-related HLH (Katano, 2004). Thus, determination of SAP and/or perforin expression is mandatory only in refractory EBV-HLH, to rule out the possibility of XLP or FHLH (Sumegi *et al.*, 2000; Ueda *et al.*, 2003). A correct diagnosis of EBV-HLH can only be achieved by a combination of thoroughly scrutinized laboratory tests for peripheral blood mononuclear cell (PBMC) subsets, bone marrow morphology, cytokine patterns, EBV serology, EBV genomes and clonality. Regarding serology at diagnosis, we observed that the majority of cases had a pattern consistent with previous exposure, whereas only 35% of EBV-HLH patients showed a pattern characteristic of first exposure or reactivation. EBV-HLH cases show a high percentage of activated (CD3$^+$HLADR$^+$) T-cells associated with an increase of CD8-positive cells, or of NK-cells, and high-serum levels of sCD25 as well as interferon-γ (Imashuku *et al.*, 1998; Imashuku, 2002a; Imashuku *et al.*, 2004). In addition, in evaluating disease activity of EBV-related disease, quantifying EBV genome copy numbers in peripheral blood (cell-free or in PBMC) is very useful (Kimura *et al.*, 1999; Teramura *et al.*, 2002) (Figure 18.6).

In typical IM, EBV genome number becomes normal in 4 weeks. In HLH, when immuno-chemo (IC) therapy is effective, the disease resolves usually by 12 weeks.

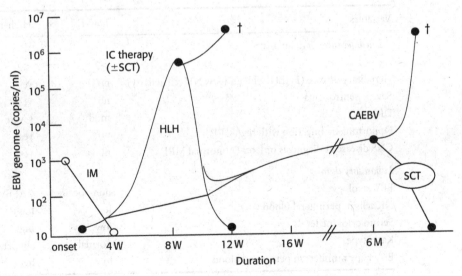

Figure 18.6 Cell-free EBV genome copy numbers reflecting the disease activity in various types of EBV-related diseases. † indicates fatal outcome

However, in fatal cases, EBV genome increases to more than 10^6 copies/ml. Although speculative, some patients develop CAEBV without showing HLH symptoms until 6 months from onset, associated with persistent increase of EBV genome copies. If CAEBV is successfully treated with SCT, the disease becomes curable. However, not appropriately managed, the disease becomes fatal, with a significant increase of EBV genome copies. Persistence of increased cell-free EBV genome copies is also noted in T/NK-LAHS.

Initial treatment

The prognosis of EBV-HLH depends on the underlying disease (hereditary or not), magnitude of the cytokine storm, cytogenetics and other factors. Patients with adverse characteristics will likely have a poor treatment response. A tentative classification of low- and high-risk EBV-HLH is shown in Table 18.2 (Imashuku, 2002a).

Supportive care is especially important at the initiation of treatment, including control of hypercytokinemia, of coagulopathy and of neutropenia-associated opportunistic infections (Imashuku *et al.*, 2000a; Imashuku *et al.*, 2001; Imashuku, 2002a). For the majority of patients with mild symptoms, prompt management of cytokine-induced symptoms by corticosteroids, IV high-dose gammaglobulin (IVIG), or CSA may be sufficient (Oyama *et al.*, 1989; Nomura *et al.*, 1992; Freeman *et al.*, 1993). If a patient needs more prompt control of hypercytokinemia, plasmapheresis could be considered (Matsumoto *et al.*, 1998).

Table 18.2 Tentative classification of low-risk and high-risk EBV–HLH

Variables	Low-risk	High-risk
Clinical features at diagnosis		
Age	>2	<2
Hereditary disease (FHLH, XLP and low NK cell activity)	no	yes
Severe neutropenia	no	yes
DIC	mild	severe
Opportunistic infection with high CRP	no	yes
CNS disease at diagnosis or later (Abnormal MRI)	no	yes
Laboratory data		
EBV serology	non-specific*	CAEBV pattern**
NK cells in peripheral blood (%)	low	high***
Serum cytokine levels	low	high
Karyotype	normal	abnormal
EBV copy numbers in peripheral blood	low	high

CRP: C-reactive protein; DIC: disseminated intravascular coagulation. *indicates previous exposure, **indicates anti-VCA-IgG >1280 and/or anti-EADR-IgG >320, *** >40%.

Specific therapy

Currently, a combination of etoposide, CSA and corticosteroids is the basic first-line treatment for severe EBV-HLH (Henter *et al.*, 1997; Imashuku *et al.*, 1999a). Etoposide is thought to be especially suitable for EBV-HLH (Imashuku *et al.*, 1999a; Imashuku *et al.*, 2001), as this agent suppresses macrophages and EBNA synthesis (Kikuta and Sakiyama, 1995). Efficacy of immunomodulatory treatment incorporating etoposide and IVIG was previously reported for EBV-HLH (Chen *et al.*, 1995; Su *et al.*, 1995). The HLH-94 protocol consisting of dexamethasone, etoposide and CSA, was found to be very effective for pediatric patients with EBV-HLH (Imashuku *et al.*, 1999a; Imashuku *et al.*, 2001), and confirmed a better prognosis for early etoposide administration in this disorder. In addition, the therapeutic results were better when CSA was added early during the initial 8 weeks especially for neutropenic patients (Imashuku *et al.*, 2001). The early death rate was also found to be significantly higher in patients who received 0–3 doses of etoposide compared to those given 4–10 doses during the first 4 weeks of treatment ($P = 0.0001$) (Imashuku *et al.*, 2002b). These data suggest a requirement for etoposide as well as CSA in the early treatment phase of EBV-HLH. Similarly, an etoposide-containing regimen has been found to be effective in the treatment of young adult patients with EBV-HLH (Imashuku *et al.*, 2003).

In the majority of EBV-HLH cases, the disease is well controlled within 4–8 weeks of treatment with a combination of etoposide, dexamethasone with/or without CSA. The patients who need treatment for longer than 8 weeks likely have refractory disease, as is also seen in XLP- or CAEBV-related HLH. For such refractory patients, salvage chemotherapy and subsequent SCT may become inevitable.

Salvage chemotherapy

ATG may be effective as salvage as previously reported (Perel *et al.*, 1997). The treatment protocols for non-Hodgkin's lymphoma or Hodgkin disease were found to be effective in some refractory EBV-HLH cases (Imashuku *et al.*, 1999b). Particularly, combination chemotherapy used for Hodgkin's disease such as adriamycin/cyclophosphamide/vincristine/procarbazine/prednisolone (ACOPP) and adriamycin/bleomycin/vinblastine/prednisolone (ABVD) was found to be effective. Such activity is not unexpected as EBV is also involved in Hodgkin's disease (Spieker *et al.*, 2000).

Hematopoietic SCT

SCT can potentially cure refractory EBV-HLH by eliminating the virus and killing proliferating cells responsible for HLH pathogenesis (Imashuku *et al.*, 1999b; Yagita *et al.*, 2001; Okamura *et al.*, 2003). SCT is also the treatment of choice for CAEBV (Fujii *et al.*, 2000; Okamura *et al.*, 2000) and XLP patients (Pracher *et al.*,

1993). As EBV-HLH and CAEBV are not considered malignant diseases, reluctance to proceed to SCT exists both in physicians and patients, even when disease is progressive. Delay of SCT often results in a poor outcome. When sibling donors are unavailable, unrelated donors are a good alternative. Although total body irradiation (TBI) containing regimens were routinely employed in the past (Imashuku *et al.*, 1999b; Yagita *et al.*, 2001; Okamura *et al.*, 2003), more recently, reduced intensity SCT with a conditioning regimen such as the combination fludarabine/L-PAM has been successfully introduced (unpublished data). To date, a survey showed successful outcomes in 9 of 12 EBV-HLH recipients of allogeneic SCT (Imashuku *et al.*, 2004).

Prognosis and late sequelae

Long-term outcome of EBV-HLH is fairly good. Of 78 EBV-HLH patients 59 (75.6%) are alive at a median of 43 (1–122) months. Of the 19 (24.4%) fatal cases, 11 (14.1%) died within 2 months of diagnosis, while eight (10.3%) died later (Imashuku *et al.*, 2004). The complications leading to early death include pulmonary infection and hemorrhage, particularly coagulopathy-associated brain hemorrhage and neutropenia-induced sepsis or fungal infections (Imashuku *et al.*, 2000a, 2004). Therapy-related AML (t-AML), has been a major concern in the treatment of HLH. Stine *et al.*, reported an 11-year-old boy treated with etoposide ($0.3 \, g/m^2$ IV and $2.8 \, g/m^2$ orally) for VAHS, who developed t-AML 26 months from diagnosis (Stine *et al.*, 1997). Takahashi *et al.* (1998) described a 19-year-old male patient with t-AML 32 months from treatment with chemotherapy including etoposide (cumulative dose $0.9 \, g/m^2$ IV) and cytarabine for VAHS. Kitazawa *et al.* (2001) documented a 5-year-old girl with EBV-HLH treated with etoposide (cumulative dose $3.15 \, g/m^2$), who developed t-AML 31 months from treatment onset. Kitazawa's case was the only t-AML among the 81 EBV-HLH patients (77 of whom were children <15 years old) whom we collected (Imashuku *et al.*, 2002). Although t-AML seems to be very rare, patients receiving high-dose etoposide should be cautiously followed.

Lymphoma-associated HLH

Lymphoma is one of the common malignancies in all age groups. However, for unknown reasons lymphoma-associated hemophagocytic syndrome (LAHS) is more a problem of adults than children. In adult patients showing typical features of HLH without known triggers such as infections or collagen diseases, LAHS should first be suspected. Many types of lymphomas are involved in development of LAHS. LAHS shows two age clusters. EBV-positive T/NK-cell lymphoma-associated disease (T/NK-LAHS) mainly seen in young adults (aged 20–40), and EBV-negative

B-cell lymphoma-associated disease (B-LAHS) diagnosed more frequently in patients older than 40 (Takahashi *et al.*, 1999). As EBV-infected T/NK-cell proliferation plays a role in the development of HLH, similarities are noted in the pathogenesis and clinical features between EBV-HLH and T/NK-LAHS (Quintanilla-Martinez *et al.*, 2000; Mitarnun *et al.*, 2002; Kawa, 2003).

Types of lymphomas and role of EBV

Of the two types of LAHS, T/NK-LAHS has characteristic pathologic features with angiocentric or angiodestructive morphology (Chan, 1989b), while in B-LAHS, the main pathologic feature is infiltration of lymphoma cells into marrow, spleen and liver (Murase and Nakamura, 1999; Allory *et al.*, 2001). These lymphomatous lesions are accompanied by an exuberant hyperplasia of benign-appearing, hemophagocytic histiocytes.

In a review of 142 adults with LAHS, 68 cases were B-LAHS and 64 cases T/NK-LAHS (Takahashi *et al.*, 1999). Thus, these two types have a nearly equal incidence. However, EBV involvement differs. The EBV genome was detected in three of 24 B-LAHS patients and 19 of 23 T/NK-LAHS patients, thus the majority of T/NK-LAHS is EBV-positive while B-LAHS is mostly EBV-negative (Ohno *et al.*, 1998). In both types, hypercytokinemia plays a role in the development of HLH. In a comparative study of serum cytokine levels between the two types of LAHS, sCD25 was equally high in both, but interferon-gamma was significantly higher in T/NK-LAHS, similar to EBV-HLH. By contrast, serum levels of interleukin-6, TNF-alpha and interleukin-10 were significantly higher in B-LAHS and these cytokines are postulated to be derived at least partly from neoplastic B-cells (Ohno *et al.*, 2003). The types of lymphomas associated with HLH reported to date are listed in Table 18.3.

In contrast to adult LAHS, reports of pediatric LAHS are very limited. Sandlund reported an 11-year-old female showing systemic hemophagocytosis masking the diagnosis of large cell non-Hodgkin's lymphoma (NHL) (Sandlund *et al.*, 1997). A 10-year-old boy with EBV-positive subcutaneous peripheral T-cell lymphoma, was refractory to specific therapy for EBV-HLH (Imashuku, unpublished observation) while a 16-year-old boy with cutaneous EBV-peripheral T-cell lymphoma and LAHS is a long-term survivor following allogeneic SCT (Weitzman, unpublished observation).

Clinical features

Most of the T/NK-LAHS patients show evidence of hemophagocytosis in bone marrow and/or within lymphoma tissue before the development of overt fatal HLH (Kadin *et al.*, 1981; Jaffe *et al.*, 1983; Falini *et al.*, 1990). In particular, cutaneous

Table 18.3 Malignant lymphomas causing hemophagocytic syndrome (LAHS)

T/NK cell lymphoma
Nasal T-cell lymphoma
Peripheral T-cell lymphoma
Immunoblastic T-cell lymphoma
Subcutaneous T-cell lymphoma
Angiocentric lymphoma
Subcutaneous panniculitic T-cell lymphoma
Hepatosplenic gammadelta T-cell lymphoma
NK cell leukemia/lymphoma
B-cell lymphoma
Diffuse large B-dell lymphoma
Hepatosplenic B-cell lymphoma
T-cell rich B-cell lymphoma
Immunoblastic B-cell lymphoma
Intravascular lymphomatosis (Asian variant)

lesions are one of the common features of T-LAHS (Su *et al.*, 1995). Similar to EBV-HLH, EBV-positive T-LAHS shows EBV-monoclonality but not necessarily associated with TCR rearrangement (Dolezal *et al.*, 1995). Most patients with B-LAHS initially show only periodic fever, pancytopenia and hemophagocytosis, causing delay of correct diagnosis (Shimazaki *et al.*, 2000; Ohno *et al.*, 2003). Particularly, diffuse large B-cell lymphoma-HLH is characterized by hemophago-cytosis in marrow in the absence of peripheral lymphadenopathy (Murase and Nakamura, 1999; Allory *et al.*, 2001). In Takahashi's review (Takahashi *et al.*, 1999), 10 of 20 Japanese B-LAHS patients were found to have intravascular lymphomato-sis, a characteristic feature of intravascular infiltration of lymphoma cells (Murase and Nakamura, 1999).

Treatment and prognosis

In LAHS, the severity of the initial magnitude of the cytokine storm and under-lying nature of the lymphoma (stage, chemo-sensitivity, etc.) determine the progno-sis (Shimazaki *et al.*, 2000; Ohno *et al.*, 2003). At onset, initial treatment described for EBV-HLH is applicable for LAHS patients. However, because of delayed diag-nosis of underlying lymphoma, timely introduction of specific therapy is always a problem. Differential diagnosis from other underlying causes can often be difficult and lack of histologic proof of malignancy in the initial stage delays definitive diag-nosis in the majority of adult patients with LAHS (Chan *et al.*, 1989a). Sometimes lymphoma may even surface later in the clinical course of HLH.

As specific therapy, various anti-NHL chemotherapeutic regimens are available for each type of LAHS, however, there are no standard treatment regimens. The prognosis of adult LAHS is very poor with a median survival of 2.5 months for T/NK-LAHS and 6–9 months for B-LAHS (Takahashi *et al.*, 1999; Shimazaki *et al.*, 2000). Prognostic data for pediatric LAHS are not available. SCT could be a curable measure for LAHS cases, if applied in a timely fashion (Imashuku *et al.*, 1999b; Takami *et al.*, 2000; Hirai *et al.*, 2001). High-dose chemotherapy followed by autologous peripheral blood SCT is expected to improve the survival rate in future (Shimazaki *et al.*, 2000).

REFERENCES

Allen, M., De Fusco, C., Legrand, F., *et al.* (2001). Familial hemophagocytic lymphohistiocytosis: how late can the onset be? *Haematologica*, **86**, 499–503.

Allory, Y., Challine, D., Haioun, C., *et al.* (2001). Bone marrow involvement in lymphomas with hemophagocytic syndrome at presentation: a clinicopathologic study of 11 patients in a Western institution. *Am J Surg Path*, **25**, 865–874.

Ambruso, D.R., Hays, T., Zwartjes, W.J., *et al.* (1980). Successful treatment of lymphohistiocytic reticulosis with phagocytosis with epipodophyllotoxin VP 16–213. *Cancer*, **45**, 2516–2520.

Aricò, M., Janka, G., Fischer, A., *et al.* (1996). Hemophagocytic lymphohistiocytosis. Report of 122 children from the International Registry. FHL Study Group of the Histiocyte Society. *Leukemia*, **10**, 197–203.

Aricò, M., Allen, M., Brusa, S., *et al.* (2002). Haemophagocytic lymphohistiocytosis: proposal of a diagnostic algorithm based on perforin expression. *Br J Haematol*, **119**, 180–188.

Baker, K.S., DeLaat, C.A., Steinbuch, M., *et al.* (1997). Successful correction of hemophagocytic lymphohistiocytosis with related or unrelated bone marrow transplantation. *Blood*, **89**, 3857–3863.

Blanche, S., Caniglia, M., Girault, D., *et al.* (1991). Treatment of hemophagocytic lymphohistiocytosis with chemotherapy and bone marrow transplantation: a single-center study of 22 cases. *Blood*, **78**, 51–54.

Chan, J.K. and Ng, C.S. (1989b). Malignant lymphoma, natural killer cells and hemophagocytic syndrome. *Pathology*, **21**, 154–155.

Chan, E.Y., Pi, D., Chan, G.T., *et al.* (1989a). Peripheral T-cell lymphoma presenting as hemophagocytic syndrome. *Hematol Oncol*, **7**, 275–285.

Chen, R.L., Lin, K.H., Lin, D.T., *et al.* (1995). Immunomodulation treatment for childhood virus-associated haemophagocytic lymphohistiocytosis. *Br J Haematol*, **89**, 282–290.

Chen, J.S., Lin, K.H., Lin, D.T., *et al.* (1998). Longitudinal observation and outcome of nonfamilial childhood haemophagocytic syndrome receiving etoposide-containing regimens. *Br J Haematol*, **103**, 756–762.

Dolezal, M.V., Kamel, O.W., van de Rijn, M., *et al.* (1995). Virus-associated hemophagocytic syndrome characterized by clonal Epstein–Barr virus genome. *Am J Clin Pathol*, **103**, 189–194.

Dufourcq-Lagelouse, R., Pastural, E., Barrat, F.J., *et al.* (1999). Genetic basis of hemophagocytic lymphohistiocytosis syndrome (Review). *Int J Molec Med*, **4**, 127–133.

Duerken, M., Horstmann, M., Bieling, P., *et al.* (1999). Improved outcome in haemophagocytic lymphohistiocytosis after bone marrow transplantation from related and unrelated donors: a single-centre experience of 12 patients. *Br J Haematol*, **106**, 1052–1058.

Duval, M., Fenneteau, O., Doireau, V., *et al.* (1999). Intermittent hemophagocytic lymphohistiocytosis is a regular feature of lysinuric protein intolerance. *J Pediatr*, **134**, 236–239.

Eife, R., Janka, G.E., Belohradsky, B.H. *et al.* (1989). Natural killer cell function and interferon production in familial hemophagocytic lymphohistiocytosis. *Pediatr Hematol Oncol*, **6**, 265–272.

Falini, B., Pileri, S., De Solas, I., *et al.* (1990). Peripheral T-cell lymphoma associated with hemophagocytic syndrome. *Blood*, **75**, 434–444.

Farquhar, J.W. and Claireaux, A.E. (1952). Familial haemophagocytic reticulosis. *Arch Dis Child*, **27**, 519–525.

Fischer, A., Virelizier, J.L., Arenzana-Seisdedos, F., *et al.* (1985). Treatment of four patients with erythrophagocytic lymphohistiocytosis by a combination of epipodophyllotoxin, steroids, intrathecal methotrexate, and cranial irradiation. *Pediatrics*, **76**, 263–268.

Fischer, A., Cerf-Bensussan, N., Blanche, S., *et al.* (1986). Allogeneic bone marrow transplantation for erythrophagocytic lymphohistiocytosis. *J Pediatr*, **108**, 267–270.

Fisman, D.N. (2000). Hemophagocytic syndromes and infection. *Emerg Infect Dis*, **6**, 601–608.

Freeman, B., Rathore, M.H., Salman, E., *et al.* (1993). Intravenously administered immune globulin for the treatment of infection-associated hemophagocytic syndrome. *J Pediatr*, **123**, 479–481.

Fujii, N., Takenaka, K., Hiraki, A., *et al.* (2000). Allogeneic peripheral blood stem cell transplantation for the treatment of chronic active Epstein–Barr virus infection. *Bone Marrow Transplant*, **26**, 805–808.

Garbagnati, E. (1993). Changes in lipid profile observed in children over the course of infectious disease. *Acta Paediatr*, **82**, 948–952.

Grom, A.A., Villanueva, J., Lee, S., *et al.* (2003). Natural killer cell dysfunction in patients with systemic-onset juvenile rheumatoid arthritis and macrophage activation syndrome. *J Pediatr*, **142**, 292–296.

Hadchouel, M., Prieur, A.M. and Griscelli, C. (1985). Acute hemorrhagic, hepatic, and neurologic manifestations in juvenile rheumatoid arthritis: possible relationship to drugs or infection. *J Pediatr*, **106**, 561–566.

Haddad, E., Sulis, M.L., Jabado, N., *et al.* (1997). Frequency and severity of central nervous system lesions in hemophagocytic lymphohistiocytosis. *Blood*, **89**, 794–800.

Henter, J.-I. and Elinder, G. (1991). Familial hemophagocytic lymphohistiocytosis. Clinical review based on the findings in seven children. *Acta Paediatr Scand*, **80**, 269–277.

Henter, J.-I. and Elinder, G. (1992). Cerebromeningeal haemophagocytic lymphohistiocytosis. *Lancet*, **339**, 104–107.

Henter, J.-I. and Nennesmo, I. (1997). Neuropathologic findings and neurologic symptoms in twenty-three children with hemophagocytic lymphohistiocytosis. *J Pediatr*, **130**, 358–365.

Henter, J.-I., Elinder, G., Soder, O. et al. (1991a). Incidence in Sweden and clinical features of familial hemophagocytic lymphohistiocytosis. *Acta Paediatr Scand*, **80**, 428–435.

Henter, J.-I., Carlson, L.A., Soeder, O., et al. (1991b). Lipoprotein alterations and plasma lipoprotein lipase reduction in familial hemophagocytic lymphohistiocytosis. *Acta Paediatr Scand*, **80**, 675–681.

Henter, J.-I., Elinder, G. and Ost, A. (1991c). Diagnostic guidelines for hemophagocytic lymphohistiocytosis. The FHL Study Group of the Histiocyte Society. *Semin Oncol*, **18**, 29–33.

Henter, J.-I., Ehrnst, A., Andersson, J., et al. (1993). Familial hemophagocytic lymphohistiocytosis and viral infections. *Acta Paediatr*, **82**, 369–372.

Henter, J.-I., Aricò, M., Egeler, R.M., et al. (1997). HLH-94: a treatment protocol for hemophagocytic lymphohistiocytosis. HLH study Group of the Histiocyte Society. *Med Pediatr Oncol*, **28**, 342–347.

Henter, J.-I., Samuelsson-Horne, A., Aricò, M., et al. (2002). Treatment of hemophagocytic lymphohistiocytosis with HLH-94 immunochemotherapy and bone marrow transplantation. *Blood*, **100**, 2367–2373.

Hirai, H., Shimazaki, C., Hatsuse, M., et al. (2001). Autologous peripheral blood stem cell transplantation for adult patients with B-cell lymphoma-associated hemophagocytic syndrome. *Leukemia*, **15**, 311–312.

Ikeda, H., Kato, M., Matsunaga, A., et al. (1998). Multiple sulphatase deficiency and haemophagocytic syndrome. *Eur J Pediatr*, **157**, 553–554.

Imashuku, S. (2002). Clinical features and treatment strategies of Epstein–Barr virus-associated hemophagocytic lymphohistiocytosis. *Crit Reviews Hematol/Oncol*, **44**, 259–272.

Imashuku, S., Hibi, S., Tabata, Y., et al. (1998). Biomarker and morphological characteristics of Epstein–Barr virus-related hemophagocytic lymphohistiocytosis. *Med Pediatr Oncol*, **31**, 131–137.

Imashuku, S., Hibi, S., Ohara, T., et al. (1999a). Effective control of Epstein–Barr virus-related hemophagocytic lymphohistiocytosis with immunochemotherapy. *Blood*, **93**, 1869–1874.

Imashuku, S., Hibi, S., Todo, S., et al. (1999b). Allogeneic hematopoietic stem cell transplantation for patients with hemophagocytic syndrome (HPS) in Japan. *Bone Marrow Transplant*, **23**, 569–572.

Imashuku, S., Hibi, S., Kuriyama, K., et al. (2000a). Management of severe neutropenia with cyclosporin during initial treatment of Epstein–Barr virus-related hemophagocytic lymphohistiocytosis. *Leuk Lymphoma*, **36**, 339–346.

Imashuku, S., Hibi, S., Tabata, Y., et al. (2000b). Outcome of clonal hemophagocytic lymphohistiocytosis: analysis of 32 cases. *Leuk Lymphoma*, **37**, 577–584.

Imashuku, S., Kuriyama, K., Teramura, T., et al. (2001). Requirement for etoposide in the treatment of Epstein–Barr virus-associated hemophagocytic lymphohistiocytosis. *J Clin Oncol*, **19**, 2665–2673.

Imashuku, S., Teramura, T., Kuriyama, K., et al. (2002). Risk of etoposide-related acute myeloid leukemia in the treatment of Epstein–Barr virus-associated hemophagocytic lymphohistiocytosis. *Int J Hematol*, **75**, 174–177.

Imashuku, S., Kuriyama, K., Sakai, R., et al. (2003). Treatment of Epstein–Barr virus-associated hemophagocytic lymphohistiocytosis (EBV-HLH) in young adults: a report from the HLH study center. *Med Pediatr Oncol*, **41**, 103–109.

Imashuku, S., Teramura, T., Tauchi, H., *et al.* (2004). Longitudinal follow-up of patients with Epstein–Barr virus-associated hemophagocytic lymphohistiocytosis. *Haematologica*, **89**, 183–188.

Ishihara, S., Okada, S., Wakiguchi, H., *et al.* (1995). Chronic active Epstein–Barr virus infection in children in Japan. *Acta Paediatr*, **84**, 1271–1275.

Jabado, N., de Graeff-Meeder, E.R., Cavazzana-Calvo, M., *et al.* (1997). Treatment of familial hemophagocytic lymphohistiocytosis with bone marrow transplantation from HLA genetically nonidentical donors. *Blood*, **90**, 4743–4748.

Jaffe, E.S., Costa, J., Fauci, A.S., *et al.* (1983). Malignant lymphoma and erythrophagocytosis simulating malignant histiocytosis. *Am J Med*, **75**, 741–749.

Janka, G.E. (1983). Familial hemophagocytic lymphohistiocytosis. *Eur J Pediatr*, **140**, 221–230.

Janka, G.E. (1989). Familial hemophagocytic lymphohistiocytosis: therapy in the German experience. *Pediatr Hematol Oncol*, **6**, 227–231.

Janka, G.E. and Schneider, E.M. (2004). Modern management of children with haemophagocytic lymphohistiocytosis. *Br J Haematol*, **124**, 4–14.

Janka, G., Imashuku, S., Elinder, G., *et al.* (1998). Infection- and malignancy-associated hemophagocytic syndromes. Secondary hemophagocytic lymphohistiocytosis. *Hematol Oncol Clin North Am*, **12**, 435–444.

Janka-Schaub, G.E., Rosenberger, M., Lorenz, I., *et al.* (1999). Hemophagocytic lymphohistiocytosis: clinical variability and usefulness of diagnostic parameters. *Med Pediatr Oncol*, **33**, 517.

Janka, G.E., Muller-Rosenberger, M. and Schneider, E.M. (2000). Persistent defect of cellular cytotoxicity after Epstein–Barr virus-associated hemophagocytic lymphohistiocytosis (HLH). *Blood*, **96**, 36b.

Kadin, M.E., Kamoun, M. and Lamberg, J. (1981). Erythrophagocytic T gamma lymphoma: a clinicopathologic entity resembling malignant histiocytosis. *New Engl J Med*, **304**, 648–653.

Kanegane, H., Nomura, K., Miyawaki, T., *et al.* (2002). Biological aspects of Epstein–Barr virus (EBV)-infected lymphocytes in chronic active EBV infection and associated malignancies. *Crit Reviews Hematol Oncol*, **44**, 239–249.

Katano, H., Ali, M.A., Patera, A.C., *et al.* (2004). Chronic active Epstein–Barr virus infection associated with mutations in perforin that impair its maturation. *Blood*, **103**, 1244–1252.

Kawa, K. (2003). Diagnosis and treatment of Epstein–Barr virus-associated natural killer lymphoproliferative disease. *Int J Hematol*, **78**, 24–31.

Kawaguchi, H., Miyashita, T., Herbst, H., *et al.* (1993). Epstein–Barr virus-infected T lymphocytes in Epstein–Barr virus-associated hemophagocytic syndrome. *J Clin Invest*, **92**, 1444–1450.

Kieslich, M., Vecchi, M., Driever, P.H., *et al.* (2001). Acute encephalopathy as a primary manifestation of haemophagocytic lymphohistiocytosis. *Develop Med Child Neurol*, **43**, 555–558.

Kikuta, H. and Sakiyama, Y. (1995). Etoposide (VP-16) inhibits Epstein–Barr virus determined nuclear antigen (EBNA) synthesis. *Br J Haematol*, **90**, 971–973.

Kikuta, H., Sakiyama, Y., Matsumoto, S., *et al.* (1993). Fatal Epstein–Barr virus-associated hemophagocytic syndrome. *Blood*, **82**, 3259–3264.

Kimura, H., Morita, M., Yabuta, Y., *et al.* (1999). Quantitative analysis of Epstein–Barr virus load by using a real-time PCR assay. *J Clin Microbiol*, **37**, 132–136.

Kitazawa, J., Ito, E., Arai, K., *et al.* (2001). Secondary acute myelocytic leukemia after successful chemotherapy with etoposide for Epstein–Barr virus-associated hemophagocytic lymphohistiocytosis. *Med Pediatr Oncol,* **37**, 153–154.

Kogawa, K., Lee, S.M., Villanueva, J., *et al.* (2002). Perforin expression in cytotoxic lymphocytes from patients with hemophagocytic lymphohistiocytosis and their family members. *Blood,* **99**, 61–66.

Komp, D.M., McNamara, J. and Buckley, P. (1989). Elevated soluble interleukin-2 receptor in childhood hemophagocytic histiocytic syndromes. *Blood,* **73**, 2128–2132.

Loechelt, B.J., Egeler, M., Filipovich, A.H., *et al.* (1994). Immunosuppression: preliminary results of alternative maintenance therapy for familial hemophagocytic lymphohistiocytosis (FHL). *Med Pediatr Oncol,* **22**, 325–328.

Mandel, H., Gozal, D., Aizin, A., *et al.* (1990). Haemophagocytosis in hereditary fructose intolerance: a diagnostic dilemma. *J Inherited Metabol Dis,* **13**, 267–269.

Matsumoto, Y., Naniwa, D., Banno, S., *et al.* (1998). The efficacy of therapeutic plasmapheresis for the treatment of fatal hemophagocytic syndrome: two case reports. *Therapeutic Apheresis,* **2**, 300–304.

Mitarnun, W., Suwiwat, S., Pradutkanchana, J., *et al.* (2002). Epstein–Barr virus-associated peripheral T-cell and NK-cell proliferative disease/lymphoma: clinicopathologic, serologic, and molecular analysis. *Am J Hematol,* **70**, 31–38.

Molleran Lee, S., Villanueva, J., Sumegi, J., *et al.* (2004). Characterisation of diverse PRF1 mutations leading to decreased natural killer cell activity in North American families with haemophagocytic lymphohistiocytosis. *J Med Genet,* **41**, 137–144.

Mouy, R., Stephan, J.L., Pillet, P., *et al.* (1996). Efficacy of cyclosporine A in the treatment of macrophage activation syndrome in juvenile arthritis: report of five cases. *J Pediatr,* **129**, 750–754.

Mroczek, E.C., Weisenburger, D.D., Grierson, H.L., *et al.* (1987). Fatal infectious mononucleosis and virus-associated hemophagocytic syndrome. *Arch Pathol Lab Med,* **111**, 530–535.

Mueller-Rosenberger, M. (2004). *Histiozytäre Hämophagozytosesyndrome bei Kindern; Klinik, Verlauf und funktionelle immunologische Diagnostik*, Thesis University Hamburg, Hamburg.

Murase, T. and Nakamura, S. (1999). An Asian variant of intravascular lymphomatosis: an updated review of malignant histiocytosis-like B-cell lymphoma. *Leuk Lymphoma,* **33**, 459–473.

Nomura, S., Koshikawa, K., Hamamoto, K., *et al.* (1992). Steroid and gamma globulin therapy against virus-associated hemophagocytic syndrome. *Rinsho Ketsueki,* **33**, 1242–1247.

Ohno, T., Miyake, N., Hada, S., *et al.* (1998). Hemophagocytic syndrome in five patients with Epstein–Barr virus negative B-cell lymphoma. *Cancer,* **82**, 1963–1972.

Ohno, T., Ueda, Y., Nagai, K., *et al.* (2003). The serum cytokine profiles of lymphoma-associated hemophagocytic syndrome: a comparative analysis of B-cell and T-cell/natural killer cell lymphomas. *Int J Hematol,* **77**, 286–294.

Okamura, T., Hatsukawa, Y., Arai, H., *et al.* (2000). Blood stem-cell transplantation for chronic active Epstein–Barr virus with lymphoproliferation. *Lancet,* **356**, 223–224.

Okamura, T., Kishimoto, T., Inoue, M., *et al.* (2003). Unrelated bone marrow transplantation for Epstein–Barr virus-associated T/NK-cell lymphoproliferative disease. *Bone Marrow Transplant,* **31**, 105–111.

Oyama, Y., Amano, T., Hirakawa, S., *et al.* (1989). Haemophagocytic syndrome treated with cyclosporin A: a T cell disorder? *Br J Haematol*, **73**, 276–278.

Parizhskaya, M., Reyes, J. and Jaffe, R. (1999). Hemophagocytic syndrome presenting as acute hepatic failure in two infants: clinical overlap with neonatal hemochromatosis. *Pediatr Develop Pathol*, **2**, 360–366.

Perel, Y., Alos, N., Ansoborlo, S., *et al.* (1997). Dramatic efficacy of antithymocyte globulins in childhood EBV-associated haemophagocytic syndrome. *Acta Paediatr*, **86**, 911.

Pracher, E., Grumayer-Panzer, E.R., Zoubek, A., *et al.* (1993). Bone marrow transplantation during fulminant EBV-infection in Duncan's syndrome. *Lancet*, **342**, 1362.

Quintanilla-Martinez, L., Kumar, S., Fend, F., *et al.* (2000). Fulminant EBV(+) T-cell lymphoproliferative disorder following acute/chronic EBV infection: a distinct clinicopathologic syndrome. *Blood*, **96**, 443–451.

Ramanan, A.V. and Baildam, E.M. (2002). Macrophage activation syndrome is hemophagocytic lymphohistiocytosis – need for the right terminology. *J Rheumatol*, **29**, 1105 (author reply).

Reiner, A.P. and Spivak, J.L. (1988). Hematophagic histiocytosis: a report of 23 new patients and a review of the literature. *Medicine (Balt)*, **67**, 369–388.

Risdall, R.J., McKenna, R.W., Nesbit, M.E., *et al.* (1979). Virus-associated hemophagocytic syndrome: a benign histiocytic proliferation distinct from malignant histiocytosis. *Cancer*, **44**, 993–1002.

Rostasy, K., Kolb, R., Pohl, D., *et al.* (2004). CNS disease as the main manifestation of hemophagocytic lymphohistiocytosis in two children. *Neuropediatrics*, **35**, 45–49.

Sandlund, J.T., Roberts, W.M., Pui, C.H., *et al.* (1997). Systemic hemophagocytosis masking the diagnosis of large cell non-Hodgkin lymphoma. *Med Pediatr Oncol*, **29**, 167–169.

Schneider, E.M., Lorenz, I., Muller-Rosenberger, M., *et al.* (2002). Hemophagocytic lymphohistiocytosis is associated with deficiencies of cellular cytolysis but normal expression of transcripts relevant to killer-cell-induced apoptosis. *Blood*, **100**, 2891–2898.

Shimazaki, C., Inaba, T. and Nakagawa, M. (2000). B-cell lymphoma-associated hemophagocytic syndrome. *Leuk Lymphoma*, **38**, 121–130.

Spieker, T., Kurth, J., Kuppers, R., *et al.* (2000). Molecular single-cell analysis of the clonal relationship of small Epstein–Barr virus-infected cells and Epstein–Barr virus-harboring Hodgkin and Reed/Sternberg cells in Hodgkin disease. *Blood*, **96**, 3133–3138.

Stephan, J.L., Donadieu, J., Ledeist, F., *et al.* (1993). Treatment of familial hemophagocytic lymphohistiocytosis with antithymocyte globulins, steroids, and cyclosporin A. *Blood*, **82**, 2319–2323.

Stephan, J.L., Kone-Paut, I., Galambrun, C., *et al.* (2001). Reactive haemophagocytic syndrome in children with inflammatory disorders: a retrospective study of 24 patients. *Rheumatology (Oxf)*, **40**, 1285–1292.

Stine, K.C., Saylors, R.L., Sawyer, J.R. *et al.* (1997). Secondary acute myelogenous leukemia following safe exposure to etoposide. *J Clin Oncol*, **15**, 1583–1586.

Su, I.J., Chen, R.L., Lin, D.T., *et al.* (1994). Epstein–Barr virus (EBV) infects T lymphocytes in childhood EBV-associated hemophagocytic syndrome in Taiwan. *Am J Pathol*, **144**, 1219–1225.

Su, I.J., Wang, C.H., Cheng, A.L., *et al.* (1995). Hemophagocytic syndrome in Epstein–Barr virus-associated T-lymphoproliferative disorders: disease spectrum, pathogenesis, and management. *Leuk Lymphoma*, **19**, 401–406.

Sullivan, K.E., Delaat, C.A., Douglas, S.D., et al. (1998). Defective natural killer cell function in patients with hemophagocytic lymphohistiocytosis and in first degree relatives. *Pediatr Res*, **44**, 465–468.

Sumazaki, R., Kanegane, H., Osaki, M., et al. (2001). SH2D1A mutations in Japanese males with severe Epstein–Barr virus – associated illnesses. *Blood*, **98**, 1268–1270.

Sumegi, J., Huang, D., Lanyi, A., et al. (2000). Correlation of mutations of the SH2D1A gene and Epstein–Barr virus infection with clinical phenotype and outcome in X-linked lymphoproliferative disease. *Blood*, **96**, 3118–3125.

Takahashi, T., Yagasaki, F., Endo, K., et al. (1998). Therapy-related AML after successful chemotherapy with low dose etoposide for virus-associated hemophagocytic syndrome. *Int J Hematol*, **68**, 333–336.

Takahashi, N., Chubachi, A., Miura, I., et al. (1999). Lymphoma-associated hemophagocytic syndrome in Japan. *Rinsho Ketsueki*, **40**, 542–549.

Takami, A., Nakao, S., Ueda, M., et al. (2000). Successful treatment of B-cell lymphoma associated with hemophagocytic syndrome using autologous peripheral blood CD34 positive cell transplantation followed by induction of autologous graft-versus-host disease. *Ann Hematol*, **79**, 389–391.

Teramura, T., Tabata, Y., Yagi, T., et al. (2002). Quantitative analysis of cell-free Epstein–Barr virus genome copy number in patients with EBV-associated hemophagocytic lymphohistiocytosis. *Leuk Lymphoma*, **43**, 173–179.

Tsuji, Y., Ayaki, H., Whitman, S.P., et al. (2000). Coordinate transcriptional and translational regulation of ferritin in response to oxidative stress. *Mol Cell Biol*, **20**, 5818–5827.

Ueda, I., Morimoto, A., Inaba, T., et al. (2003). Characteristic perforin gene mutations of haemophagocytic lymphohistiocytosis patients in Japan. *Br J Haematol*, **121**, 503–510.

Wulffraat, N.M., Rijkers, G.T., Elst, E., et al. (2003). Reduced perforin expression in systemic juvenile idiopathic arthritis is restored by autologous stem-cell transplantation. *Rheumatology (Oxf)*, **42**, 375–379.

Yagita, M., Iwakura, H., Kishimoto, T., et al. (2001). Successful allogeneic stem cell transplantation from an unrelated donor for aggressive Epstein–Barr virus-associated clonal T-cell proliferation with hemophagocytosis. *Int J Hematol*, **74**, 451–454.

Zheng, C., Schneider, E.M., Samuelsson-Horne, A.C., et al. (2004). Natural killer cell activity subtypes provide therapeutic guidance in hemophagocytic lymphohistiocytosis. *Pediatr Blood Cancer*, **43**, 200.

19

Secondary haemophagocytic syndromes associated with rheumatic diseases

Athimalaipet Ramanan, Ronald Laxer and Rayfel Schneider

Macrophage activation syndrome (MAS) is a term used by rheumatologists to describe a form of secondary haemophagocytic lymphohistiocytosis (HLH) in association with chronic rheumatic diseases of childhood. It occurs most commonly with systemic-onset juvenile rheumatoid arthritis (SoJRA), but has also been reported with other rheumatic diseases. MAS manifestations may be seen at the onset of the rheumatic disease, during periods of active disease or even when the underlying rheumatic disease is quiescent.

Historical perspective and issues with nomenclature

The earliest description of MAS in the paediatric rheumatology literature may be the report of deaths from hepatic failure in patients with SoJRA at the first American Rheumatism Association(ARA) conference on rheumatic diseases of childhood (Boone, 1977). In 1983, Silverman described seven patients with 'consumptive coagulopathy' in children with SoJRA, either following the second dose of intramuscular gold or in the face of active disease (Silverman et al., 1983). The prominent clinical feature seen was a coagulopathy resembling disseminated intravascular coagulation (DIC), which most likely was a manifestation of secondary HLH. Subsequently, Jacobs reported five children (four with SoJRA, one with polyarticular juvenile rheumatic arthritis (JRA)) with a fatal outcome from a similar coagulopathy following the second gold injection (Jacobs et al., 1984). Hadchouel in 1985 described seven patients with SoJRA who developed a clinical syndrome characterized by haemorrhagic and neurological manifestations and hepatic, haematological and metabolic derangements (Hadchouel et al., 1985). These authors were the first to hypothesise that the syndrome was secondary to excessive activation of macrophages, which may have been precipitated by the second injection of gold. Haemophagocytic syndromes following coxsackie and varicella zoster virus infections were described in 1985 in two children with SoJRA (Heaton and Moller, 1985; Morris et al., 1985).

The term 'macrophage activation syndrome' (abbreviated as MAS) was first used by Stephan et al. who described four children with chronic rheumatic disease

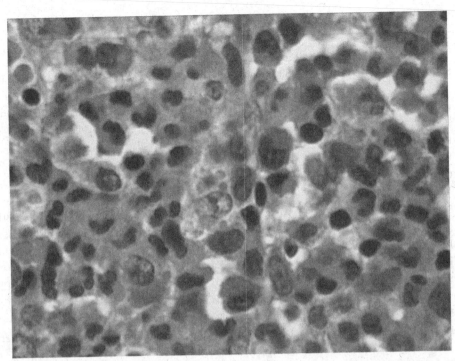

Figure 19.1   Hemophagocytosis in bone marrow of a 13-year-old girl who developed MAS when her SoJRA was in remission without medications

who developed a coagulopathy and features of a haemophagocytic syndrome (Stephan *et al.*, 1993). They identified the most characteristic feature of this syndrome to be the presence in the bone marrow of well-differentiated macrophages showing active hemophagocytosis (Figure 19.1). MAS has been the term used to describe secondary HLH in patients with rheumatic disease, since this description. Numerous case reports of MAS in children have been published over the last decade and a wide variety of potential triggers have been identified. However, in many cases, no identifiable trigger can be found.

The issue of a universally accepted nomenclature has not been resolved. The recognition of MAS as a form of secondary HLH and adoption of common terminology might alleviate some of the confusion surrounding this diagnosis (Athreya, 2002; Ramanan and Schneider, 2003a) and may lead to better understanding of the pathogenesis and treatment of this potentially fatal complication.

Classification of MAS among histiocyte disorders

MAS falls into the category of macrophage-related disorders and along with other forms of HLH accounts for most patients in the category of Class II histiocytosis.

Table 19.1 Rheumatic diseases associated with MAS/HLH

Rheumatic diseases	References
SoJRA	Silverman *et al.* (1983); Jacobs *et al.* (1984); Hadchouel *et al.* (1985); Morris *et al.* (1985); Stephan *et al.* 1993, (2001); Sawhney *et al.* (2001); Ramanan and Schneider, (2003); Ravelli *et al.* (2001); Cuende *et al.* (2001); Ramanan *et al.* (2003); Yamanouchi *et al.* (1998)
Polyarticular JRA	Davies *et al.* (1994); Stephan *et al.* (2001)
ERA	Sawhney *et al.* (2001)
CINCA	Sawhney *et al.* (2001)
AOSD	Coffernils *et al.* (1992); Dhote *et al.* (2003)
SLE	Wong *et al.* (1991); Takahashi *et al.* (1998); Sawhney *et al.* (2001); Stephan *et al.* (2001); Tsuji *et al.* (2002); Dhote *et al.* (2003);
Juvenile dermatomyositis	Kobayashi *et al.* (2000); Madaule *et al.* (2000)
Kawasaki disease	al-Eid, (2000); Kaneko, (1998)
Systemic sclerosis	Dhote *et al.* (2003); Katsumata *et al.* (2002); Tochimoto *et al.* (2001); Kumakura *et al.* (1997)
Mixed connective tissue disease	Dhote *et al.* (2003); Kumakura *et al.* (1997)
Rheumatoid arthritis	Dhote *et al.* (2003); Onishi and Namiuchi, (1994); Yamanouchi *et al.* (1998); Vecer *et al.* (2000)
Sarcoidosis	Dhote *et al.* (2003); Kobayashi *et al.* (2000)
Sjogren's syndrome	Dhote *et al.* (2003)
Polyarteritis nodosa	Dhote *et al.* (2003)

ERA: enthesitis-related arthritis; CINCA: chronic infantile neurological and cutaneous syndrome; AOSD: adult Still's disease; SLE: Systemic lupus erythematosus.

However, the current classification of histiocytic disorders does not specifically include rheumatic disease-associated MAS/HLH and it's addition as a distinct entity within the macrophage-related disorders (Class II-non-Langerhans cell histiocytosis) would be appropriate (Athreya, 2002; Ramanan and Baildam, 2002).

Rheumatic diseases associated with MAS (Table 19.1)

Systemic-onset JRA (SoJRA)

SoJRA is a systemic disease characterized by fever, rash, hepatosplenomegaly, lymphadenopathy, serositis, anaemia, leucocytosis, thrombocytosis and arthritis. When this disease begins after the age of 16, it is referred to as adult-onset Still's disease (AOSD). Although SoJRA constitutes only 10–20% of JRA, it accounts for more than two-thirds of the mortality in children with JRA. One of the major causes of morbidity and mortality seen in SoJRA is MAS. The incidence of SoJRA is estimated to be about 0.4–0.8/100,000. The true incidence of MAS in childhood SoJRA is

Table 19.2 Potential triggers of MAS/HLH in rheumatic diseases

Triggers	References
Drugs	
Aspirin	Silverman *et al.* (1983); Hadchouel *et al.* (1985); Stephan *et al.* (2001)
Non steroidal anti-inflammatory drugs	Silverman *et al.* (1983)
Methotrexate	Ravelli *et al.* (2001)
Gold salts (particularly second dose of IM gold)	Silverman *et al.* (1983); Hadchouel *et al.* (1985)
Etanercept	Ramanan and Schneider, (2003)
Sulfasalazine	Ravelli *et al.* (2001); Stephan *et al.* (2001)
Morniflumate	Stephan *et al.* (2001)
ASCT	Barron *et al.* (2001)
Viruses	
EBV	Sawhney *et al.* (2001); Davies *et al.* (1994); Stephan *et al.* (2001)
Varicella zoster virus	Morris *et al.* (1985); Stephan *et al.* (2001)
Coxsackie virus	Heaton and Moller, (1985); Stephan *et al.* (2001)
Parvovirus B19	Stephan *et al.* (2001)
Hepatitis A virus	McPeake *et al.* (1993)
Salmonella enteritidis	Stephan *et al.* (2001)
Pneumocystis carinii	Stephan *et al.* (2001)
Enterococcal sepsis	Sawhney *et al.* (2001)

ASCT: autologous stem cell transplant; IM: intramuscular.

unknown. In one retrospective study from a tertiary institution, seven of the 103 children diagnosed with SoJRA over a 20-year period developed MAS (6.7%) (Sawhney *et al.*, 2001).

As with other forms of MAS, a variety of triggers have been implicated in the pathogenesis of MAS associated with SoJRA, including viral infections, non-steroidal anti-inflammatory drug therapy, gold salts, sulphasalazine, methotrexate and etanercept (Table 19.2). MAS in SoJRA can be seen at the initial diagnosis, during a flare of the disease or even when the disease is in remission (Davies *et al.*, 1994; Cuende *et al.*, 2001; Prahalad *et al.*, 2001).

The hallmark manifestation of MAS in these patients appears to be a haemorrhagic syndrome resembling DIC. The clinical manifestations of the coagulopathy may range from simple petechiae to extensive ecchymotic lesions, epistaxis, and major upper and lower gastrointestinal bleeds with haematemesis and rectal bleeding. Children are usually acutely unwell with unremitting high fever and the relatively rapid development of hepatosplenomegaly and lymphadenopathy. Neurological symptoms may include headache, lethargy and irritability, and may progress to more severe encephalopathy with confusion, seizures and coma. Children with the most severe forms may have multiorgan involvement with cardiac, respiratory and renal failure. In the face of severe systemic illness, a paradoxical improvement in the symptoms and signs of arthritis has been noted in some patients (Sawhney *et al.*, 2001). There may be a range of clinical severity with some children having relatively mild symptoms in association with the typical laboratory derangements.

Laboratory investigations characteristically reveal prolonged clotting profiles as measured by prothrombin time, partial thromboplastin time, international normalized ratios (INR) and marked hypofibrinogenemia (which contributes to the low erythrocyte sedimentation rate (ESR) that is seen). The fibrin degradation products (D-dimers) are also elevated to a much greater degree than expected with active systemic disease. Liver transaminases are typically elevated, sometimes progressing to frank hepatic failure. Cerebrospinal fluid (CSF) analysis may reveal pleocytosis and elevation of the CSF protein. Hyponatremia may also occur. Renal involvement is infrequent but haematuria, proteinuria and renal failure may be seen.

One of the major difficulties in diagnosis is distinguishing signs and symptoms of the underlying active disease from MAS, since several clinical features (including fever, hepatosplenomegaly and lymphadenopathy) and several laboratory features (including anaemia, elevated transaminases and elevated D-dimers) may be seen in both conditions. Table 19.3 highlights the differences between active systemic disease and MAS in patients with SoJRA. Children with SoJRA typically have fever spikes once or twice each day, often with exacerbation of a maculopapular rash and might appear rather well with defervescence of the fever. The fever with MAS is more often sustained. The key distinguishing laboratory features of MAS include hypofibrinogenemia (rather than hyperfibrinogenemia as in active systemic onset juvenile idiopathic arthritis (SoJIA)) and a sudden and sharp drop in the white cell, neutrophil and platelet counts (as opposed to the neutrophilic leucocytosis and thrombocytosis that is typically seen with active SoJRA). Anaemia is an important manifestation of MAS but is also frequently seen with active systemic disease. In addition to a flare of SoJRA, differential or concurrent diagnoses that need to be considered include infections, the evolution of a new malignancy and the toxicities of medications. Low-dose weekly methotrexate, a commonly used immunosuppressive agent in JRA, can cause cytopaenias as well as elevated transaminases.

Systemic lupus erythematosus

Among the other pediatric rheumatic diseases (systemic lupus erythematosus, SLE) is most often associated with a haemophagocytic syndrome. In 1991, Wong showed that the bone marrow of SLE patients manifested a reactive haemophagocytosis and proposed the term 'lupus haemophagocytic syndrome' (Wong *et al.*, 1991). There have since been several reports of MAS with SLE in both children and

Table 19.3 Comparison of clinical and laboratory features of SoJRA and MAS

	SoJRA	MAS
Fever pattern	Quotidian	Unremitting
Rash	Evanescent, maculopapular	Petechial or purpuric
Hepatosplenomegaly	+	+
Lymphadenopathy	+	+
Arthritis	+	−
Serositis	+	−
Encephalopathy	−	+
WCC and neutrophil count	↑↑	↓
Hb	N or ↓	↓
Platelets	↑↑	↓
ESR	↑↑	N or sudden decrease
Bilirubin	N	N or ↑
ALT/AST	N or ↑	↑↑
PT	N	↑
PTT	N	↑
D-dimers	↑	↑↑
Fibrinogen	↑	↓
Ferritin	N or ↑	↑↑

ALT: alanine aminotransferase; AST: asparate aminotransferase; Hb: haemoglobin; N: normal; PT: prothrombin time; PTT: partial thromboplastin time.

adults (Takahashi et al., 1998; Ravelli et al., 2001a; Stephan et al., 2001; Tsuji et al., 2002). In one study of 80 adult patients with SLE, 73/80 had elevated liver enzymes; 7/73 patients (9.6%) were considered to have a haemophagocytic syndrome and it was emphasized that a haemophagocytic syndrome complicating SLE is not infrequent (Tsuji et al., 2002). The diagnosis of MAS in SLE patients may also be difficult since manifestations of active lupus include fever, lymphadenopathy, hepatosplenomegaly and sometimes petechiae and purpura. Laboratory investigations characteristically reveal cytopaenias and not infrequently elevated liver enzymes. Distinguishing active SLE from MAS relies on identifying typical clinical features of active disease, such as malar rash, mucositis, arthritis and serositis aided by laboratory evidence of nephritis, low complement levels and elevated titres of autoantibodies. The toxicities of immunosuppressive agents used to treat SLE, such as azathioprine and cyclophosphamide, can also mimic some of the laboratory features of MAS, especially cytopaenias and elevated transaminases.

Other rheumatic diseases associated with MAS include dermatomyositis, Kawasaki disease, mixed connective tissue disease, adult rheumatoid arthritis and systemic sclerosis (Table 19.1).

Etiopathogenesis of MAS associated with rheumatic diseases

The features common to all cases of HLH are thought to be attributable to hyper-activation of T-cells and macrophages, and the resulting hypercytokinemia.

It is unclear why some patients with rheumatic disease, particularly children with SoJRA, develop macrophage hyperactivation while others do not, even when exposed to the same potential triggers. Subsequent to studies in children with familial HLH, where defects in perforin genes are thought to account for 20–40% of all cases (Goransdotter Ericson *et al.*, 2001), several investigators have looked at the role of perforin in cases of rheumatic disease-associated HLH.

In a study by Grom *et al.*, natural killer (NK) cell activity was low in some patients with MAS (Grom *et al.*, 2003). Some of these patients also had low levels of perforin expression but genetic analysis did not identify known perforin mutations. Wulffraat demonstrated that four patients with SoJRA with low levels of perforin expression had a clear increase in perforin expression 12 months after autologous stem cell transplantation (Wulffraat *et al.*, 2003). Defective perforin expression and low NK cell activity may potentially explain why some children with SoJRA develop MAS when incited with a triggering agent. As only 20–40% of primary HLH cases have an identified genetic defect, there may be as yet unidentified genes associated with primary HLH which may also predispose some children with rheumatic diseases to develop MAS.

A link with defective apoptosis may be further suggested by the association of MAS and Kikuchi's disease, a necrotizing lymphadenitis, in patients with SoJRA. There are reports of at least nine patients in the literature with SoJRA, AOSD or SLE, with lymph node pathology suggesting Kikuchi's disease, who later went on to develop MAS and it is possible that these two diseases represent underlying defects in apoptotic pathways and share common pathogenic mechanisms (Ohta *et al.*, 1988; Wong *et al.*, 1991; Cousin *et al.*, 1999; Oliveira *et al.*, 2000; Grom *et al.*, 2003; Ramanan *et al.*, 2003a). The importance of identifying the underlying defects lies not only in potential early diagnosis of MAS, but also in the ability to identify these children at the time of diagnosis of their rheumatic disease, when different management may potentially avert the development of MAS.

Hypercytokinemia in MAS

A cytokine storm is known to be responsible for most of the clinical manifestations of MAS/HLH. Among the cytokines implicated are tumour necrosis factor-alpha (TNF-α), interleukin (IL-6) and interferon-gamma (IFN-γ). TNF-α is possibly the major cytokine since many features of MAS including hypertriglyceridemia and DIC may be attributed to TNF hypersecretion (Henter *et al.*, 1991b). Although a single case report documented effectiveness of the anti-TNF agent, etanercept in MAS and SoJRA, at least four patients have developed MAS either secondary to an anti-TNF agent as a trigger, or while being maintained on anti-TNF agents for their underlying systemic disease (Prahalad *et al.*, 2001; Aouba *et al.*, 2003; Grom *et al.*, 2003; Ramanan and Schneider, 2003b).

Diagnostic criteria

There are currently no validated diagnostic criteria for MAS secondary to rheumatic diseases. Diagnostic criteria for HLH established in 1991 (Henter *et al.*, 1991a) and revised for the Second International HLH Study – 2004 were designed for the diagnosis of primary HLH, but many clinicians in practice use the same criteria for secondary HLH/MAS. It is now well established that not all patients with HLH will fulfill the diagnostic criteria at initial presentation, and that therapy may need to be started on the basis of a high index of suspicion, even when patients do not satisfy the suggested criteria (see Chapter 18).

The existing criteria pose particular problems for the diagnosis of MAS in association with SoJRA. Low haemoglobin (Hb) raised white cell count (WCC) and raised platelet count are characteristic of active systemic disease in SoJRA. Relative cytopaenia (reduction in Hb, WCC and platelets by a certain fraction as compared to the initial levels in a particular patient) may be more useful than the absolute cytopaenia required by the criteria, in the early diagnosis of MAS in children with SoJRA. Other laboratory parameters, such as serum ferritin and lactate dehydrogenase (LDH), deserve special consideration as diagnostic markers. In a large series of secondary HLH patients, Imashuku *et al.* have shown that hyperferritinemia (>1000 μg/l) and elevated blood levels of LDH (>1000 IU/l) were observed in 90% and 89.7% of patients, respectively. In contrast, hypertriglyceridemia (>2 mmol/l) and hypofibrinogenemia (<1.5 gm/L) which are part of the diagnostic criteria were seen in only 50% and 57.4% of patients. Serum ferritin and LDH may, therefore, be more sensitive parameters for HLH compared with serum triglyceride and fibrinogen (Imashuku *et al.*, 1997). There has recently been a great deal of interest in the role of serum ferritin as a potential marker for MAS. The revised diagnostic guidelines for HLH-2004 propose that ferritin equal to or more than 500 mg/l should be a diagnostic criterion. Mild elevation of serum ferritin is frequently seen in active SoJRA, along with elevations of acute phase reactants. Some authors suggest that serum ferritin $>10,000$ μg/l is a sensitive and specific marker for MAS (Emmenegger *et al.*, 2001, 2002; Ravelli *et al.*, 2001b), but this is not confirmed by our experience. We determined the diagnoses of all children with a serum ferritin >5000 μg/l over a 7-year period. Hyperferritinemia (>5000 μg/l) was not only associated with HLH but also with SoJRA without MAS, liver disease and infections. Fewer than 50% of patients with serum ferritin $>10,000$ μg/l had a diagnosis of HLH or MAS (Ramanan *et al.*, 2003b). There are also reports that the combination of high serum ferritin with a low percentage of glycosylation could be a potential marker of excessive macrophage activation. Whilst hyperferritinemia is a promising potential marker for MAS, it is probably most useful in conjunction with other clinical and laboratory markers.

Another significant problem with the existing criteria for HLH is the need for tissue demonstration of haemophagocytosis. It is well recognized that haemophago-cytosis is not always demonstrable early in the course of HLH (Janka, 1983; Ost *et al.*, 1998). In one series of 27 children with primary HLH, autopsy studies revealed haemophagocytosis in the bone marrow in only 39% (9/23). In contrast, 71% and 74% showed haemophagocytosis in the spleen and lymph nodes respectively, but biopsies of spleen and lymph nodes constitute a much greater risk in the face of a severe coagulopathy (Ost *et al.*, 1998). Also, the presence of mild haemophagocy-tosis does not always imply HLH, as haemophagocytosis can be seen as a normal physiological phenomenon in the reticuloendothelial system, which can be enhanced after transfusion or following cytostatic treatments (Tiab *et al.*, 2000). It has been suggested that ≥3% of haemophagocytic histiocytes or 2500 cell/ml, associated with otherwise unexplained cytopaenia involving at least 2 cell lines, be considered one of the diagnostic criteria for HLH. There is a need for criteria which take into account these difficulties, yet provide a robust framework for early diagnosis of MAS (Ramanan and Schneider, 2003a).

Prognostic factors

MAS is a potentially fatal condition with a reported mortality of 8–22% in the two largest paediatric series (Sawhney *et al.*, 2001; Stephan *et al.*, 2001). Most children who survive have a single episode of MAS, but recurrences do occur. There do not appear to be any reliable predictors for recurrence.

It has been suggested that delayed diagnosis and severe multiorgan involvement are associated with a poor prognosis. The influence of renal involvement on outcome is controversial. In two case series of MAS, renal involvement was associated with a poor prognosis (Sawhney *et al.*, 2001; Stephan *et al.*, 2001). In another series of 57 adult patients with reactive MAS (23 had AOSD or SoJRA), 62% (35/57) had evidence of renal impairment with 17% (10/57) requiring dialysis. The authors concluded that patients with more severe renal impairment had a worse outcome (Emmenegger *et al.*, 2002). However, we recently reported three children with varying severity of renal involvement who had a favourable outcome (Ramanan *et al.*, 2003c). It appears that renal involvement, like other manifestations of MAS, has a spectrum of severity and even severe renal involvement does not always portend a poor outcome. Other factors thought to indicate a poor prognosis are the presence of severe neutropenia particu-larly with an opportunistic infection, severe coagulation abnormalities, the presence of central nervous system (CNS) disease and a poor response to initial therapy.

Treatment

In 2001, Imashuku outlined measures necessary for effective therapy of HLH. These include control of hypercytokinemia, treatment of underlying disease, correction of haemorrhagic diathesis and appropriate supportive care including therapy of febrile neutropenia (Imashuku et al., 2001). In MAS associated with rheumatic diseases, supportive care may include elimination of potential triggering medications and the use of antimicrobial agents for suspected triggering or associated opportunistic infections.

Control of hypercytokinemia is an essential part of early management of HLH. In the Histiocyte Society Protocol HLH 2004, suggested induction therapy for all severely ill HLH patients, including those with primary HLH, is corticosteroids, etoposide and cyclosporine-A (CSA) (see Chapter 18). Rheumatic-disease associated HLH/MAS, on the contrary, has been conventionally managed with corticosteroids alone along with appropriate supportive management, and further immunosuppressive treatment has been reserved for resistant cases or severe manifestations. In the two largest paediatric series of rheumatic disease-associated MAS close to half the patients were treated only with corticosteroids (Table 19.4) and one of the features distinguishing rheumatic disease-associated MAS from other forms of HLH may be this response of a proportion of patients to corticosteroids alone. Second-line immunosuppressive medications, including CSA, etoposide and intravenous gamma immunoglobin (IVIG), have been used in only a proportion of patients.

Stephan et al. (1993) in their original description of MAS, demonstrated that CSA was effective in two of the four patients in whom it was used. CSA acts by suppressing T-cell activation and proliferation (Schreiber and Crabtree, 1992; Faulds et al., 1993) and down-modulating the cytokine storm. In combination with corticosteroids, CSA was reported to be useful in five patients with MAS associated with rheumatic diseases (Mouy et al., 1996), and there have since been several additional reports of the efficacy of CSA in conjunction with corticosteroids (Ravelli et al., 1996; Quesnel et al., 1997; Ravelli et al., 2001c; Sawhney et al., 2001; Stephan et al., 2001).

Other therapies including etoposide and cyclophosphamide have been used in anecdotal case reports of MAS (Stephan et al., 1993, 2001; Fishman et al., 1995; Sawhney et al., 2001). IVIG therapy had also been found to be useful in various forms of secondary HLH, used alone, or in combination with corticosteroids or etoposide. In one series, 7/20 MAS patients were treated with IVIG. Seven of 20 had a diagnosis of AOSD, 2/20 had SoJRA and 1/20 had SLE. One patient with AOSD and one patient with SoJRA died (Emmenegger et al., 2001). The same authors also published their experience using IVIG for reactive MAS in 57 patients of whom 23 had Still's disease (Emmenegger et al., 2002). From their paper it is unclear what percentage responded, which factors distinguished responders from non-responders and

Table 19.4 Clinical features of MAS/HLH. These are features set as table footnotes in two paediatric series of rheumatic disease-related MAS/HLH (Sawhney *et al.*, 2001; Stephan *et al.*, 2001)

	Stephan *et al.* (n = 24)	Sawhney *et al.* (n = 9)
Clinical features	No (%)	No (%)
Fever	24/24 (100)	9/9 (100)
Splenomegaly	24/24 (100)	8/9 (100)
Hepatomegaly	24/24 (100)	8/9 (100)
Lymphadenopathy	8/24 (33)	6/9 (66)
Renal involvement	3/24 (13)	3/9 (33)
ICU admission	10/24 (42)	3/9 (33)
Laboratory features		
Hypofibrinogenemia	24/24 (100)	1/6 (16)
Hypertriglyceridemia	24/24 (100)	NA
Coagulopathy	NA	5/8 (63)
Low Hb	NA	8/9 (89)
Low neutrophils	NA	NA
Low platelets	24/24 (100)	NA
Hemophagocytosis on bone marrow	14/17 (82)	5/7 (71)
Treatment and outcome		
Treatment: steroids	24/24 (100)	9/9 (100)
Cyclosporine	12/24 (50)	5/9 (55)
Etoposide	1/24 (4)	1/9 (11)
IVIG	1/24 (4)	–
Cyclophosphamide	–	2/9 (22)
Haematological recovery (mean)	NA	17.3 days
Biochemical recovery (mean)	NA	30.0 days
Median time to recovery	NA	23.6 days
Recurrence rate of MAS	4/24 (17)	
Death	2/24 (8)	2/9 (22)

Percentages in parenthesis. ICU: intensive care unit; NA: not applicable.

whether patients received any other therapy including corticosteroids. IVIG has been postulated to have a wide range of anti-inflammatory effects, but the precise mechanism of action in MAS is unclear (Kazatchkine and Kaveri, 2001).

Antithymocyte globulin (ATG), combined, with corticosteroids, has also been reported as effective therapy in familial (Stephan *et al.*, 1993) and refractory Epstein–Barr Virus (EBV)-related HLH (Perel *et al.*, 1997), and the combination may prove to be useful in patients with MAS who do not respond to front-line therapy. Since TNF has been considered as a key cytokine in the pathogenesis of MAS, anti-TNF agents have been thought to be potentially useful in therapy. Although there

Table 19.5 Suggested management according to risk groups at initial diagnosis

Risk group	Suggested therapy
Low-risk group	
MAS in the absence of high-risk features	Corticosteroids
	Supportive care
High-risk group	
CNS involvement	Corticosteroids + CSA ± etoposide
Severe bleeding diathesis (DIC)	Supportive care
Severe renal impairment	
Multiorgan failure	
Failure to respond to initial therapy	

was one report of successful use of etanercept in a child with SoJRA who developed MAS at onset of the disease, there have been other reports of etanercept being implicated as a potential trigger or of patients developing MAS while being maintained on anti-TNF agents (Grom *et al.*, 2003; Ramanan and Schneider, 2003b).

There are currently no large trials and thus no clear consensus or evidence to suggest any particular therapeutic strategy in MAS. The authors' approach has been to use corticosteroids alone initially (starting with pulse methylprednisone) in patients who do not have severe multiorgan involvement at onset and those who do not require intensive care admission. If there is a poor response to corticosteroids, worsening or severe multiorgan involvement, we have a low threshold to initiate second-line medications including cyclosporine and/or etoposide. In line with suggested management for EBV-induced HLH (Imashuku *et al.*, 2001) it seems reasonable to divide patients with MAS into a low-risk and a high-risk group at initial diagnosis (Table 19.5), and to institute treatment accordingly. Therapy for low-risk patients would be with corticosteroids alone plus careful observation, while high-risk patients would receive corticosteroids in combination with CSA, with early addition of etoposide for poor responders. Both groups would have prompt institution of supportive care. The suggested strategy minimises potentially harmful treatments for patients with low-risk disease and allows early institution of intensive therapy for those at higher risk. While this approach may be theoretically reasonable, an international cooperative trial to fully evaluate this strategy is strongly recommended.

Summary and conclusion

MAS appears to occur in up to 7% of patients with SoJRA, often in response to a triggering event. Disease manifestations vary from mild to severe multiorgan failure with a reported fatality rate of 8–22%. In the face of the symptoms, signs and laboratory features associated with the underlying rheumatological condition, the diagnosis of MAS may be difficult and not always clear cut. A high index of suspicion is needed. Based on the severity of the disease, a step-wise approach to therapy is suggested, aimed at alleviating the effects of the macrophage activation and the resulting cytokine storm, while reducing the potential toxicity of therapy.

REFERENCES

al-Eid, W., al-Jefri, A., Bahabri, S., *et al.* (2000). Hemophagocytosis complicating Kawasaki disease. *Pediatr Hematol Oncol*, **17**, 323–329.

Aouba, A., De Bandt, M., Aslangul, E., *et al.* (2003). Haemophagocytic syndrome in a rheumatoid arthritis patient treated with infliximab. *Rheumatol (Oxf)*, **42**, 800–802.

Athreya, B.H. (2002). Is macrophage activation syndrome a new entity? *Clin Exp Rheumatol*, **20**, 121–123.

Barron, K.S., Wallace, C., Woolfrey, C.E.A., *et al.* (2001). Autologous stem cell transplantation for pediatric rheumatic diseases. *J Rheumatol*, **28**, 2337–2358.

Boone, J.E. (1977). Hepatic disease and mortality in juvenile rheumatoid arthritis. *Arthritis Rheum*, **20**, 257–258.

Coffernils, M., Soupart, A., Pradier, O., *et al.* (1992). Hyperferritinemia in adult onset Still's disease and the haemophagocytic syndrome. *J Rheumatol*, **19**, 1425–1427.

Cousin, F., Grezard, P., Roth, B., Balme. B., *et al.* (1999). Kikuchi disease associated with Still disease. *Int J Dermatol*, **38**, 464–467.

Cuende, E., Vesga, J.C., Perez, L.B., *et al.* (2001). Macrophage activation syndrome as the initial manifestation of systemic onset juvenile idiopathic arthritis. *Clin Exp Rheumatol*, **19**, 764–765.

Davies, S.V., Dean, J.D., Wardrop, C.A., *et al.* (1994). Epstein–Barr virus-associated haemophagocytic syndrome in a patient with juvenile chronic arthritis. *Br J Rheumatol*, **33**, 495–497.

Dhote, R., Simon, J., Papo, T., *et al.* (2003). Reactive haemophagocytic syndrome in adult systemic disease: report of twenty-six cases and literature review. *Arthritis Rheum*, **49**, 633–639.

Emmenegger, U., Frey, U., Reimers, A., *et al.* (2001). Hyperferritinemia as indicator for intravenous immunoglobulin treatment in reactive macrophage activation syndromes. *Am J Hematol*, **68**, 4–10.

Emmenegger, U., Reimers, A., Frey, U., *et al.* (2002). Reactive macrophage activation syndrome: a simple screening strategy and its potential in early treatment initiation. *Swiss Med Weekly*, **132**, 230–236.

Faulds, D., Goa, K.L. and Benfield, P. (1993). Cyclosporin. A review of its pharmacodynamic and pharmacokinetic properties, and therapeutic use in immunoregulatory disorders. *Drugs*, **45**, 953–1040.

Fishman, D., Rooney, M. and Woo, P. (1995). Successful management of reactive haemophagocytic syndrome in systemic-onset juvenile chronic arthritis. *Br J Rheumatol*, **34**, 888.

Goransdotter Ericson, K., Fadeel, B., Nilsson-Ardnor, S., *et al.* (2001). Spectrum of perforin gene mutations in familial haemophagocytic lymphohistiocytosis. *Am J Hum Genet*, **68**, 590–597.

Grom, A.A., Villanueva, J., Lee, S., *et al.* (2003). Natural killer cell dysfunction in patients with systemic-onset juvenile rheumatoid arthritis and macrophage activation syndrome. *J Pediatr*, **142**, 292–296.

Hadchouel, M., Prieur, A.M., *et al.* (1985). Acute hemorrhagic, hepatic, and neurologic manifestations in juvenile rheumatoid arthritis: possible relationship to drugs or infection. *J Pediatr*, **106**, 561–566.

Heaton, D.C. and Moller, P.W. (1985). Still's disease associated with coxsackie infection and haemophagocytic syndrome. *Ann Rheum Dis*, **44**, 341–344.

Henter, J.-I., Elinder, G. and Ost, A. (1991a). Diagnostic guidelines for haemophagocytic lymphohistiocytosis. The FHL Study Group of the Histiocyte Society. *Semin Oncol*, **18**, 29–33.

Henter, J.-I., Elinder, G., Soder, O., *et al.* (1991b). Hypercytokinemia in familial haemophagocytic lymphohistiocytosis. *Blood*, **78**, 2918–2922.

Imashuku, S., Hibi, S. and Todo, S. (1997). Haemophagocytic lymphohistiocytosis in infancy and childhood. *J Pediatr*, **130**, 352–357.

Imashuku, S., Teramura, T., Morimoto, A., *et al.* (2001). Recent developments in the management of haemophagocytic lymphohistiocytosis. *Expert Opin Pharmacother*, **2**, 1437–1448.

Janka, G.E. (1983), Familial haemophagocytic lymphohistiocytosis. *Eur J Pediatr*, **140**, 221–230.

Jacobs, J.C., Gorin, L.J., Hanissian, A.S., *et al.* (1984). Consumption coagulopathy after gold therapy for JRA. *J Pediatr*, **105**, 674–675.

Kaneko, K., Takahashi, K., Fujiwara, S., *et al.* (1998). Kawasaki disease followed by haemophagocytic syndrome. *Eur J Pediatr*, **157**, 610–611.

Katsumata, Y., Okamoto, H., Harigai, M., *et al.* (2002). Etoposide ameliorated refractory haemophagocytic syndrome in a patient with systemic sclerosis. *Ryumachi*, **42**, 820–826.

Kazatchkine, M.D. and Kaveri, S.V. (2001). Immunomodulation of autoimmune and inflammatory diseases with intravenous immune globulin. *New Engl J Med*, **345**, 747–755.

Kobayashi, I., Yamada, M., Kawamura, N., *et al.* (2000). Platelet-specific hemophagocytosis in a patient with juvenile dermatomyositis. *Acta Paediatr*, **89**, 617–619.

Kumakura, S., Ishikura, H., Umegae, N., *et al.* (1997). Autoimmune-associated haemophagocytic syndrome. *Am J Med*, **102**, 113–115.

Madaule, S., Porte, L., Couret, B., *et al.* (2000). Fatal haemophagocytic syndrome in the course of dermatomyositis with anti-Mi2 antibodies. *Rheumatol (Oxf)*, **39**, 1157–1158.

McPeake, J.R., Hirst, W.J., Brind, A.M., *et al.* (1993). Hepatitis A causing a second episode of virus-associated haemophagocytic lymphohistiocytosis in a patient with Still's disease. *J Med Virol*, **39**, 173–175.

Morris, J.A., Adamson, A.R., Holt, P.J., *et al.* (1985). Still's disease and the virus-associated haemophagocytic syndrome. *Ann Rheum Dis*, **44**, 349–353.

Mouy, R., Stephan, J.L., Pillet, P., *et al.* (1996). Efficacy of cyclosporine A in the treatment of macrophage activation syndrome in juvenile arthritis: report of five cases. *J Pediatr*, **129**, 750–754.

Ohta, A., Matsumoto, Y., Ohta, T., *et al.* (1988). Still's disease associated with necrotizing lymphadenitis (Kikuchi's disease): report of 3 cases. *J Rheumatol*, **15**, 981–983.

Oliveira, S., Destri, U.B.W., Vasquez., L.C.O., *et al.* (2000). Systemic juvenile idiopathic arthritis associated with Kikuchi's disease. *Ann Rheum Dis*, **59**(Suppl), 731.

Onishi, R. and Namiuchi, S. (1994). Haemophagocytic syndrome in a patient with rheumatoid arthritis. *Intern Med*, **33**, 607–611.

Perel, Y., Alos, N., Ansoborlo, S., *et al.* (1997). Dramatic efficacy of antithymocyte globulins in childhood EBV-associated haemophagocytic syndrome. *Acta Paediatr*, **86**, 911.

Prahalad, S., Bove, K.E., Dickens, D., *et al.* (2001). Etanercept in the treatment of macrophage activation syndrome. *J Rheumatol*, **28**, 2120–2124.

Ost, A., Nilsson-Ardnor, S. and Henter, J-I. (1998). Autopsy findings in 27 children with haemophagocytic lymphohistiocytosis. *Histopathology*, **32**, 310–316.

Quesnel, B., Catteau, B., Aznar, V., *et al.* (1997). Successful treatment of juvenile rheumatoid arthritis associated haemophagocytic syndrome by cyclosporin A with transient exacerbation by conventional-dose G-CSF. *Br J Haematol*, **97**, 508–510.

Ramanan, A.V. and Baildam, E.M. (2002). Macrophage activation syndrome is haemophagocytic lymphohistiocytosis – need for the right terminology. *J Rheumatol*, **29**, 1105; discussion 1105.

Ramanan, A.V. and Schneider, R. (2003a). Macrophage activation syndrome – what's in a name! *J Rheumatol*, **30**, 2513–2516.

Ramanan, A.V. and Schneider, R. (2003b) Macrophage activation syndrome following initiation of etanercept in a child with systemic onset juvenile rheumatoid arthritis. *J Rheumatol*, **30**, 401–403.

Ramanan, A.V., Wynn, R.F., Kelsey, A., *et al.* (2003a). Systemic juvenile idiopathic arthritis, Kikuchi's disease and haemophagocytic lymphohistiocytosis – is there a link? Case report and literature review. *Rheumatol (Oxf)*, **42**, 596–598.

Ramanan, A.V., Akikusa, J.D., Silverman, E.D., *et al.* (2003b). Extreme hyperferritinemia in childhood. *Clin Exp Rheumatol*, **21**, 559.

Ramanan, A.V., Rosenblum, N.D., Feldman, B.M., *et al.* (2003c). Favorable outcome in patients with renal involvement complicating macrophage activation syndrome (MAS) in systemic onset JIA (SoJIA). *Pediatr Rheumatol Online J*, **1**, 15.

Ravelli, A., De Benedetti, F., Viola, S., *et al.* (1996). Macrophage activation syndrome in systemic juvenile rheumatoid arthritis successfully treated with cyclosporine. *J Pediatr*, **128**, 275–278.

Ravelli, A., Caria, M.C., Buratti, S., *et al.* (2001a). Methotrexate as a possible trigger of macrophage activation syndrome in systemic juvenile idiopathic arthritis. *J Rheumatol*, **28**, 865–867.

Ravelli, A., Magni-Manzoni, S., Foti, T., *et al* . (2001b). Macrophage activation syndrome in juvenile idiopathic arthritis: towards the development of diagnostic guidelines. *Arthritis Rheum*, **44**, S166.

Ravelli, A., Viola, S., De Benedetti, F., *et al.* (2001c). Dramatic efficacy of cyclosporin A in macrophage activation syndrome. *Clin Exp Rheumatol*, **19**, 108.

Sawhney, S., Woo, P. and Murray, K.J. (2001). Macrophage activation syndrome: a potentially fatal complication of rheumatic disorders. *Arch Dis Child*, **85**, 421–426.

Schreiber, S.L. and Crabtree, G.R. (1992). The mechanism of action of cyclosporin A and FK506. *Immunol Today*, **13**, 136–142.

Silverman, E.D., Miller 3rd, J.J. , Bernstein, B., *et al.* (1983). Consumption coagulopathy associated with systemic juvenile rheumatoid arthritis. *J Pediatr*, **103**, 872–876.

Stephan, J.L., Kone-Paut, I., Galambrun, C., *et al.* (2001). Reactive haemophagocytic syndrome in children with inflammatory disorders. A retrospective study of 24 patients. *Rheumatol (Oxf)*, **40**, 1285–1292.

Stephan, J.L., Zeller, J., Hubert, P., *et al.* (1993). Macrophage activation syndrome and rheumatic disease in childhood: a report of four new cases. *Clin Exp Rheumatol*, **11**, 451–456.

Takahashi, K., Kumakura, S., Ishikura, H., *et al.* (1998). Reactive hemophagocytosis in systemic lupus erythematosus. *Intern Med*, **37**, 550–553.

Tiab, M., Mechinaud, F. and Harousseau, J.L. (2000). Haemophagocytic syndrome associated with infections. *Baillieres Best Pract Res Clin Haematol*, **13**, 163–178.

Tochimoto, A., Nishimagi, E., Kawaguchi, Y., *et al.* (2001). A case of recurrent haemophagocytic syndrome complicated with systemic sclerosis: relationship between disease activity and serum level of IL-18. *Ryumachi*, **41**, 659–664.

Tsuji, T., Ohno, S. and Ishigatsubo, Y. (2002). Liver manifestations in systemic lupus erythematosus: high incidence of haemophagocytic syndrome. *J Rheumatol*, **29**, 1576–1577.

Vecer, J., Charvat, J., Kubatova, H., *et al.* (2000). Secondary haemophagocytic syndrome in a systemic disease. *Cas Lek Cesk*, **139**, 379–381.

Wong, K.F., Hui, P.K., Chan, J.K., *et al.* (1991). The acute lupus haemophagocytic syndrome. *Ann Intern Med*, **114**, 387–390.

Wulffraat, N.M., Rijkers, G.T., Elst, E., *et al.* (2003). Reduced perforin expression in systemic juvenile idiopathic arthritis is restored by autologous stem-cell transplantation. *Rheumatol (Oxf)*, **42**, 375–379.

Yamanouchi, J., Yamauchi, Y., Yokota, E., *et al.* (1998). Haemophagocytic syndrome in a patient with rheumatoid arthritis. *Ryumachi*, **38**, 731–734.

20

Malignancies of the monocyte/macrophage system

David K.H. Webb

Introduction

Historically, there has been much confusion regarding the spectrum and classification of malignancies of the monocyte/macrophage system, largely as original classifications were based on morphological appearance alone or with histochemical stains. This approach resulted in misinterpretation of cell lineage in a substantial proportion of cases, especially amongst the lymphomas. More recently, the widespread availability of immunohistochemistry plus cytogenetics to inform and support diagnosis, has established cell lineage in the majority of cases and allowed greater accuracy in classification of these tumours. Based on current knowledge, an appropriate classification is to divide these malignancies between tumours of dendritic cells (follicular dendritic cell (FDC) and interdigitating reticulum cell sarcomas) and tumours of monocyte/macrophage lineage (acute myelomonocytic leukaemia, acute monocytic leukaemia, chronic myelomonocytic leukaemia (CMML) and juvenile myelomonocytic leukaemia (JMML)).

Acute myeloid leukaemia (AML) with involvement of the monocyte lineage has been well defined for many years and classified as AML M4 (myelomonocytic) and M5 (monocytic) under the French–American–British (FAB) system. Originally identified by morphological criteria and cytochemistry, these entities have become better defined by immunophenotyping and the identification of associated cytogenetic changes (see below). Localized tumour masses comprised of these cells are well recognized, and may occur with or without clinically apparent bone marrow disease. In apparently isolated tumour masses, eventual detection of bone marrow involvement is usual in patients who have not received comprehensive systemic therapy.

With the introduction of modern histochemical techniques and the identification of tumour-specific translocations, it was recognized that most cases previously diagnosed as malignant histiocytosis were truly anaplastic large cell lymphoma (Koh et al., 1980; Egeler et al., 1995; Favara et al., 1997; Gogusev and

Nezelhof, 1998; Schmidt *et al.*, 2001). These patients had fever, weight loss, enlargement of liver, spleen and lymph nodes, pulmonary and skin infiltrates. Demonstration of T-lymphocyte antigens, rearrangement of the T-cell receptor genes, the CD30 antigen, the translocation between chromosomes 2 and 5, t(2;5)(p23;q35), and the anaplastic lymphoma kinase (ALK) protein confirmed the true nature of the disease. The t(2;5) translocation involves the ALK and nucleophosmin (NPM) genes, resulting in expression of a novel NPM–ALK fusion protein which can be demonstrated immunohistochemically. Rappaport introduced the term histiocytic lymphoma to describe localized proliferations of large cells which were misinterpreted to be histiocytic in origin (Rappaport, 1966). Studies of cell suspensions and immunohistochemistry indicated that this group comprised a wide variety of malignancies of B- or T-cell lineages. As a result, there are now very few new reports of malignant histiocytosis/histiocytic lymphoma.

AML involving cells of monocyte/macrophage lineage

The World Health Organization (WHO) classification requires over 20% leukaemic blasts in the bone marrow for a diagnosis of AML. In the FAB system, patients in whom 20–80% of non-erythroid bone marrow cells are monoblasts are classified as having AML M4, whilst those with over 80% monoblasts have AML M5. AML M4 and M5 respectively, account for 20% and 9% of patients with AML (Hann *et al.*, 1997). Despite some overlap, there are distinct biological and clinical differences between these two FAB types (Figure 20.1). The prevalence of different FAB types in a series of children treated in two consecutive UK trials (AML 10 and 12) between 1988 and 1995 is shown in Table 20.1.

Table 20.1 FAB types in children with AML – MRC AML 10 and 12 trials (Webb *et al.*, 2001)

FAB type	Number (total = 589) (%)
M0	19 (3)
M1	81 (14)
M2	186 (32)
M3	50 (9)
M4	87 (15)
M5	98 (17)
M6	12 (2)
M7	39 (7)

MRC: Medical Research Council.

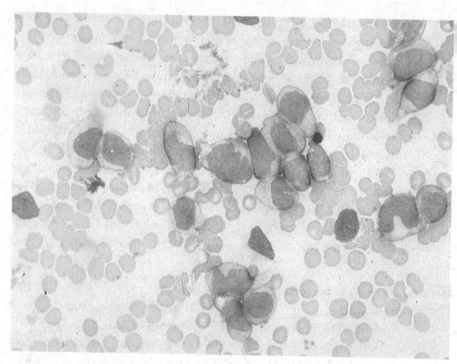

Figure 20.1 Blood film in child with acute monocytic leukaemia, FAB type AML M5

Monoblasts are large cells measuring 30–40 μm in diameter. The nucleus is round to oval with prominent nucleoli and lacy chromatin. The cytoplasm is abundant and basophilic, with fine azurophilic granules. Auer rods are not a feature. The cells contain high concentrations of lysozyme. Cytochemistry for Sudan Black and myeloperoxidase is negative or weakly positive, and the cells show strong positivity for nonspecific esterase which is inhibited by sodium fluoride. The leukaemic blasts variably express the myeloid antigens CD13 and CD33, and the monocytic antigens CD14 and CD11c. Leukaemic monoblasts are characterized by greater adhesiveness, deformability and motility compared with other subtypes of AML (Odom et al., 1990). Monoblasts can undergo partial differentiation and develop characteristics which enable tissue infiltration. AML M4 shows a mixed population of myeloid and monocytic cells, and eosinophils (the M4Eo subtype) may be prominent. AML M5 is subdivided into M5a (undifferentiated) and M5b (differentiated). In M5b the predominant promonocyte is similar to the monoblast but has a large, cerebriform nucleus, less prominent nucleoli, and reduced cytoplasm.

AML M5 is most common in children under 10 and adults over 40 years of age. The peak incidence in childhood occurs in very young children reaching 40% in

Table 20.2 Prevalence of FAB types M4 and M5 by age in children treated in the MRC AML 10 and 12 trials (Webb *et al.*, 2001)

FAB type	0–1 year (%)	1–2 years (%)	2–4 years (%)	5–9 years (%)	10–15 years (%)	P-value test for trend
M4	12	10	13	15	16	0.2
M5	41	27	18	6	10	<0.001

MRC: Medical Research Council.

the first year, and contributes a low proportion of cases after 5 years of age (Webb *et al.*, 2001) (Table 20.2). Patients with AML M5 often have a high presenting white cell count (WCC), which often exceeds $100 \times 10^9/l$ (Tobelem *et al.*, 1980; Janvier *et al.*, 1984). The ability of monoblasts to migrate to tissues may result in pulmonary infiltrates and respiratory failure. Serum and urine lysozyme levels are high in over 50% of patients and may result in renal tubular leak of potassium and hypokalaemia, which may be life-threatening (Janvier *et al.*, 1984). Pro-coagulant activity of monoblast granules results in a relatively high risk of coagulopathy during induction chemotherapy and around 20% of patients have disseminated intravascular coagulation at presentation. The combination of high WCC, blast size, and deformability can result in leucostasis, and severe brain damage due to leucostasis and bleeding is described. The likelihood of renal impairment, leucostasis in lung and brain, hypokalaemia, and coagulopathy is proportional to the presenting WCC. Extramedullary disease is a common feature, especially affecting skin, gingiva, orbit, abdomen, thorax, and central nervous system (CNS) (Johansson *et al.*, 2000; Dusenbery *et al.*, 2003). Isolated tumour masses may be the only evidence of disease, although eventual bone marrow involvement has occurred on follow-up of patients treated with local therapies or chemotherapy. The incidence of CNS disease at diagnosis is higher than other subtypes of AML, reaching 10% in some series (Janvier *et al.*, 1984). Rare cases of congenital AML are almost uniformly monocytic in nature. Congenital acute monocytic leukaemia may undergo spontaneous remission, but may also recur months later (Van Eys *et al.*, 1969), arguing for a period of observation prior to therapy wherever possible (Francis *et al.*, 1989).

Characteristic cytogenetic changes are features of both AML M4 and M5. Inversion of chromosome 16 occurs with M4, and carries a favourable prognosis (Grimwade *et al.*, 1998, Wheatley *et al.*, 1999). Several studies relate prognosis to morphology rather than cytogenetics (Creutzig *et al.*, 1985), and in these the M4 with eosinophilia subtype (M4Eo) is associated with a favourable outcome. Most

Table 20.3 Outcome of therapy in 1,857 adults and children treated in the MRC AML 10 trial by FAB type (Hann *et al.* 1997)

FAB type	CR rate (%)	OS at 5 years (%)	DFS at 5 years (%)
M0	55	20	40
M1	78	33	34
M2	86	42	42
M3	83	59	57
M4	**80**	**38**	**44**
M5	**86**	**38**	**43**
M6	87	34	32
M7	68	28	34

Tests for heterogeneity: CR, rate $P = 0.8$; OS, $P = 0.9$; DFS, $P = 0.9$.
Tests for interactions M4/M5 versus other FAB types: CR rate, $P = 0.4$; OS, $P = 0.7$; DFS, $P = 0.6$.
CR: complete remission; DFS: disease-free survival; MRC: Medical Research Council.

inversion 16 occurs in M4Eo, so that both favourable features identify similar patients. AML M5 is associated with translocations with breakpoints on the long arm of chromosome 11, usually at 11q23, and less often at q13–14. Breakpoints at 11q23 involve rearrangement of the mixed-lineage leukaemia (MLL) gene. This change has been described both in *de novo* disease, and in secondary AML following prior therapy with epipodophyllotoxins (Whitlock *et al.*, 1991, Ratain Rowley, 1992; and Nichols *et al.*, 1993). Partner chromosomes (breakpoints) involved in these translocations with chromosome 11 include 9(p21–22), 19(p13), 10(p11–15), and 17(q21–25) with chromosome 9 the commonest partner. Translocations involving chromosome 4 with chromosome 11 are typical of acute lymphoblastic leukaemia (ALL) in infancy, but not AML.

There has been much debate regarding the prognostic significance of 11q23 translocations in AML, especially given the known adverse influence of MLL gene rearrangements in ALL. However, in large groups of adults and children treated with modern therapy, neither an adverse nor favourable effect on survival has been demonstrated (Hann *et al.*, 1997; Wheatley *et al.*, 1999) (Table 20.3), and these patients are considered to have an intermediate prognosis. Similarly studies using morphology rather than cytogenetics to define prognostic subgroups show M5 to carry an intermediate prognosis (Creutzig *et al.*, 1990). Excess deaths in induction therapy (Creutzig *et al.*, 1985) have been reduced by improved supportive care, and early effective reduction of blast count by chemotherapy. Leucophoresis is rarely necessary provided chemotherapy is started promptly. Although bone marrow transplantation (BMT) may reduce relapse in these patients, the procedure-related mortality is significant, resulting in similar overall survival (OS) to chemotherapy alone. Accordingly these children should receive intensive standard chemotherapy as first-line therapy. Early studies of AML therapy reported increased extramedullary relapse, including CNS, in AML M5, but this is no longer true since the introduction of modern, effective, intensive therapy. The hypothesis that epipodophyllotoxins are especially effective in monocytic leukaemia (Chard *et al.*, 1979; Odom *et al.*, 1984; Nishikawa *et al.*, 1987) has not been substantiated (Hann *et al.*, 1997) in the setting of modern chemotherapy. Isolated tumour masses (chloroma, granulocytic sarcoma) of monocytic/myelomonocytic cells should be treated with standard AML protocols. There is no evidence for routine addition of local radiotherapy.

CMML and JMML

CMML is a haematological malignancy with wide heterogenicity of presentation and clinical course. Clinical features include hepatosplenomegaly, lymphadenopathy, anaemia, thrombocytopaenia and leucocytosis. The disorder has both myelodysplastic and myeloproliferative features, and is presently classified as a form of myelodysplasia (MDS), identified by the FAB criteria as MDS with blood monocytes above $1 \times 10^9/l$, with less than 5% blasts in the blood and less than 20% blasts in the bone marrow. The FAB classification subdivides CMML into two forms; patients with presenting WCC less than $13 \times 10^9/l$ are considered primarily dysplastic, whereas those with higher WCC are classified as being predominantly proliferative. Around 50% of patients with initial dysplastic disease evolve to become proliferative. The distinction may thus appear inappropriate, but several studies indicated poorer survival for the proliferative form, although differences in median survival were measured in months only. Median OS for patients with CMML is 14–18 months. The WHO suggested subdividing CMML patients according to whether the percentage of bone marrow blasts is above or below 10%, with poorer survival in patients with 10–20% blasts. Numerous studies have been undertaken to identify or confirm prognostic factors, but the patient populations included have varied and have failed to conform to uniform diagnostic criteria. In one recent large study of 213 patients with stringent diagnostic criteria in line with the FAB classification, haemoglobin below 12 g/dl, immature myeloid cells in blood, lymphocyte count over $2.5 \times 10^9/l$, and bone marrow blasts over 10% were adverse features (Onida *et al.*, 2002).

Chromosome studies are normal in up to 60% of patients. Cytogenetic abnormalities seen in CMML include monosomy 7, deletions of the long arm of chromosome 7, and balanced translocations such as t(5;12), t(9;12), and t(5;7). Fusion proteins involving the tyrosine kinase family are seen in some cases, and may affect the platelet-derived growth factor receptor beta. Possible responses to the kinase inhibitor imatinib have been observed in this group. The natural course of CMML is variable with survival ranging from months to years. Deaths are due to infection, bleeding, or transformation to AML. Around 20% of patients experience evolution

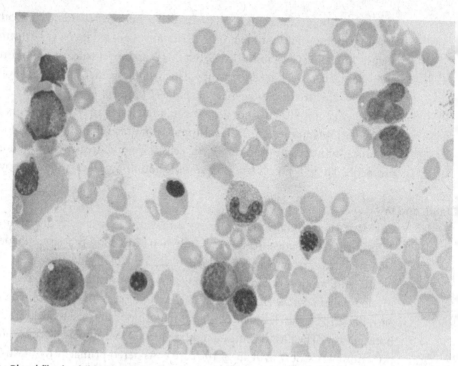

Figure 20.2   Blood film in child with JMML showing leucoerythroblastic change and dysplastic monocytes

of disease to AML within 5 years from diagnosis. Chemotherapy is not curative, although hydroxyurea is used in the proliferative form to control WCC, and may extend survival. Treatment for the dysplastic form is similar to that in other types of MDS, with supportive care, and selective use of erythropoietin and chemotherapy. BMT is the only therapy with the potential for cure of CMML, although the elderly age of many patients limits this approach. However, event-free survival rates of up to 50% are described in selected patient groups treated with BMT.

Childhood cases generally fit the FAB criteria poorly, and this has led to description of a distinct, if rare, entity of childhood, JMML. JMML is a proliferative dysplastic disorder which is heterogenous in clinical features and behaviour (Niemeyer et al., 1997). Diagnostic criteria require blood monocytosis over 1×10^9/l (Figure 20.2), less than 20% blasts in the marrow, and negativity for bcr-abl, the product of the t(9;22) translocation of chronic myeloid leukaemia. Patients should also have two of the following features:

- leucocytosis above 10×10^9/l,
- elevated haemoglobin F (HbF) for age,
- myeloid precursors on the blood film,
- evidence of hypersensitivity to granulocyte/macrophage colony-stimulating factor (GM-CSF) in bone marrow culture.

High HbF, often above 10%, is a characteristic feature of the disorder, and reflects a foetal pattern of haematopoiesis. Some children manifest autoimmune features and immune dysregulation. The disease is typified clinically by hepatosplenomegaly, fever, skin rash, anemia, thrombocytopaenia and leucocytosis. The blood film shows dysplastic features, leucoerythroblastic change, and monocytosis. Most often, affected children have or develop a wasting disease with transfusion requirement, respiratory infections and weight loss. Transformation to acute leukaemia is uncommon, but both AML and ALL have been observed rarely. The clonal nature of JMML was demonstrated by X-inactivation studies and by transmission of the disease by transplantation to immune deficient mice. Bone marrow cells from JMML patients exhibit *in vitro* hypersensitivity to GM-CSF. This hypersensitivity is specific, and no abnormality is found with other cytokines (Emanuel *et al.*, 1996). The role of tumour necrosis factor in generating some of the features of the disease (fever, weight loss) is thought to be due to secondary production from activated monocytes. The hypersensitivity to GM-CSF is thought to be due to abnormalities of the intracellular signalling pathways, and mutations in several genes involved in these pathways have been identified in JMML. Mutations in ras, the neurofibromatosis gene (NF1), the Noonan gene (NPTN 11) and SHP-1 have all been identified. All these gene products have regulatory functions in cell signalling. As a result, hypersensitivity to GM-CSF results in cell proliferation, tissue infiltration, and cytokine release giving the typical clinical features.

Cytogenetic abnormalities are found in 40% of children with JMML, with monosomy 7 the most common. In distinction from other MDS and AML, monosomy 7 in JMML does not confer an adverse prognosis. The reasons for this are unclear, but JMML patients with monosomy 7 tend to be infants, and have low HbF levels, both of which are favourable prognostic features.

Most children with JMML have rapid deterioration, either from the time of diagnosis or after a period of relative stability. A small proportion of patients, usually with onset of disease in the first year of life, have an indolent course however, and survive long term with limited or no therapy. The biological differences between these subgroups remain to be determined. For children with the typical, aggressive form of the disease, BMT is curative, although treatment failure is common, mostly due to relapse which may be aggressive and early (Locatelli *et al.*, 1997). The role of chemotherapy is limited to the debulking of disease and stabilization of the ill child before BMT. The spleen is a highly active site of disease proliferation in these children and splenectomy is also often useful in stabilization before BMT. The importance of a graft-versus-leukaemia effect in the cure of this disease has been clearly demonstrated in a number of case reports. Early withdrawal of immune suppression and donor lymphocyte infusions post relapse, have been effective on occasion, but the pace of deterioration may preclude further response.

Dendritic cell malignancies

Neoplasms of dendritic cells are extremely rare, and two are of monocyte/macrophage lineage – Follicular Dendritic Cell (FDC) sarcoma and interdigitating reticulum cell sarcoma (Fonseca et al., 1998).

FDC sarcoma

FDCs are localized to the germinal centre of the lymph node, in close proximity to follicular centre cells to which they present antigen–antibody complexes. In health, FDCs are large, 70–10 μm cells with long cytoplasmic processes, and often have two nuclei. They interact closely with each other, and attach to each other via desmosomes. The lineage of origin of FDCs is uncertain, although both CD45 (the common leucocyte antigen), and CD14 (a monocytic marker) are frequently positive. Expression of HLA-DR is variable. A range of lymphoid markers may also be expressed including CD19, CD20, CD21, CD23, and CD24. The cells are positive for 5-nucleotidase, but negative for ATP-ase. Other typical markers on immunostaining are r4/23, KiM4, KiM4p, and Ki-FDC1p (Chan et al., 1997).

The neoplastic cells in FDC sarcoma display the characteristic spindle shape and multinucleation of normal FDCs, together with a similar antigenic profile.

The disease usually presents with cervical or axillary lymphadenopathy, but extranodal sites are well described, including mouth, liver, spleen, bowel, pancreas and, peritoneum. This is a disease of late teenage and adult life. The youngest patient in the literature was 17 years at diagnosis, median age at presentation is 41 years. The disease may progress rapidly, or be indolent with long survival with limited therapy. Treatment has been based on local excision alone or combined with adjuvant radiotherapy and/or chemotherapy. In a comprehensive literature review, 31 patients were treated by excision alone, of whom 19 stayed disease-free (Fonseca et al., 1998). Eight patients underwent surgery plus radiotherapy; six were alive free of disease. Twelve patients were given chemotherapy following local therapy due to bulky or residual disease, with follow-up in nine cases. Four were disease-free, three died of disease, and two were alive with disease. Radiotherapy appears to have been effective in some cases with incomplete resection of the primary tumour, but recurrence occurred in other patients despite local irradiation. In contrast, chemotherapy has no proven role, despite administration of cyclophosphamide, prednisolone, doxorubicin and vincristine (CHOP), cytarabine, dexamethasone and cisplatin (DHAP), 2-chlorodeoxyadenosine, or bleomycin, doxorubicin, cyclophosphamide, vincristine and prednisone, and has certainly failed in patients with recurrent disease or measurable residual tumour after local treatment. Accordingly, local excision alone or with radiotherapy appears appropriate current choices.

Interdigitating dendritic cell sarcoma

Interdigitating dendritic cells (IDDCs) have a similar antigen-presenting role to FDCs, but primarily interact with T-cells, and IDDCs are accordingly localized to T-cell rich areas of lymph nodes. They have a single, folded nucleus, have long fine cytoplasmic processes, and lack desmosomes. IDDCs express CD45, HLA-DR, and S-100. The cells are strongly positive for ATP-ase, but negative for 5-nucleotidase.

Interdigitating cell (IDC) sarcoma grows in a whorl-shaped pattern of spindle cells. Immunohistochemistry fits the pattern of IDCs in health. The usual presentation is with lymphadenopathy, but extranodal sites occur. Median age at diagnosis is 52 years, but the disease has been diagnosed as early as 8 years of age. The disease has been treated successfully by excision alone. Similarly, local radiotherapy has been effective, producing disease-free survival as a single treatment modality. Chemotherapy, used for extensive or recurrent disease, has been of limited benefit, whether given in conventional doses, or myeloablative doses with autologous stem cell rescue. In one review, the median survival of all 21 reported cases was 15 months (Fonseca *et al.*, 1998), 10 died of disease, two were alive with disease, six were alive and disease free, two died of unrelated causes, and one was lost to follow up.

REFERENCES

Chan, J.K., Fletcher, C.D., Nayler, S.J., *et al.* (1997). Follicular dendritic cell sarcoma. Clinicopathological analysis of 17 cases suggesting a malignant potential higher than currently recognized. *Cancer*, **79**, 294–313.

Chard, R.L., Krivit, W., Bleyer, A., *et al.* (1979). Phase II study of VP-16 in childhood malignant disease: a Children's Cancer Study Group report. *Cancer Treat Reports*, **63**, 1755–1759.

Creutzig, U., Ritter, J. and Schellong, G. (1990). Identification of two risk groups in childhood acute myelogenous leukaemia after therapy intensification in the study AML BFM-83 as compared with study AML BFM-78. *Blood*, **75**, 1932–1940.

Creutzig, U., Ritter, J., Riehm, H., *et al.* (1985). Improved treatment results in childhood acute myelogenous leukaemia: a report of the German Cooperative Study AML BFM-78. *Blood*, **65**, 298–306.

Dusenbery, K.E., Howells, W.B., Arthur, D.C., *et al.* (2003). Extramedullary leukaemia in children with newly diagnosed acute myeloid leukaemia: a report from the children's cancer group. *J Pediatr Hematol Oncol*, **25**, 760–768.

Egeler, R.M., Schmitz, L., Sonneveld, P., *et al.* (1995). Malignant histiocytosis: a reassessment of cases formerly classified as histiocytic neoplasms and review of the literature. *Med Pediatr Oncol*, **25**, 1–7.

Emanuel, P.D., Shannon, K.M. and Castlebury, R.P. (1996). Juvenile myelomonocytic leukemia: molecular understanding and prospects for therapy. *Molec Med Today*, **2**, 468–475.

Favara, B.E., Feller, A.C., Pauli, M., *et al.* (1997). Contemporary classification of histiocyte disorders. The WHO committee on histiocytic/reticulum cell proliferations. Reclassification working group of the Histiocyte Society. *Med Pediatr Oncol*, **29**, 157–166.

Fonseca, R., Yamakawa, M., Nakamura, S., *et al.* (1998). Follicular dendritic cell and interdigitating reticulum cell sarcoma: a review. *Am J Hematol*, **59**, 161–167.

Francis, J.S., Sybert, V.P. and Benjamin, D.R. (1989). Congenital monocytic leukemia: a report of a case with cutaneous involvement and review of the literature. *Pediatr Dermatol*, **6**, 306–311.

Gogusev, J. and Nezelhof, C. (1998). Malignant histiocytosis. Histologic, cytochemical, chromosomal, and molecular data with a nosologic discussion. *Hematol Oncol Clin North Am*, **12**, 445–463.

Grimwade, D., Walker, H., Oliver, F., *et al.* (1998). The importance of diagnostic cytogenetics on outcome in AML: analysis of 1,612 patients entered into the MRC AML 10 trial. *Blood*, **96**, 2322–2333.

Hann, I.M., Stevens, R.F., Goldstone, A.H., *et al.* (1997). Randomized comparison of DAT versus ADE as induction chemotherapy in children and younger adults with acute myeloid leukemia. Results of the Medical Research Council's 10th AML trial (MRC AML10). *Blood*, **89**, 2311–2318.

Janvier, M., Tobelem, G., Daniel, M., *et al.* (1984). Acute monoblastic leukemia. Clinical, biological data and survival in 45 cases. *Scand J Haematol*, **32**, 385–390.

Johansson, B., Fioretos, T., Kullendorff, C.M., *et al.* (2000). Granulocytic sarcomas in body cavities in childhood acute myeloid leukemias with 11q23/MLL rearrangements. Genes chromosomes. *Cancer*, **27**, 136–142.

Koh, S.J., Vargas, G.F., Caces, J.N., *et al.* (1980). Malignant 'histiocytic' lymphoma in childhood. *Am J Clin Pathol*, **74**, 417–426.

Locatelli, F., Niemeyer, C. and Angelucci, E. (1997). Allogeneic bone marrow transplantation for chronic myelomonocytic leukemia of childhood: a report from the European Working Group on Myelodysplasia. *J Clin Oncol*, **15**, 566–573.

Nichols, C.R., Breeden, E.S., Loehrer, P.J., *et al.* (1993). Secondary leukemia associated with a conventional dose of etoposide: review of serial germ cell tumour protocols. *J Natl Cancer Instit*, **85**, 36–40.

Niemeyer, C.M., Arico, M. and Basso, A. (1997). Chronic myelomonocytic leukemia of childhood: a retrospective analysis of 110 cases. *Blood*, **89**, 3534–3543.

Nishikawa, A., Nakamura, Y., Noborim U., *et al.* (1987). Acute monocytic leukemia in children. Response to VP-16–21 as a single agent. *Cancer*, **60**, 2146–2149.

Odom, L.F., Lampkin, B.C., Tannous, R., *et al.* (1990). Acute monoblastic leukemia: a unique subtype – a review from the children's cancer study group. *Leuk Res*, **14**, 1–10.

Onida, F., Kantarjian, H.M., Smith, T.L., *et al.* (2002). Prognostic factors and scoring systems in chronic myelomonocytic leukemia: a retrospective analysis of 213 patients. *Blood*, **99**, 840–849.

Rappaport, H. (1966). Tumors of the hematopoietic system. In *Atlas of tumor pathology*, Armed Forces Institute of Pathology; Section 3, Fasc 8.

Ratain, M.J. and Rowley, J.D. (1992). Therapy-related acute myeloid leukemia secondary to inhibitors of topoisomerase II: from the bedside to the target genes. *Ann Oncol*, **3**, 107–111.

Schmidt, D. (2001). Malignant histiocytosis. *Curr Opin Hematol*, **8**, 1–4.

Tobelem, G., Jacquillat, C., Chastang ,C., *et al.* (1980). Acute monoblastic leukemia: a clinical and biological study of 74 cases. *Blood*, **55**, 71–76.

Van Eys, J. and Flexner, J.M. (1969). Transient spontaneous remission in a case of untreated congenital leukemia. *Am J Dis Child*, **118**, 507–514.

Webb, D.K., Harrison, G., Stevens, R.F., *et al.* (2001). Relationships between age at diagnosis, clinical features and outcome of therapy in children treated in the Medical Research Council AML 10 and 12 trials for acute myeloid leukemia. *Blood*, **98**, 1714–1720.

Wheatley, K., Burnett, A.K., Goldstone, A.H., *et al.* (1999). A simple, robust, validated and highly predictive index for the determination of risk-directed therapy in acute myeloid leukaemia derived from the MRC AML 10 trial. *Br J Haematol*, **107**, 69–79.

Whitlock, J.A., Greer, J.P. and Lukens, J.N. (1991). Epipodophyllotoxin-related leukemia. Identification of a new subset of secondary leukemia. *Cancer*, **68**, 600–604.

21

Psychosocial aspects of the histiocytic disorders: staying on course under challenging clinical circumstances

Steve Simms, Elizabeth Kuh and Giulio John D'Angio

The course of the histiocytic disorders is unpredictable. The natural history and response to treatment is variable and uncertain. As development proceeds, the impact of the illness and its treatment can range from negligible to increasingly complex. Each patient and family brings a unique complement of strengths and vulnerabilities to dealing with a life-threatening illness. Children and adults with permanent severe late effects pose unique and, sometimes, disheartening challenges. These challenges include neuropsychologic deficits (Whitsett *et al.*, 1999; Nanduri *et al.*, 2003), in particular, retardation, and neuropsychiatric conditions, such as uncontrollable sexual excitement or emotional lability. Unfortunately, these patients may respond sub-optimally or not at all to specialized medical or psychologic management approaches.

In a previous publication, Simms and Warner (1998) describe a framework for understanding and responding to the psychosocial needs of children with the commonest of the histiocytic disorders, Langerhans cell histiocytosis (LCH), and their families. Providers are encouraged to use five cardinal points when addressing psychosocial concerns. The five points are:

1 Attend to the provider–family relationship.
2 Emphasize that LCH imposes changes on family life.
3 Recognize that LCH can affect normal development.
4 Build collaborative relationships with family members.
5 Focus on competence (i.e. the ability to cope).

This framework is applicable to difficult clinical situations associated with the histiocytic disorders, in particular, noncompliance, permanent severe consequences, and death. Although this framework does not help control noncompliant patients or symptoms linked to permanent severe consequences, it does help patients, families, and providers contain them and adaptively cope. Despite this broad applicability, difficult clinical situations (in particular, those outside of the family and provider's control) can undercut everybody's confidence to creatively apply the principles. In this chapter, we explain how to stay on course under challenging clinical circumstances. Two cases not amenable to standard medical and psychologic approaches are used to illustrate the application of this framework, with aliases and fictitious age given to avoid identification.

Case reports

Case A

Greg is a 16-year-old high school student. At 2 years of age, he experienced numerous fevers and intermittent strabismus. After 6 months, the pediatrician referred him to a children's hospital where LCH was diagnosed. Lesions in the frontal, parietal, and temporal regions received 600-cGy radiation therapy. Two LCH relapses responded to chemotherapy (prednisone and vinblastine) and two relapses (skull lesions) spontaneously resolved. Visual, speech, and motor problems were noted during follow-up visits. Radiographic studies revealed white matter changes in the cerebellum, medulla, pons, and midbrain. He struggled with initiating, sustaining interest in, and completing classroom and homework assignments. Psycho-educational testing documented low-average intellectual functioning, fine motor development and academic achievement, and average memory functioning. His parents assiduously advocated for in-class accommodations. During the latency years, Greg and his parents effectively used psychosocial consultations to help him contain intense emotional reactions that interfered with sleep, peer relationships, and community activities. This case study picks up at an annual follow-up visit to the oncology clinic.

Case B

Anna is an 18-year-old college student. At 4 years of age she was diagnosed with LCH. At 17 years of age, after starting to smoke, she developed pulmonary LCH that failed to respond to chemotherapy and corticosteroids. This case study picks up after she was admitted to the hospital for rapidly declining pulmonary functioning.

Point 1: Attend to the provider–family relationship

Patients and their families want providers to use their knowledge and experience to treat the disease, relieve pain and suffering, and prevent late complications. Each contact and conversation is a very personal and meaningful experience. The patient–family–provider relationship can evolve effortlessly and require little attention when the disease responds to treatment and all are soothed by the provider's special touch. These relationships may be considerably more challenging when the clinical course is less smooth. When noncompliance, permanent severe late effects, or threat of death occur, the relationship encounters a turning point. Although the patient or the medical situation may appear uncontrollable, a key task for staying on track is to remember that *the patient–family–provider relationship has the capacity to contain and channel intense emotions into productive responses* (Brendler *et al.*, 1991). Talking openly about intense emotions and conflicting perspectives from a genuinely caring, empathic position is essential. Expert psychologic and psychiatric advice, when needed, is a concrete way to channel intense emotions into productive rather confrontational channels (Table 21.1).

Case A

The oncologist warmly greets Greg and his mother and asks, 'How are you feeling?' Greg responds, 'Fine. No problems.' His mother drops a bombshell, 'Greg is smoking cigarettes. He knows this is the worst thing for his histiocytosis but he does it anyway.' She pleads, 'Get him to quit.' Greg lashes back, 'Mind your own damn business. It's my life. Nobody can stop me from doing what I want to do.' His mother then described an escalating pattern of academic underachievement, negativistic and defiant behavior at home, and a drift to a deviant peer group. Greg clams up.

Rather than focusing on Greg's worrisome behaviors, the oncologist stays on track by focusing on their relationship, 'Greg, we have worked together for 11 years. How can I help you today?' Greg mutters, 'I'm fine. I don't want to be here. She made

Table 21.1 Key tasks for staying on track

Point 1: Attend to the provider–family relationship
- Believe that the patient–family–provider relationship has the capacity to contain and channel intense emotions into productive responses.

Point 2: Emphasize that LCH imposes changes on family life
- Resist the temptation to underestimate the capacity of the patient or family to reorganize, adapt, and respond competently to disease-imposed changes.

Point 3: Recognize that LCH can affect normal development
- Remember that the patients and family's behaviors as understandable and predictable responses to the specific developmental challenges imposed by LCH.

Point 4: Build collaborative relationships with family members
- Persistence is the key to staying on track. Problem solving with ARCH helps the provider persist.

Point 5: Focus on competence
- Remember that each person has a reservoir of skills and capacities they have developed in response to prior life experiences on which to build.

---

me come.' The oncologist turns to Greg's mother and expresses an appreciation for the parents' long time struggle. He states, 'Greg knows my position on tobacco use. We disagree. You are worried about a preventable death. We faced four relapses. We can work with Greg's decision to smoke.'

Case B

The oncology fellow asked the psychologist to join the team. She believed Anna was 'depressed' and her parents were 'emotionally unavailable because they are in denial.' She requested supportive counseling.

The psychologist conducted an assessment. The mental status examination was normal. Anna described significant distress over disease-imposed disruptions in her life, but denied predominant manifestations of a mood disorder. The psychologist asked her about death and dying. She thoughtfully acknowledged that death was a possibility but quickly offered, 'I will get better.' In a conjoint interview, her mother indicated that her daughter and family were coping well. She indicated that Anna would respond to treatment and return to a normal life. Anna tacitly agreed that counseling was unnecessary.

The psychologist told the fellow that Anna rejected counseling. She expressed concern over the family's ability to face an adverse event, much less support Anna in that eventually. She indicated that the LCH was not responding to aggressive therapy and expressed concern that a rapid deterioration in pulmonary functioning was likely. Although a transplant was the only life-saving treatment option, the transplant team was not optimistic about expediently obtaining a donor. She stated, 'This family does not get it. Maybe they need to hear it from the transplant team.'

The psychologist suggested that conflicting perspectives over predicted medical outcomes were inadvertently driving a wedge in the provider–family relationship. The fellow non-defensively agreed, 'I do not know how to get them to understand that Anna will probably die.' The psychologist suggested organizing conversations around the five cardinal points rather than remaining locked into the goal of soliciting agreement with her perspective. He offered to participate in each conversation. They role-played how to use each point.

After a physical examination, the fellow stated, 'We are at a turning point. The LCH is not responding. Our intent is to proceed with a double-lung transplant, but factors beyond our control may quickly make palliative care our only option.' The mother stated, 'She will make it. Anna is strong.' Anna and her father nodded. Rather than attempting to secure an agreement, the fellow emphasized the relationship, 'I have asked the psychologist to join us. He will help *me* guide *us* down whatever road LCH takes us.' Anna's mother reiterated, 'Don't worry. She will make it.'

Point 2: Emphasize that LCH imposes changes on family life

LCH is an unpredictable disease with an uncertain course and outcome. Some face few problems, but others navigate many LCH-imposed challenges. As the current volume indicates, recent advances in disease management offer hope for controlling new symptoms or even eliminating progressive disease. In the face of hope, however, noncompliance, neuropsychiatric dysfunction, and relapses force everyone to consider the possibility of a poor quality of life and even death. Direct and immediate control of intense emotional reactions to these terrifying events is unlikely. In the face of worrisome symptoms or escalating family distress, a provider may believe that the patient or family lacks the resources to cope. In turn, they may too quickly offer referrals for expert help. The second key task for staying on track is *to resist the temptation to underestimate the capacity* of patient or family to reorganize, adapt, and respond competently to disease-imposed changes (Micucci, 1998). By identifying and naming the change, the provider helps the family acknowledge the turning point (Logan and Simms, 2002). This sets the stage for collaborative problem solving.

Case A

Greg's mother responds, 'I want Greg to understand that smoking could kill him.' The oncologist states, 'Greg, you will smoke; or you will stop. This I accept.' Respecting Greg's burgeoning independence while addressing the mother's concern, he adds, 'You did not want to come today. You came because of your mother. I get it. Let's focus on what we can do today, rather than what you will do tomorrow. As your doctor, I am curious how you are doing *now*. A physical exam helps me understand you and your body. OK?' Greg grunts, 'Alright.' Although Greg is marginally involved in the conversation, the provider has a foothold to move to the next point.

Case B

The fellow conducts a physical examination and then offers, 'Anna, the laprascopic procedure shows that LCH has extensively invaded your lungs. Your lung functioning is deteriorating. The transplant team does not believe that a donor will be available any time soon and even if a transplant is successful, the disease may recur'. Anna asked, and the fellow answered, a series of poignant questions. The mother lashes out, 'This can't be true. I cannot handle this.' Borrowing directly from the role-play, the fellow emphasizes change rather than agreement, 'Histiocytosis turned your family upside down. Of course you are not prepared. You faced other challenges. We will figure out how to face this one.'

Point 3: Recognize that LCH can affect normal development

LCH can temporally derail or even reroute developmental trajectories. Children and adults grow and develop by creatively solving problems and weathering failure within secure attachments with family and trusted friends (Simms, 1995). Families, too, have a developmental trajectory that unfolds in response to both predictable and unforeseen shifts in family membership and status (Rolland, 1994). Severe learning problems, neuropsychiatric dysfunction, relapses, aggressive therapies, and progressive disease have significant impact on these individual and family processes. Psychosocial symptoms or family dysfunction are signs that disease-related adversities have taxed coping mechanisms beyond their capacities and development is disrupted (Logan and Simms, 2002). For example, an accumulation of frustration with academics or ostracism by peers over changes in physical appearance and aberrant behaviors, such as uncontrollable crying or laughter, may propel patients into dysfunctional behavior patterns or deviant lifestyles. By denying cognitive deficits or an impending death, a family avoids an intolerable grief. Because symptomatic behaviors or dysfunctional patterns may complicate medical care or even appear dangerous, providers may shift abruptly to symptom management to 'fix the problem.' The provider can stay on track by *seeing the patients and family's behaviors as understandable and predictable responses to the specific developmental challenges* imposed by LCH.

Case A

After completing the physical examination, the oncologist states, 'LCH got in the way of school and making friends. Of course you are angry.' He turns to Greg's mother, 'LCH even got in the way of family life.' He looks at both of them, 'For the past 11 years, I have watched you and your parents walk this difficult road.'

Case B

As the mother turns away, the fellow looks at Anna. Drawing on key phrases from the role-play, the fellow states, 'Histiocytosis turned your life upside down too. I have seen you go from an active college student to a very sick person. I agree with the psychologist. Your sadness is about your losses.' Anna agreed, but quickly reframed her experience, 'I think I am better off than my friends. They do not know what life is about. They take it for granted. I don't. Yeah, they are out there having fun. I have been with my family. That is the most important thing.'

Point 4: Build collaborative relationships with family members

Psychosocial symptoms and family dysfunction are more likely to occur when people feel alone, isolated, and cut off (Brendler *et al.*, 1991; Micucci, 1998). Rather than taking responsibility for other's psychologic well-being, providers are encouraged to help patients/family members see that they have choices, make plans *with* rather than *for* the patient/family, and define treatment goals as a joint process. At a time when they feel helpless and overwhelmed, families need the provider to partner with them. When they know they can rely on the provider's support and expert guidance, patients/family are more likely to access the ability to rise to the challenges. Conversely, those who feel isolated may respond to the patient's apathy, troublemaking, or neuropsychiatric symptoms with benevolent pity rather than resolve for teamwork. A family overwhelmed by intense emotions may avoid the provider by politely scheduling, then canceling, follow-up meetings.

Providers may be tempted to 'lay down the law' with 'difficult' patients and unilaterally make referrals to child welfare agencies and mental health providers to 'make them get help.' *Persistence* is the key to staying on track. Problem solving with ARCH (*Acceptance*, *Respect*, *Curiosity*, *Honesty*) helps the provider persist (Micucci, 1998). Acceptance signals a commitment to the relationship: 'I will take you exactly as you are and are not'. Respect conveys the expectation that everyone value the relationship: 'I will honor your (position, wishes, beliefs) and expect you to honor mine'. Curiosity allows the provider to show interest and a desire for collaboration: 'How can *we* make this work?' Honesty helps the provider to communicate clearly, unapologetically and empathically whatever information is necessary and relevant. 'I'm sorry to give you bad news, but this is really important.'

Case A

The oncologist continues, 'Greg, I have good news. Your physical exam was normal.' Greg shrugs his shoulders as his mother breathes a sigh of relief. The oncologist uses ARCH to organize a plan and set goals. He states, 'Greg, our relationship is a two-way street. Because of this, I expect you to respect my perspective.' In an unexpected flash of warmth Greg responds, 'I do respect what you think. It's just that I am not ready to quit.' Curiosity then allows the oncologist to direct attention to securing agreement, 'I am not sure how smoking will affect you. I want to stay on top of this. 'The provider then uses honesty to modify the plan, 'Tobacco use is serious risk factor for relapse. Rather than once a year, I want you return to clinic in either three or four months.'

Case B

The fellow and psychologist enter a dark room. Anna is unconscious and breathing is labored. Her mother sits silently and her father is next to the bed. The fellow assesses breathing, then states, 'I am sorry. Anna will die soon. We need to make a palliative care plan. These measures will maximize Anna's comfort and minimize her suffering.' Her mother lashes out, 'Nothing will help now'. Relying on ARCH, the fellow states 'I agree, but Anna needs your help more than ever. I need your help more than ever.'

Point 5: Focus on competence

When facing quality of life challenges, relapse, and death, patients and families may present 'at their worst.' Rather than focusing exclusively on psychopathology, providers are encouraged to believe that people bring obscured strengths to the bedside. This orientation helps motivate people to stop underestimating themselves and rediscover hidden assets (Kazak *et al.*, 2001; Blackall and Simms, 2002). Providers get off track when they exclusively see patients or families as disturbed. This perspective assumes that the individual or family is helpless and therefore not responsible for their actions (Haley, 1980). Here, the provider is at risk to assume too much responsibility for finding a solution. Regardless of disease-imposed limitations and adverse circumstances, stay on track by *remembering that each person has a reservoir of skills and capacities they have developed in response to prior life experiences on which to build* (Erickson, 1985). Providers help spark competent responses to adversity by directly and indirectly suggesting that these patients and families find and then use their personal resources to respond to temporary or permanent changes.

Case A

As his mother enthusiastically agrees, Greg balks by stating, 'Three months! No way.' The provider transforms the situation into one that is not a contest, 'Come back in 3 months. Sit in this room. Stare at the clock. Just listen to what I have to say about histiocytosis and smoking.' Greg responds, 'I will come back and listen … in 4 months.' Highlighting Greg's competence, the provider states, 'See you in 4 months. By the way, do not let anything happen to this willful side. You may need it when you decide to quit smoking.' Greg smiles.

Case B

The fellow states, 'If Anna were conscious, what would she be doing now?' Her mother states, 'Listening to music'. The fellow responds, 'Would you play her favorite song?' Her mother selected a popular female recording artist. While listening, the fellow asked questions about Anna's likes and dislikes. The mother slowly shifted from answering questions to telling stories about her daughter and was encouraged to continue to fill the room with Anna's interests. Later that night, the fellow received a call that Anna died peacefully with her parents at her side. At the funeral, the parents expressed their sincere appreciation to the fellow for 'all your help.'

Conclusion

The histiocytic disorders, in particular those that cause permanent severe late effects and threaten death, can undermine coping skills and leave individuals and families less functional or more rigid than normal. Providers who lose sight of patient/family strengths and key relationships as a source of containment and healing can inadvertently and unintentionally engender anger, frustration, and desire to control people on both sides of the relationship. In this chapter, we have offered ideas for staying on course under challenging clinical circumstances.

REFERENCES

Blackall, G. and Simms, S. (2002). Principles for seeking and using professional consultation to resolve therapeutic impasses in medical settings. *Fam Syst Health*, **20**, 253–264.

Brendler, J., Silver, M., Haber, M., *et al.* (1991). *Madness, Chaos, and Violence: Therapy for Families at the Brink*, Basic Books, New York.

Erickson, M. (1985). *Life Reframing in Hypnosis: The Seminars, Workshops, and Lectures of Milton H. Erickson*, Irvington Publishers, New York.

Haley, J. (1980). *Leaving Home: The Therapy of Disturbed Young People*, McGraw-Hill Book Company. New York.

Kazak, A.E., Simms, S. and Rourke, M. (2001). Family systems practice in pediatric psychology. *J Pediatr Psychol*, **27**, 133–143.

Logan, D.E. and Simms, S. (2002). Using relational themes to design interventions for crisis and conflicts in pediatric settings. *Families, Systems, and Health*, **20**, 61–73.

Micucci, J. (1998). *The Adolescent in Family Therapy; Breaking the Cycle of Conflict and Control*, Guilford Press, New York.

Nanduri, V.A., Lillywhite, L., Chapman, C., *et al.* (2003). Cognitive outcome of long-term survivors of multisystem Langerhans cell histiocytosis: a single-institution, cross-sectional study. *J Clin Oncol*, **21**, 2961–2967.

Rolland, J.S. (1994). *Families, Illness, and Disability*, HarperCollins, New York.

Simms, S.G. (1995). A protocol for seriously ill children with severe psychosocial symptoms: avoiding potential disasters. *Fam Syst Med*, **13**, 245–257.

Simms, S. and Warner, N. (1998). A framework for understanding and responding to the psychosocial needs of children with Langerhans cell histiocytosis and their families. *Hematol/Oncol Clin N Am*, **12**, 359–367.

Whitsett, S.F., Kneppers, K. and Coppes, M.J. (1999). Neuropsychological deficits in children with Langerhans cell histiocytosis. *Med Pediatr Oncol*, **33**, 486–492.

Index